MD ANDERSON
CANCER CARE
SERIES

Series Editors

Aman U. Buzdar, MD   **Ralph S. Freedman, MD, PhD**

For further volumes:
http://www.springer.com/series/4596

MD ANDERSON CANCER CARE SERIES

Series Editors: Aman U. Buzdar, MD
Ralph S. Freedman, MD, PhD

K. K. Hunt, G. L. Robb, E. A. Strom, and N. T. Ueno, Eds., *Breast Cancer*

F. V. Fossella, R. Komaki, and J. B. Putnam, Jr., Eds., *Lung Cancer*

J. A. Ajani, S. A. Curley, N. A. Janjan, and P. M. Lynch, Eds., *Gastrointestinal Cancer*

K. W. Chan and R. B. Raney, Jr., Eds., *Pediatric Oncology*

P. J. Eifel, D. M. Gershenson, J. J. Kavanagh, and E. G. Silva, Eds., *Gynecologic Cancer*

F. DeMonte, M. R. Gilbert, A. Mahajan, and I. E. McCutcheon, Eds., *Tumors of the Brain and Spine*

Patrick P. Lin • Shreyaskumar Patel
Editors

The University of Texas MD Anderson Cancer Center, Houston, Texas

Bone Sarcoma

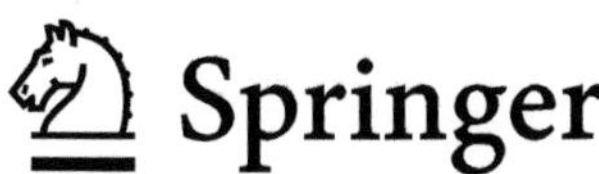 Springer

Editors
Patrick P. Lin, MD
Department of Orthopaedic Oncology
Division of Surgery
The University of Texas MD Anderson
  Cancer Center
Houston, TX, USA

Shreyaskumar Patel, MD
Department of Sarcoma Medical Oncology
Division of Cancer Medicine
The University of Texas MD Anderson
  Cancer Center
Houston, TX, USA

Series Editors
Aman U. Buzdar, MD
Department of Breast Medical Oncology
Division of Cancer Medicine
The University of Texas MD Anderson
  Cancer Center
Houston, TX, USA

Ralph S. Freedman, MD, PhD
Department of Gynecologic Oncology
  and Reproductive Medicine
Division of Surgery
The University of Texas MD Anderson
  Cancer Center
Houston, TX, USA

ISBN 978-1-4614-5193-8   ISBN 978-1-4614-5194-5 (eBook)
DOI 10.1007/978-1-4614-5194-5
Springer New York Heidelberg Dordrecht London

Library of Congress Control Number: 2012951843

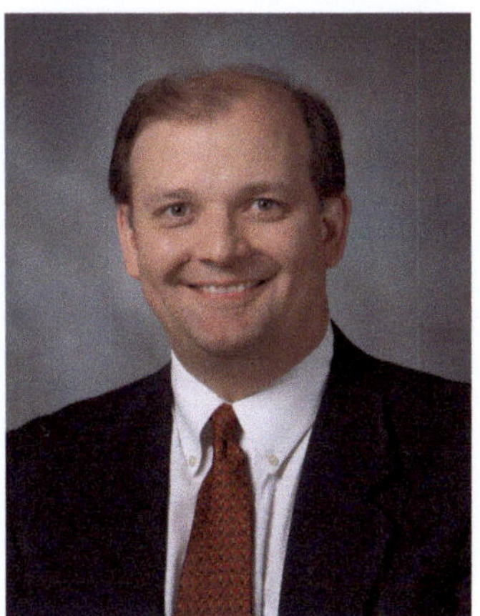

Alan William Yasko, MD
1958–2010

Foreword

During the past 40 years, major advances have been forged in the oncologic management of malignant bone tumors. These improvements derive from therapeutic discoveries in chemotherapy, better surgical techniques, progress in the delivery of radiation therapy, improved supportive care, and new imaging methodologies. As a consequence, an increasing number of survivors of both childhood and adult bone sarcomas are being observed.

The quality of life of these patients has been improved, particularly by advances achieved in innovative surgical techniques and procedures. Amputation has been reduced to a minimum, and limb-salvage procedures have become viable options for the majority of patients. These limb-preserving procedures appear to have great potential for the treatment of the different types of skeletal defects arising from tumor resection. Better implant materials and design configurations have been developed and are being discovered; they will probably reduce the incidence of complications in the future. The improvements have been facilitated by new approaches to enhance bone transplantation procedures, special systems for internal fixation of implants, and composite reconstructions that incorporate both biological and metallic materials. The surgical advances have been integrated with advances in chemotherapy, compounding the success of both.

The first series of osteoarticular allografts in the USA were reported in 1968 by Frank Parrish from MD Anderson Cancer Center. During the subsequent years, the techniques for treating patients with bone sarcomas at MD Anderson were developed by a team of dedicated clinicians, which included two notable orthopedic surgeons. The late John A. Murray, MD, a partner in Frank Parrish's practice and a founding member of the Musculoskeletal Tumor Society, was one of the early pioneers in the treatment of osteosarcoma. His ideas were advanced and extended by the late Alan W. Yasko, MD. I had the privilege of working with both of these remarkable individuals, and their contributions, particularly to the concept of multidisciplinary care, cannot be understated. The present-day staff at MD Anderson, under the direction of Valerae O. Lewis, MD, with whom I have also had the privilege of working, has continued the work of early pioneers, with ongoing, broad research efforts that are yielding significant results in many diverse areas.

A compendium of tactics and strategies is provided in this monograph, and it serves as an invaluable guide for the optimum treatment of patients with malignant bone tumors. The volume is intended to facilitate multidisciplinary care by offering a practical, portable resource for health professionals in many different medical fields who participate in the treatment of patients with musculoskeletal tumors. The MD Anderson approach described here demonstrates effective interaction between the different disciplines deployed in the management of patients with bone sarcomas and strives to develop safe, effective, and superior forms of care for these patients.

Norman Jaffe, MD, DSc
Houston, TX, USA

Preface

Sarcomas of bone form a unique topic in oncology. Apart from obvious differences in histology and etiology, a number of characteristics set this group of tumors apart from all other malignancies, including sarcomas of soft tissue. Involvement of the skeletal system creates a host of surgical, functional, and emotional issues that are not encountered in other diseases. Moreover, the response to chemotherapy, radiologic analysis, and pathologic evaluation of bone sarcomas are distinctly different from those of other malignancies. For these reasons, it seems vital to devote a book to these uncommon but fascinating neoplasms.

A multidisciplinary team approach is essential to maximize a patient's chances of having a successful outcome. Success in any one area is not sufficient. A patient may have an excellent response to chemotherapy and be rendered disease free, yet have a poor outcome because of stiffness, weakness, and pain in a limb. Many different specialties and services are involved in the care of patients with bone sarcomas. As each of these fields becomes more technologically advanced, it becomes increasingly difficult for workers in one field to understand what their coworkers do in other fields. Many team members have a surprisingly limited knowledge of what the rest of the team does.

In an effort to foster collaboration and teamwork, we have written a succinct volume that summarizes the key elements of different specialties as they pertain to bone sarcomas. The book is not meant for any one branch of medicine but rather for all who have an interest in how the entire enterprise operates and how their efforts are intimately intertwined with those of their colleagues. The first chapter focuses upon the multidisciplinary nature of bone sarcomas. The next three chapters discuss diagnostic techniques, which include essential aspects of radiology, biopsy, and pathology. The following chapters explore in detail the three main diseases in the field—osteosarcoma, Ewing sarcoma, and chondrosarcoma. Treatment modalities, including surgery, chemotherapy, and radiation therapy, are discussed within the context of each of these diseases, since the treatment is quite different for each diagnosis. A special chapter is devoted to very rare sarcomas that arise in bone. The next portion of the book addresses important issues related to reconstruction and function.

These include growth of the skeleton in pediatric patients, soft tissue reconstruction, techniques for restoring skeletal defects, and physical rehabilitation of the patient. Finally, two chapters are more globally oriented toward algorithms for perioperative management and follow-up of patients.

It is hoped that this book will facilitate communication between health-care providers who are involved in the care of bone sarcoma patients. Through mutual understanding of each other's work, the practice of each professional can be refined, and the overall care of the patient with bone sarcoma can be optimized. Quite possibly, as a result of cross-fertilization of ideas, we may find fresh new ways to achieve a cure for our patients.

We thank Walter Pagel, Sunita Patterson, Joe Munch, and Kristi Speights of MD Anderson's Department of Scientific Publications for their encouragement, expertise, and outstanding editorial support. We are also indebted to Terri Robinson and Maribel Martinez of the Department of Orthopaedic Oncology for their invaluable assistance in the preparation of the manuscript.

Patrick P. Lin, MD
Shreyaskumar Patel, MD
Houston, TX, USA

Contents

Contributors

Kamran Ahrar, MD Professor, Section of Interventional Radiology, Department of Diagnostic Radiology, Division of Diagnostic Imaging

Christopher P. Cannon, MD Assistant Professor, Department of Orthopaedic Oncology, Division of Surgery (current position: Orthopedic Surgeon, The Polyclinic, Seattle, WA)

David W. Chang, MD Professor, Department of Plastic Surgery, Division of Surgery

Colleen M. Costelloe, MD Associate Professor, Section of Musculoskeletal Imaging, Department of Diagnostic Radiology, Division of Diagnostic Imaging

Ashleigh Guadagnolo, MD, MPH Associate Professor, Department of Radiation Oncology, Division of Radiation Oncology

Tamara Miner Haygood, PhD, MD Associate Professor, Department of Diagnostic Radiology, Division of Diagnostic Imaging

Cynthia E. Herzog, MD Professor, Department of Pediatrics, Division of Pediatrics

Norman Jaffe, MD Professor Emeritus, Department of Pediatrics, Division of Pediatrics

Benedict Konzen, MD Associate Professor, Department of Palliative Care and Rehabilitation Medicine, Division of Cancer Medicine

Rajendra Kumar, MD Professor, Department of Diagnostic Radiology, Division of Diagnostic Imaging

Alexander J. Lazar, MD, PhD Associate Professor, Department of Pathology, Division of Pathology and Laboratory Medicine; and Department of Dermatology, Division of Internal Medicine

Valerae O. Lewis, MD Associate Professor, Chief, Department of Orthopaedic Oncology, Division of Surgery

Patrick P. Lin, MD Associate Professor, Department of Orthopaedic Oncology, Division of Surgery

John E. Madewell, MD Professor, Chief, Section of Musculoskeletal Imaging, Department of Diagnostic Radiology, Division of Diagnostic Imaging

Bryan S. Moon, MD Associate Professor, Department of Orthopaedic Oncology, Division of Surgery

William A. Murphy Jr., MD Professor, John S. Dunn Sr., Distinguished Chair, Department of Diagnostic Radiology, Division of Diagnostic Imaging

Scott D. Oates, MD Professor, Department of Plastic Surgery, Division of Surgery

Shreyaskumar Patel, MD Professor, Deputy Chair, Department of Sarcoma Medical Oncology, Division of Cancer Medicine

Mark S. Pilarczyk, PA-C Physician Assistant, Department of Orthopaedic Oncology, Division of Surgery

Vinod Ravi, MD Assistant Professor, Department of Sarcoma Medical Oncology, Division of Cancer Medicine

A. Kevin Raymond, MD Associate Professor, Chief, Section of Orthopaedic Pathology, Department of Pathology, Division of Laboratory Medicine (retired)

Laurence D. Rhines, MD Professor, Department of Neurosurgery, Division of Surgery

Janie Rutledge, MSN, RN-C, ANP Advanced Practice Nurse, Department of Orthopaedic Oncology, Division of Surgery

Alan W. Yasko, MD Associate Professor, Chief, Section of Orthopaedic Oncology, Department of Orthopaedic Oncology, Division of Surgery (now deceased; position at the time of his death: Professor, Department of Orthopaedic Surgery, Northwestern University Feinberg School of Medicine, Chicago, IL)

Chapter 1
A Multidisciplinary Approach
to the Management of Sarcomas of Bone

Bryan S. Moon

Chapter Overview The treatment of bone sarcomas has changed dramatically over the past 30 years. Appropriate diagnosis and adequate treatment depend on a multidisciplinary approach. MD Anderson Cancer Center has designed a unique clinic system devoted to the complex treatment of bone sarcomas. Multidisciplinary providers see patients side by side. Multidisciplinary team conferences, as well as surgery-specific conferences, enable agreement on and coordination of treatment. Pathologist and physician expertise specific to bone sarcomas is crucial.

With an incidence in the USA of only approximately 2,500 cases a year, bone sarcomas are quite rare, and it can be difficult to find a team of physicians who have adequate experience and expertise in their treatment. Although there are many cancer centers across the country at which bone sarcomas can be treated, only a few of these centers have physicians from different disciplines whose practice is focused primarily on the treatment of sarcomas. At MD Anderson Cancer Center, there are not only physicians dedicated to the care of patients with sarcomas but also a unique clinic system that was designed specifically to provide a multidisciplinary team approach to the complex care of these patients.

Historically, the management of sarcomas was not so complicated. As recently as the 1970s, the majority of bone sarcomas were treated with amputation; occasionally, radiation therapy was also used. The results of this type of management

B.S. Moon (✉)
Department of Orthopaedic Oncology, Unit 1448, Division of Surgery,
The University of Texas MD Anderson Cancer Center, P.O. Box 301402,
Houston, TX 77230, USA
e-mail: bsmoon@mdanderson.org

P.P. Lin and S. Patel (eds.), *Bone Sarcoma*, MD Anderson Cancer Care Series,
DOI 10.1007/978-1-4614-5194-5_1,

were dismal, and survival rates were less than 20%. The use of modern chemotherapy and advanced imaging techniques has markedly changed the treatment and prognosis of patients with bone sarcomas, such that survival rates have increased dramatically and most patients are limb-salvage candidates.

The experience of the past few decades has demonstrated that the management of the majority of bone sarcomas requires multidisciplinary input from clinicians, musculoskeletal radiologists, and bone pathologists. The therapy for bone sarcomas is also multimodal and frequently includes chemotherapy, surgery, and/or radiation therapy. Although such multimodal therapy is required for a variety of cancers, the severity of disease and need for aggressive management seen with bone sarcomas make them a distinct entity. For these reasons, the importance of physician experience in the treatment of bone sarcomas cannot be overstated.

MD Anderson has had a Sarcoma Center since 1996. All disciplines that are involved in the care of a patient with sarcoma are represented, and providers see patients side by side, which enables close interactions among the providers and simplifies the patient's visit. Referrals to the Sarcoma Center can be made by telephone or online by physicians or by patients themselves. These referrals may be for patients with imaging results suggestive of sarcoma, patients with newly diagnosed sarcomas who are seeking definitive treatment, or those who are seeking second opinions but will be treated closer to home. Once the referral is initiated, each patient is assigned a primary physician and an advanced nurse practitioner who will coordinate the patient's care.

One of the most critical aspects of coordinating the patient's care is obtaining complete medical records and pathologic specimens. Initially, this may seem to be an onerous task, but it is critical because it enables the multidisciplinary team to review the patient's previous workup and determine whether further testing will be required. In some instances, needed tests or imaging can be scheduled in advance and coordinated with the physician's evaluation. If imaging is done far enough in advance, the images can be submitted to the radiology team and an interpretation can be rendered even prior to the patient's arrival. Clinicians can then make sure that outside imaging is adequate in scope and quality and can verify the outside radiographic interpretations. This review can significantly expedite the workup during the patient's initial evaluation period.

A review of the biopsy specimen and pathology slides is essential. At MD Anderson, prior to the initiation of any treatment, all outside biopsies must undergo review by an MD Anderson pathologist who specializes in sarcomas. Since bone sarcomas are rare, it is mandatory that a pathologist with significant sarcoma experience evaluates the specimen. It is not at all uncommon for this review to result in a change in the diagnosed grade or type of sarcoma, and occasionally a sarcoma diagnosis will be completely overturned. As will be discussed in later chapters, bone sarcomas are not all treated alike, and the correct diagnosis is critical to appropriate management.

Once the patient has been evaluated, imaging reviewed, and pathologic diagnosis confirmed, a specific treatment plan must be designed, and a team of clinicians must be assembled to carry out the plan. In some cases, this process can be straightforward, but quite often complex factors and considerations may influence the management of the case. Presentation at a tumor board or similar conference can be quite beneficial to address these issues and ensure that all members of the multidisciplinary team are working in concert. At MD Anderson, cases are routinely presented and discussed at the Sarcoma Multidisciplinary Conference. The conference is devoted solely to sarcomas and is attended by the appropriate specialists in the fields of orthopedic oncology, surgical oncology, medical oncology, radiation oncology, diagnostic imaging, and pathology. In addition to the attending physicians, many other health care providers participate in the conference, including clinic nurses, research nurses, physician assistants, advanced practice nurses, fellows, residents, medical students, and other trainees. The inclusion of many different disciplines and health care professionals helps foster teamwork, facilitate communication, and provide continuing education for all attendees. Another beneficial effect of having a regular forum such as this conference for discussion of cases is the development of a consistent, effective treatment philosophy and approach to these rare diseases. This approach, in essence, reflects the distilled experience of many years of practice of many specialized physicians.

Presentation of a patient's case at the conference involves a synopsis of the medical history, projection of the pertinent radiologic findings by a radiologist, review of the histologic diagnosis by a musculoskeletal pathologist, and discussion of different treatment options. Whenever appropriate, the patient's eligibility for clinical trials is also discussed. The patient's primary team (the primary provider and advanced nurse practitioner) then discuss the conference recommendations with the patient, and appropriate care is initiated.

The following case is a good illustration of the effectiveness of the Sarcoma Multidisciplinary Conference and demonstrates how different clinicians can work together to improve the care of a patient. The patient was a 72-year-old woman who presented with right shoulder pain. A workup by her local physician had revealed a lesion in the right proximal humerus. Plain radiographs showed a calcified lesion suggestive of a cartilaginous tumor (Fig. 1.1), and magnetic resonance imaging (MRI) scans revealed erosion of the tumor through the cortical bone, which would be compatible with a radiologic diagnosis of chondrosarcoma. However, surprisingly, a needle biopsy did not confirm the presence of malignant chondrocytes or cartilaginous tissue. Instead, the biopsy showed epithelioid cells with large nuclei and scattered mitotic figures. The pathologic findings alone clearly did not support the diagnosis of a conventional chondrosarcoma. With the additional input from clinicians in orthopedics and radiology, it was determined that the appropriate diagnosis was a dedifferentiated chondrosarcoma, a rare type of chondrosarcoma characterized by components of low-grade cartilaginous tumor juxtaposed with malignant, high-grade spindle cell sarcoma. The important aspect of this multidisciplinary case is that dedifferentiated chondrosarcoma is treated with chemotherapy and surgery, whereas conventional chondrosarcoma is treated with surgery alone. If not for the collaboration of the multiple teams, the patient could have been at risk of misdiagnosis and inadequate treatment.

The majority of bone sarcomas will require surgical intervention. These surgeries, which are typically very complex, range from limb salvage to amputation. In

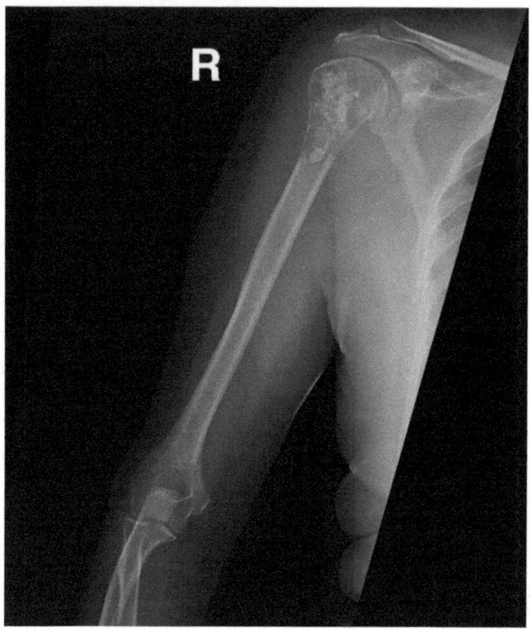

Fig. 1.1 A radiograph of the humerus demonstrates calcifications in the proximal end of the bone that are typical of a benign cartilaginous tumor. However, there is also seen lytic destruction of the surrounding cancellous bone and thinning of the overlying cortical bone. Subsequent workup revealed this tumor to be a dedifferentiated chondrosarcoma arising from an old benign enchondroma.

addition to the Sarcoma Multidisciplinary Conference, a separate surgical conference meets weekly to discuss cases that require surgery. It is attended primarily by orthopedic surgeons and musculoskeletal radiologists. At this conference, the images are again reviewed, and surgical options are discussed among the faculty. Given their rarity and heterogeneous nature, bone sarcomas can present unique challenges that may be encountered by a surgeon only a limited number of times during a surgical career. By combining the knowledge, experience, and expertise of several faculty members, the surgical conference creates a synergy that benefits the patient. It also assists in maintaining a standard of care and promotes the development of innovative surgical plans.

In summary, the major advances that have occurred in bone sarcoma management over the past 30 years demand a well-integrated, multidisciplinary approach. The chapters that follow will discuss in detail various aspects of sarcoma management and will illustrate amply how optimal treatment requires the input of many highly specialized health care professionals. Although outcomes for patients with bone sarcomas have improved over the years, there is still room for improvement. It is only through a focused, multidisciplinary approach that future improvements will emerge.

Key Practice Points

- Survival rates for patients treated for bone sarcomas have increased dramatically, and most patients are now limb-salvage candidates.
- The therapy for bone sarcomas is multimodal and frequently includes chemotherapy, surgery, and/or radiation therapy.
- Multidisciplinary conferences enable health care providers to optimize a patient's care.
- Because these diseases are rare and aggressive, we recommend evaluation and treatment by physicians and pathologists with expertise in bone sarcomas.

Suggested Readings

Federman N, Bernthal N, Eilber FC, Tap WD. The multidisciplinary management of osteosarcoma. Curr Treat Options Oncol. 2009;10:82–93.

Ludwig JA. Ewing sarcoma: historical perspectives, current state-of-the-art, and opportunities for targeted therapy in the future. Curr Opin Oncol. 2008;20:412–8.

Mirabello L, Troisi RJ, Savage SA. Osteosarcoma incidence and survival rates from 1973 to 2004: data from the Surveillance, Epidemiology, and End Results Program. Cancer. 2009;115:1531–43.

Weber K, Damron TA, Frassica FJ, Sim FH. Malignant bone tumors. Instr Course Lect. 2008;57: 673–88.

Chapter 2
Bone Sarcoma Imaging

John E. Madewell, Colleen M. Costelloe, Tamara Miner Haygood, Rajendra Kumar, and William A. Murphy, Jr.

Contents

Chapter Overview Imaging studies are invaluable in the diagnosis, staging, and evaluation of response to treatment of bone sarcomas. At MD Anderson Cancer Center, the most essential initial imaging studies performed for diagnosis and staging are plain film radiography and magnetic resonance imaging (MRI), respectively.

J.E. Madewell (✉) • C.M. Costelloe
Section of Musculoskeletal Imaging, Department of Diagnostic Radiology, Unit 1475,
Division of Diagnostic Imaging, The University of Texas MD Anderson Cancer Center,
1400 Pressler Street, Houston TX 77030-4009, USA
e-mail: jmadewell@mdanderson.org; ccostelloe@mdanderson.org

T.M. Haygood • R. Kumar • W.A. Murphy, Jr.
Department of Diagnostic Radiology, Division of Diagnostic Imaging,
The University of Texas MD Anderson Cancer Center, Houston, TX, USA
e-mail: tamara.haygood@mdanderson.org; rajkumar@mdanderson.org;
wmurphy@mdanderson.org

P.P. Lin and S. Patel (eds.), *Bone Sarcoma*, MD Anderson Cancer Care Series,
DOI 10.1007/978-1-4614-5194-5_2,

To answer specific questions, these studies are often augmented by other imaging modalities, such as computed tomography (CT), skeletal scintigraphy, positron emission tomography (PET) with fused CT (PET/CT), and ultrasonography. After treatment, plain radiography, MRI, and PET/CT may be used to evaluate tumor response. One cannot overemphasize the importance of these modalities in the comprehensive evaluation of patients with bone sarcomas. Accurate characterization of the primary lesion is key to the diagnosis, while precise identification of local, regional, and distant disease is critical to staging and treatment.

Introduction

The radiographic appearance of a tumor indicates its degree of aggressiveness, thereby suggesting whether the tumor is benign or malignant. As a standard of practice at MD Anderson Cancer Center, findings from plain radiographs are coupled with clinical information; decisions are then made about the need for additional imaging studies and procedures. Over time, as imaging studies advance into functional and metabolic realms, their impact will be incorporated more fully into the practice of radiology. Even at present, diagnosis of and treatment planning for bone sarcomas involve a multidisciplinary correlation of clinical, radiologic, and pathologic data (Morrison et al. 2005).

The multidisciplinary approach necessitates cooperation among the medical oncologist, radiologist, pathologist, radiation oncologist, and orthopedic oncologist. At our institution, the radiologist participates in the initial patient evaluation, so that imaging studies are interpreted within the clinical context.

The initial analysis of imaging features of bone sarcomas, derived mostly from plain radiographs, includes consideration of the location of the lesion within a bone, the appearance of its margins, the pattern of periosteal reaction (if present), the pattern of osteolysis (bone destruction), and the type of matrix mineralization. The data about the bone lesion derived from the plain radiographs facilitate the radiographic diagnosis and at times even influence the pathologic diagnosis. After the radiographic diagnosis, further radiologic imaging becomes essential for staging the local disease. During preoperative treatment (usually with chemotherapy), imaging of the tumor is important for evaluating response and can help guide the oncologist in deciding whether to continue or alter treatment. Specific considerations for the role of imaging in diagnosis, in assessing extent of disease, and in evaluating response to treatment are described in this chapter.

Lesion Location

Bone sarcomas occur in predictable locations; most arise in the metaphysis of a long bone, especially around the knee in either the distal femur or the proximal tibia. The dominant anatomic sites of many bone tumors have been described (Johnson 1953; Madewell et al. 1981). The locations in which these tumors arise (Fig. 2.1) reflect

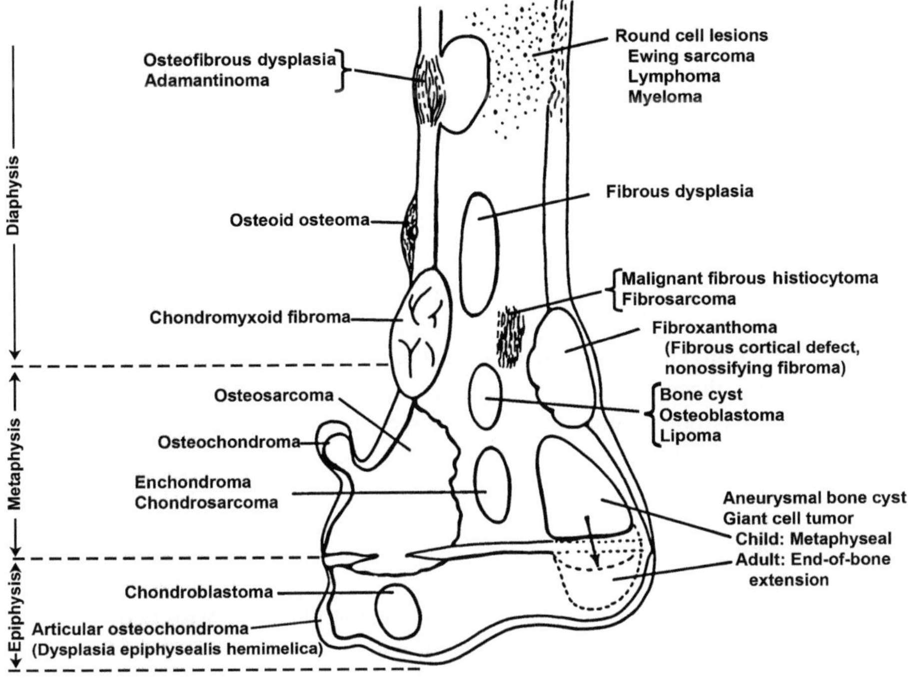

Fig. 2.1 Frequent sites of common primary bone tumors, depicted in the end of a long bone, which is divided into the epiphysis, metaphysis, and diaphysis. Adapted from Madewell et al. (1981).

increased underlying cellular activity. Because the distal femur and proximal tibia are the most rapidly growing areas of the skeleton, it is understandable that they are the most common sites for many bone neoplasms. However, bone sarcomas may arise at other sites in a long bone, and any bone in the body may be involved.

An important aspect of imaging bone sarcomas is the relationship of the tumor to the adjoining normal soft tissues and other vital structures, such as the neurovascular bundle. Description of the relationship between the tumor and these adjacent normal structures is critical to local staging of the bone sarcoma and to the planning of surgical intervention.

Diagnostic Imaging

As described below, plain radiography remains the primary imaging modality for the initial evaluation of skeletal neoplasms because of its utility for detecting, characterizing, and quantifying bone alterations. Magnetic resonance imaging (MRI) has distinct advantages in detection of bone marrow and soft tissue extension, and computed tomography (CT) is useful in certain circumstances, especially in instances of complex bony anatomy. Skeletal scintigraphy (radionuclide bone scanning) can help in the detection of multiple lesions, either within a single anatomic compartment (skip lesions) or in distant sites. Other modalities used on occasion in workup of patients with potential bone sarcomas are positron emission tomography (PET), fluoroscopy, and ultrasonography.

Radiography

At the time of presentation, primary bone sarcomas usually are characterized by fairly extensive local disease. Plain radiographs usually demonstrate osteolysis, periosteal reaction, and even matrix mineralization, depending on the type of bone tumor. Besides these tumor characteristics, radiographs also show the specific location of the tumor within the bone: whether it is located in the epiphysis, the metaphysis, the diaphysis, or a combination of these sites (Fig. 2.1).

Osteolytic Margin Pattern

One of the important types of diagnostic information identified with radiography is the nature of the tumor margins. A lytic lesion's appearance on radiographs depends on the structure of the underlying bone, whether it is cancellous (trabecular) or cortical (compact) bone, the degree of adjoining bone loss, and the amount of contrast between the lesion and the surrounding bone (Madewell et al. 1981). For example, a small, focal area of bone loss within the dense cortical bone is easily seen with radiography, but a similar focus of destruction in the cancellous bone of the marrow may be difficult to see because there is less adjacent bone to produce visual contrast. Thus, a greater volume of osteolysis is needed for perceiving abnormalities in cancellous bone than for perceiving them in cortical bone. An example of this background contrast effect can be seen in the elderly patient with osteoporosis, in whom early destructive lesions are more difficult to detect; even advanced infiltrative destructive processes may not be appreciated because of lack of contrast due to density loss within the cancellous bone. In such radiographic settings, other more sensitive imaging modalities, such as MRI, CT, or skeletal scintigraphy, are most helpful in detection of the lesion.

The growth of bone sarcomas induces host osteoclastic activity and modifies bone structure locally and regionally to produce the fundamental radiographic patterns referred to as *geographic* (type I), *moth-eaten* (type II), and *permeative* (type III) bone destruction (Fig. 2.2). These lucency patterns serve as an index of tumor growth rates (Lodwick et al. 1980; Oudenhoven et al. 2006).

Geographic osteolysis creates a well-circumscribed lesion with a narrow zone of transition. Arcuate, lobulated, or scalloped borders are commonly associated with slow-growing, benign lesions, such as enchondroma, fibrous dysplasia, fibroxanthoma, chronic osteomyelitis (Brodie abscess), and bone cysts. These non-aggressive types of margin are also sometimes associated with low-grade (grade 1)

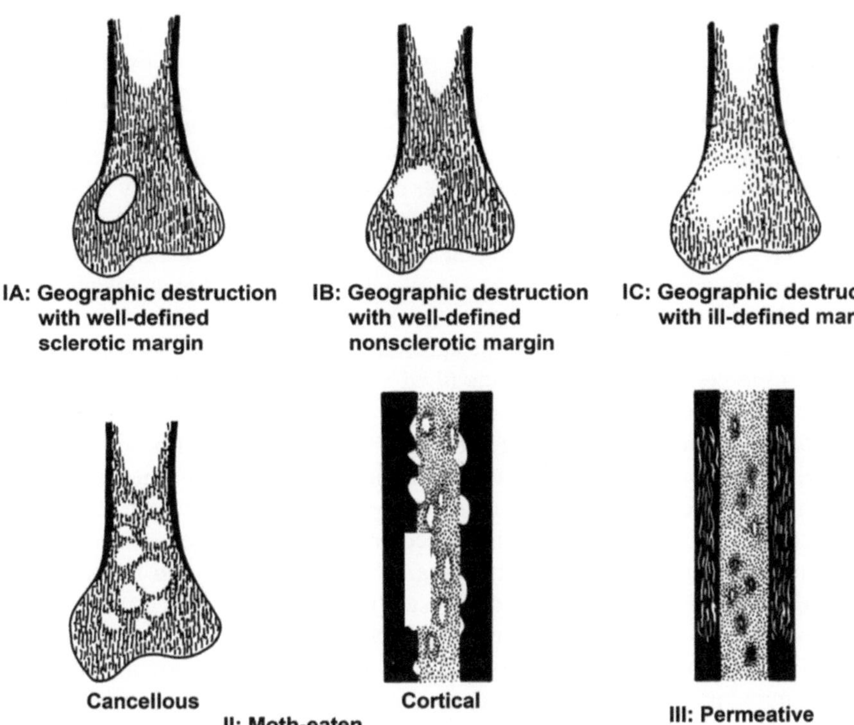

Fig. 2.2 Patterns of osteolysis (types IA, IB, IC, II, and III) and their margins. Transitions from a lower numbered pattern to a higher numbered pattern imply increased activity and a greater probability of an aggressive process or malignancy. Adapted from Madewell et al. (1981).

malignancies. Tumors with the geographic pattern of radiolucency may have rims with margins that are *sclerotic* (IA), *nonsclerotic* (IB), or *ill defined* (IC). These three different phases of the geographic pattern, described below, correspond to progressive tumor aggression.

Geographic lesions with sclerotic and nonsclerotic margins represent a narrow zone of transition. In both these margin types, the normal cancellous bone is present up to the peripheral edge of the tumor, but the degrees of remodeling vary. Lesions with nonsclerotic margins are more aggressive but are still generally associated with benign bone tumors, such as giant cell tumor, chondromyxoid fibroma, enchondroma, and chondroblastoma. Occasionally, deceptive low-grade sarcomas, such as chondrosarcoma, may exhibit a similar radiographic appearance. Hence, the possibility of a bone sarcoma increases when the geographic pattern with nonsclerotic margins is detected. The likelihood of malignancy increases even further when the tumor margin is ill defined or fuzzy. This type of geographic lesion represents a locally infiltrating, poorly contained lytic process and is indicative of local aggression. The tumor usually extends into the bone marrow beyond the main, perceived margin of the lytic lesion, and the true extent of the lesion is best appreciated with MRI. Such locally invasive tumors may include giant cell tumor, osteosarcoma, fibrosarcoma, malignant fibrous histiocytoma, and chondrosarcoma.

Moth-eaten osteolysis consists of multiple scattered holes that vary in size and may arise separately or originate from the edge of a major central, lytic component. They can coalesce into a more focal or larger destructive lesion and may affect cancellous bone, cortical bone, or both. In the cancellous bone, the normal trabecular markings can usually be seen between the holes. The holes are caused by regional infiltration from more aggressive processes, which tend to spare the intervening normal bone. In the cortical bone, the destructive holes that create this moth-eaten pattern usually begin on the endosteal surface and progress along the cortical axis outward to the periosteum. The defects filled with neoplasm are usually oval and represent active osteoclastic resorption at the cancellous and cortical bone. Bone lesions with a moth-eaten pattern of osteolysis may have cortical penetration and soft tissue extension. Evaluation for such extension is best accomplished with MRI. The moth-eaten osteolytic pattern is frequently seen in malignant neoplasms such as osteosarcoma, chondrosarcoma, Ewing sarcoma, malignant fibrous histiocytoma, fibrosarcoma, and primary bone lymphoma. This pattern may also be seen with osteomyelitis, which may cause aggressive osteolysis, especially in its acute/subacute form. However, osteomyelitis is usually associated with clinical and laboratory findings indicative of an inflammatory process. Subacute/chronic osteomyelitis and other inflammatory diseases, such as Langerhans cell histiocytosis, may masquerade as neoplasms, and biopsy of the lesion may be the only way to differentiate them from bone sarcomas.

Permeative osteolysis is predominantly cortical bone destruction in which multiple uniform, tiny, oval areas of lucency or streaks are seen within the cortex. These streaks are created by cortical tunneling from osteoclastic cutting cones in an accelerated phase of normal cortical remodeling that is stimulated by hypervascularity and tumor extension. These cortical permeations are usually seen with highly aggressive neoplasms such as Ewing sarcoma and osteosarcoma. However, they can also be seen with aggressive benign bone lesions, such as stress fractures and acute osteomyelitis. Again, clinical and laboratory features are helpful in excluding malignancy in such cases. Even metabolic diseases with active cortical remodeling, such as hyperparathyroidism, can exhibit this permeative lytic pattern, usually in metaphyseal cutback areas such as the concave portion of the metaphysis or at points of greatest stress. Cortical permeation caused by metabolic disease is usually more generalized and multifocal than the focal cortical permeation caused by a bone sarcoma.

Bone sarcomas may simultaneously exhibit more than one type of osteolytic margin pattern. The area of most aggressive destruction is the most ominous and relevant in regard to patient management and prediction of the biologic activity of the tumor. Such areas of aggressive osteolysis should be biopsied to obtain representative tissue samples from the tumor. Another important feature of margin evaluation is its change over time. A prior radiograph that shows a well-defined or sclerotic rim of a bone lesion, paired with a follow-up radiograph that shows aggressive destruction, suggests biological change and a more malignant neoplasm.

Table 2.1 Relationship of biologic activity to osteolytic margin pattern and periosteal reaction

Growth rate	Osteolytic margin pattern	Periosteal reaction
Slow	Geographic (I)	Solid
	IA	
	IB	
	IC	
Intermediate	Moth-eaten (II)	Shells
		Ridged
		Lobulated
		Smooth
Fast	Permeative (III)	Lamellated
Fastest	Nonvisible	Spiculated or none

IA, well-defined sclerotic margin; IB, well-defined nonsclerotic margin; IC, ill-defined margin. Adapted from Madewell et al. (1981).

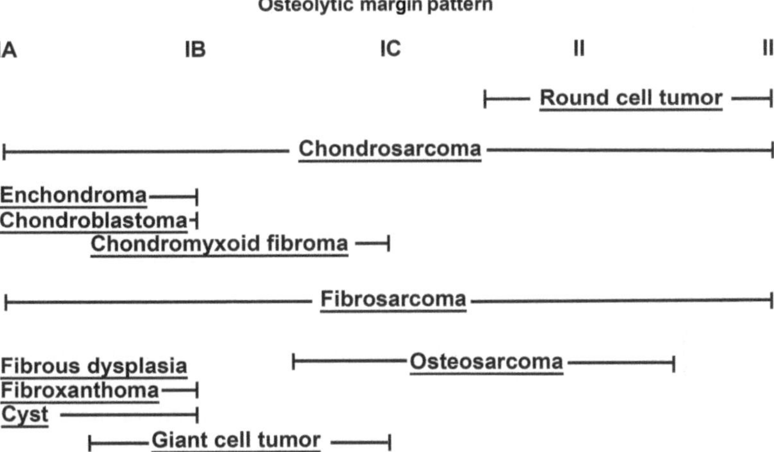

Fig. 2.3 Common bone tumors classified by their typical patterns of osteolysis. IA, geographic destruction with well-defined sclerotic margin; IB, geographic destruction with well-defined nonsclerotic margin; IC, geographic destruction with ill-defined margin; II, moth-eaten destruction (regionally invasive); III, permeative destruction (diffusely invasive). Note that most benign tumors occur on the left side of this spectrum, with patterns from IA to IC, whereas most malignant tumors occur on the right side, with patterns from IC to III. This distribution illustrates the general principle that the biologic activity and probability of malignancy increase from left to right. Adapted from Madewell et al. (1981).

To summarize, the defining margin or interface between the tumor and adjacent normal bone in cortical and/or cancellous locations is an indicator of the underlying biologic process of the tumor and its aggressiveness (Table 2.1, Fig. 2.3). The radiographic image shows best the location in bone and represents a summation of bone osteolysis (osteoclastic activity) and osteosclerosis (osteoblastic activity). Sarcomas may arise in preexisting benign lesions or may be lower-grade tumors. In such cases, the radiographic pattern may lag behind the histologic activity, producing a radiographic discrepancy (a lesion that appears to be growing slowly but has a malignant histologic type). A careful analysis of these radiographic patterns, when integrated with clinical data, will enable accurate diagnosis in the initial evaluation of suspected bone sarcomas in most patients.

Periosteal Reactions

The periosteum is traditionally defined as an envelope consisting of inner cellular and outer fibrous components that separate the bone from surrounding soft tissue. In the child, it is a rich source of uncommitted mesenchymal stem cells and preosteoblasts. In the adult, even though the periosteum may not be as substantial as it is in children, periosteal reactions are common sequelae of underlying bone marrow processes, including bone sarcomas, and are helpful in predicting the biologic activity of the bone lesions.

The various patterns of periosteal reactions in a bone (Fig. 2.4) represent the periosteum's attempt to contain a bone lesion, and the radiographic appearance of the periosteal reaction relates to the manner, time, and course of periosteal bone production and mineralization (Ragsdale et al. 1981). Periosteal reactions are biologic measures of the intensity, aggression, and duration of the inciting underlying bone processes. These reactions involve the reawakening and acceleration of mechanisms that modify the surface of bone in normal growth by production of new bone from the cambian layer of the periosteum. The periosteal reaction must be mineralized in order for radiography to demonstrate its presence. This mineralization may require as much as 10 days to 3 weeks from the initial stimulus, depending on the nature of the stimulus and the age of the patient. When the periosteal reaction is continuous and solid, it is an indicator of slow underlying biologic activity and is commonly associated with benign or slow-growing processes. However, if the periosteal reaction is interrupted, spiculated, or lamellated or demonstrates a Codman angle or buttress angle, it is indicative of an aggressive process, and, with the exclusion of certain conditions such as infection and trauma, it is associated with a high probability of a malignant bone tumor.

Matrix Production and Mineralization

The term *matrix* refers to an acellular intercellular substance produced by mesenchymal cells and may include osteoid, chondroid, myxomatous material, and/or collagen. Bone tumors may be divided into matrix-producing and non-matrix-producing lesions. When radiographic mineralized matrix patterns of increased density (Fig. 2.5) are present, their significance in predicting the specific diagnosis of bone tumors is well recognized (Sweet et al. 1981). Specific patterns of mineralized matrix can indicate the underlying histologic composition of either chondroid- or osteoid-producing bone tumors (Figs. 2.6b, c, 2.7, and 2.8). These patterns may also be helpful to the

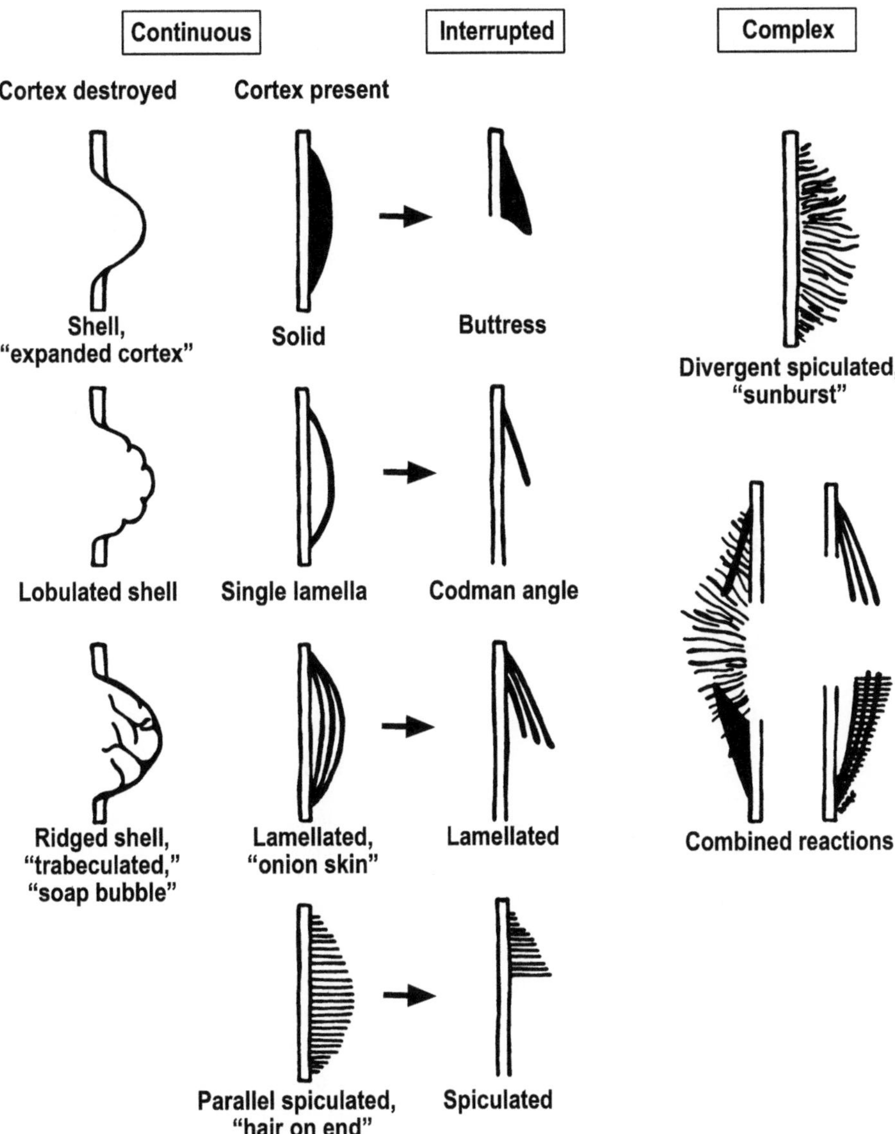

Fig. 2.4 Patterns of periosteal reactions. The arrows indicate that the continuous reaction patterns may become interrupted. Reproduced from Ragsdale et al. (1981).

pathologist in rendering specific diagnoses. For instance, "chicken wire" calcification in a chondroid bone tumor is often seen in chondroblastoma.

For a matrix to be appreciated on radiographs, there must be adequate mineralization. Calcification within biologic systems generally occurs in the form of calcium hydroxyapatite. Because other inorganic salts and trace elements are usually incorporated, *mineralization,* rather than *calcification,* is the preferred term

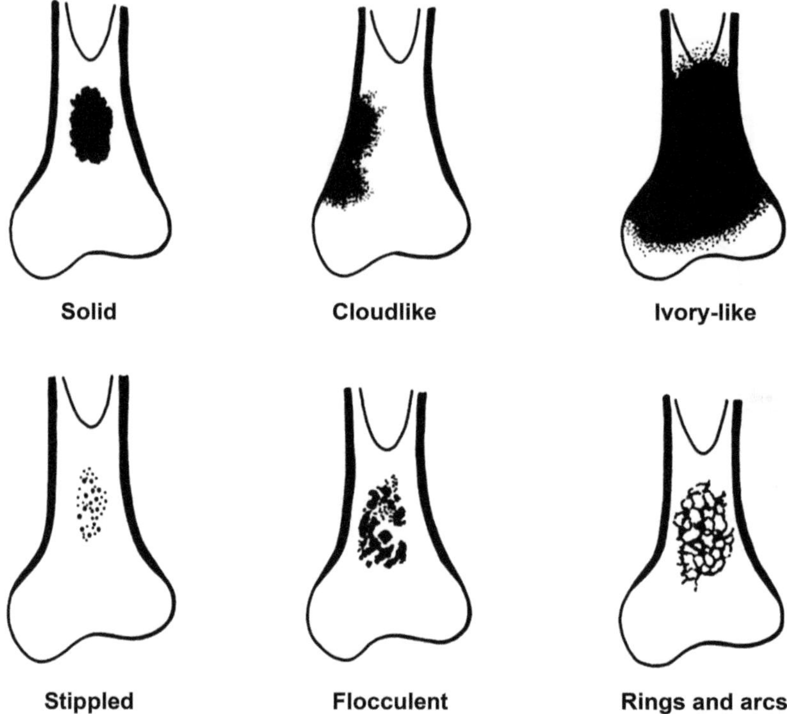

Fig. 2.5 Mineralized matrix patterns. Tumor osteoid (*top row*) appears as increased density with a solid (sharp edge) or cloudlike to ivory-like (ill-defined edge) pattern. Tumor cartilage (*bottom row*) creates stippled, flocculent, and solid density patterns. Rings and arcs represent bony rims around tumor cartilage lobules. Dystrophic mineralization and ischemic osteoid tend to mimic the stippled, flocculent, or patchy solid density patterns. "Ground glass" density can occur from faint osteoid production in fibrous dysplasia and is not depicted. Reproduced from Sweet et al. (1981).

for these areas of density. Mineralization almost invariably occurs within some form of preexisting organic background substance. In the case of tumors, the production of matrix may be osteoid, chondroid, fibrous (collagen), myxolipoid, or a mixture of these tissue types. Unless mineralized to a radiographically detectable threshold, bone tumors will appear as non–matrix producing. However, when sufficiently mineralized, the matrix can be further classified as either osteoid- or chondroid-producing matrix.

Because bone formation is a function of osteoblasts, the demonstration of mineralized osteoid matrix in a bone tumor indicates that it is osteoblastic. Radiographically, such osteoid matrix appears as a homogeneous area of increased density in the bone lesion. The degree of density may range in appearance from diffuse and hazy ("ground glass") to cloudlike or even ivory-like (Fig. 2.5). Osteoid formation, when associated with aggressive periosteal reactions or bone destruction, implies that the bony lesion is an osteosarcoma. Osteoid-producing tumors most commonly occur within the metaphysis of growing long bones (e.g., conventional osteosarcoma) but may occasionally be seen on the bone surface (e.g., osteoid

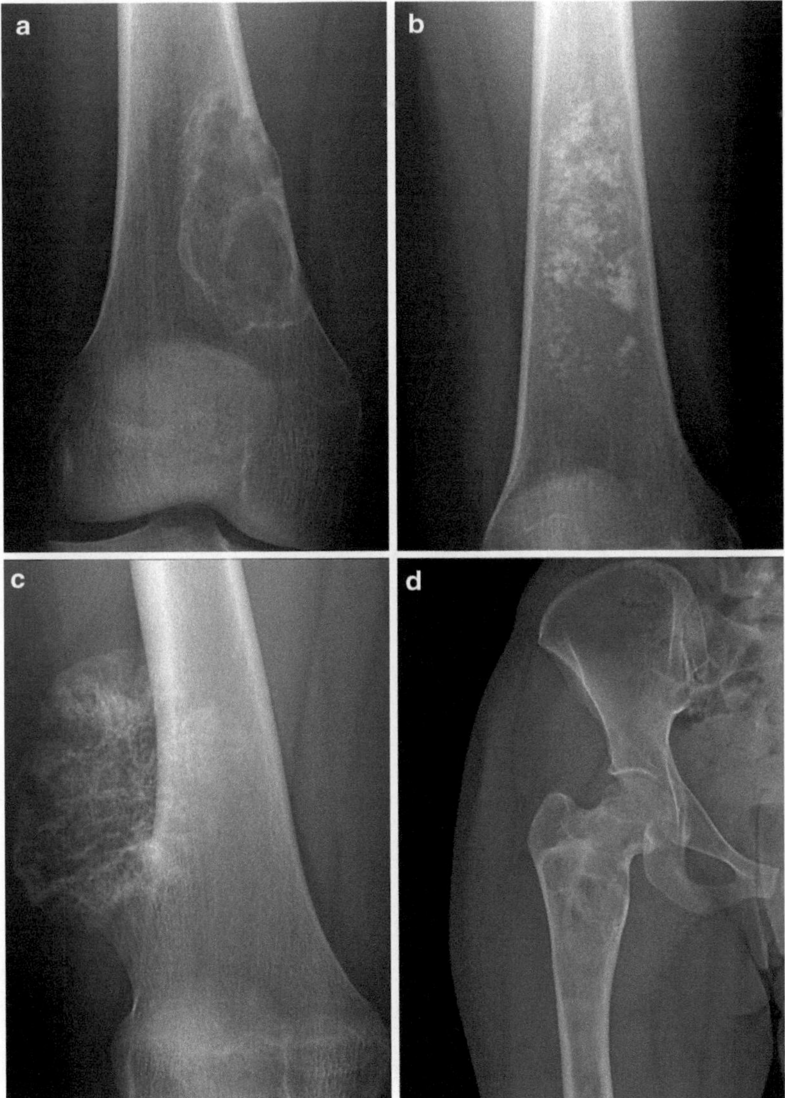

Fig. 2.6 The radiographic patterns of a spectrum of benign bone lesions. (**a**) A nonossifying fibroma/fibroxanthoma located eccentrically in a metadiaphysis. The tumor has a sclerotic rim that is slightly lobulated and expanded. (**b**) An enchondroma with typical rings and arcs, stipples, and flocculent mineralization. (**c**) An osteochondroma with trabeculated marrow extending into the stalk, a slight deformity of the femur, and a large cap formed from cartilage/endochondral bone. (**d**) Fibrous dysplasia with "ground glass" and more dense mineralization.

osteoma, parosteal osteosarcoma). The essential histologic and radiographic pattern in either of these circumstances is the predominance of neoplastic osteoid production by the sarcoma cells and increased density caused by subsequent mineralization of this new neoplastic bone.

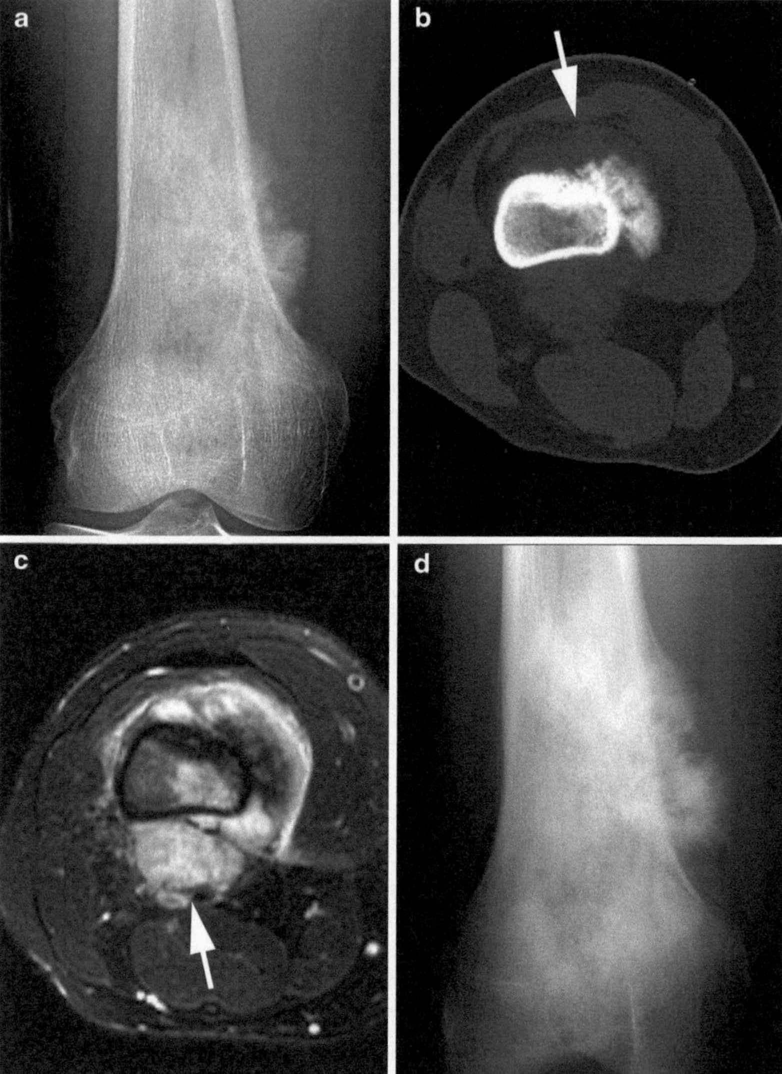

Fig. 2.7 Osteosarcoma in a femur. (**a**) Radiography shows osteoid matrix inside and outside the femur. (**b**) CT confirms the presence of osteoid matrix inside and outside the femur with a soft tissue mass (*arrow*) around the femur that is not mineralized and with anterior cortical destruction. (**c**) MRI (T2-weighted with fat saturation) shows extensive soft tissue involvement, but the neurovascular bundle (*arrow*) is intact on the surface of the posterior extension. (**d**) Radiography after intra-arterial chemotherapy shows progressive sclerosis inside and outside the femur compared with the amount seen in (**a**). The resected tumor had a histologic necrosis rate of 97%.

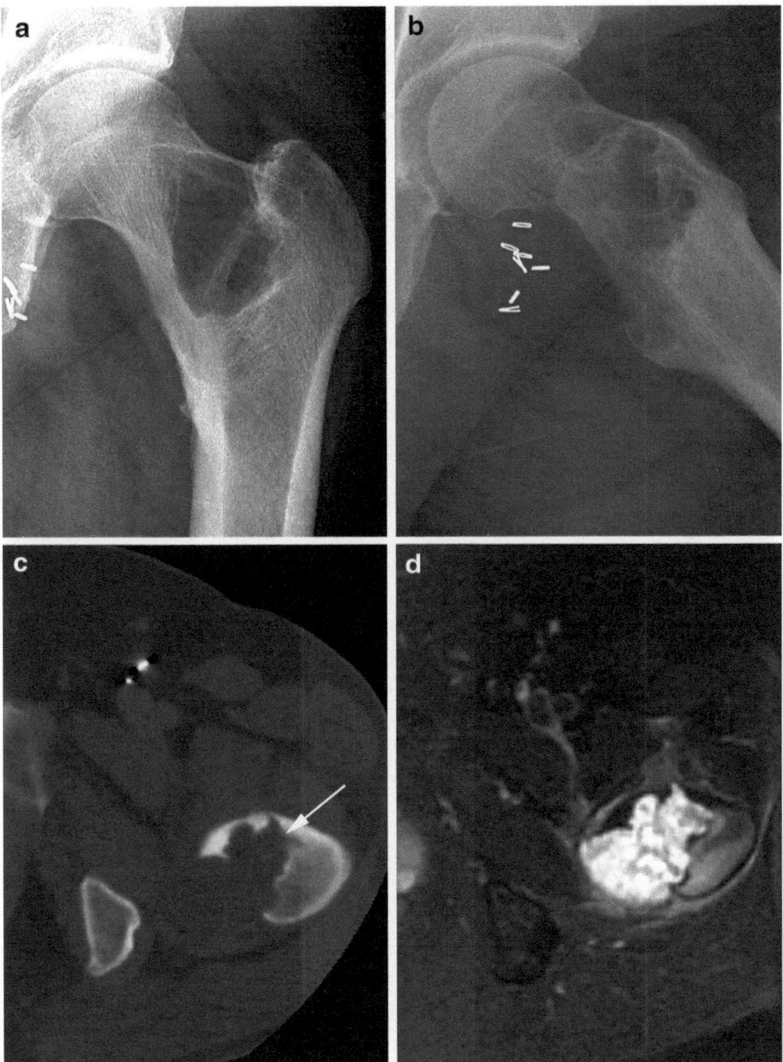

Fig. 2.8 Chondrosarcoma in a femur with vascular clips from a previous surgery. (**a**) Radiography shows a geographic lesion with a combination of sclerotic, nonsclerotic, and ill-defined margins. (**b**) Oblique radiography better demonstrates the posterior medial ill-defined margin and its aggressive cortical destruction. (**c**) CT shows cortical destruction, a soft tissue mass, a small area of chondroid mineralization (*arrow*), and varied margins, some with sclerotic and nonsclerotic rims. (**d**) MRI confirms the extent of posterior medial soft tissue extension but also shows anterior cortical penetration.

During normal cartilage formation, cell proliferation is followed by matrix secretion, hypertrophy, and the death of cartilage cells. Provisional calcification of chondroid matrix then occurs, followed by chondrolysis and replacement by endochondral bone. Cartilaginous tumors are capable of undergoing complete cartilage maturation, including provisional calcification and induction of endochondral bone formation. It is the architecture of the cartilaginous bone formation that produces the unique appearance of the chondroid matrix (Fig. 2.5, bottom row). The familiar parallel and linear shapes of normal growth-plate provisional calcification and endochondral bone are distorted in the chondroid development of a cartilaginous tumor, resulting in a lack of uniform maturation with varying sizes of proliferating cartilage lobules that may then mineralize. A caricature of provisional calcification occurs in the form of stipples, which can be coalescent or flocculent. Endochondral bone formation also occurs with mineralization, seen as rings and arcs within the cartilaginous tumor. The typical radiographic patterns are stipples or floccules of patchy, solid areas of density plus rings and/or arcs of increased density.

Frequently associated with these types of intramedullary chondroid-producing tumors is endosteal scalloping. The cartilaginous tumor favors lobular growth, and endosteal erosion is a common finding. However, as with many lytic patterns, endosteal scalloping is not specific to a cartilaginous bone tumor; it may also be seen in other tumors, such as metastases and myeloma. Further, endosteal scalloping (although it does suggest some degree of intramedullary growth) and chondroid matrix mineralization are not in and of themselves indicative of malignancy, being most commonly seen in benign cartilaginous lesions. However, when accompanied by aggressive periosteal reactions and/or bone destruction, endosteal scalloping is a strong indicator of malignancy. Thus, in the setting of endosteal erosion when there is osteolysis, aggressive periosteal reaction, or worrisome clinical signs and symptoms, the diagnosis of chondrosarcoma should be considered (Fig. 2.8).

Magnetic Resonance Imaging

MRI is the most comprehensive imaging modality for local staging of bone tumors. Its strengths are spatial resolution, contrast resolution, multiplanar display, flow sensitivity, contrast enhancement, and lack of ionizing radiation. The soft tissue contrast produced by MRI is greater than that seen with other imaging modalities, allowing differentiation between adjacent structures (Fig. 2.9). This contrast makes MRI invaluable for assessment of the local extent of bone tumors, including intramedullary and soft tissue extension. Generally, MRI does not permit an initial specific diagnosis of a bone sarcoma. MRI with and without intravenous gadolinium contrast can distinguish some benign bone lesions, such as lipomas (through the identification of fat signal) and simple or aneurysmal bone cysts (through lack of internal enhancement); however, for the most part, the signal characteristics of different types of sarcomas are too similar to be of much use in distinguishing one from another (Kransdorf et al. 1989), and these features may also be shared with many benign and nontumorous conditions. Interpretation of MRI scans of suspected or undiagnosed bone tumors must therefore always be accompanied by radiography.

Bone sarcomas typically demonstrate hypo- to isointense T1 signal intensity in comparison with muscle and heterogeneously hyperintense T2 signal intensity

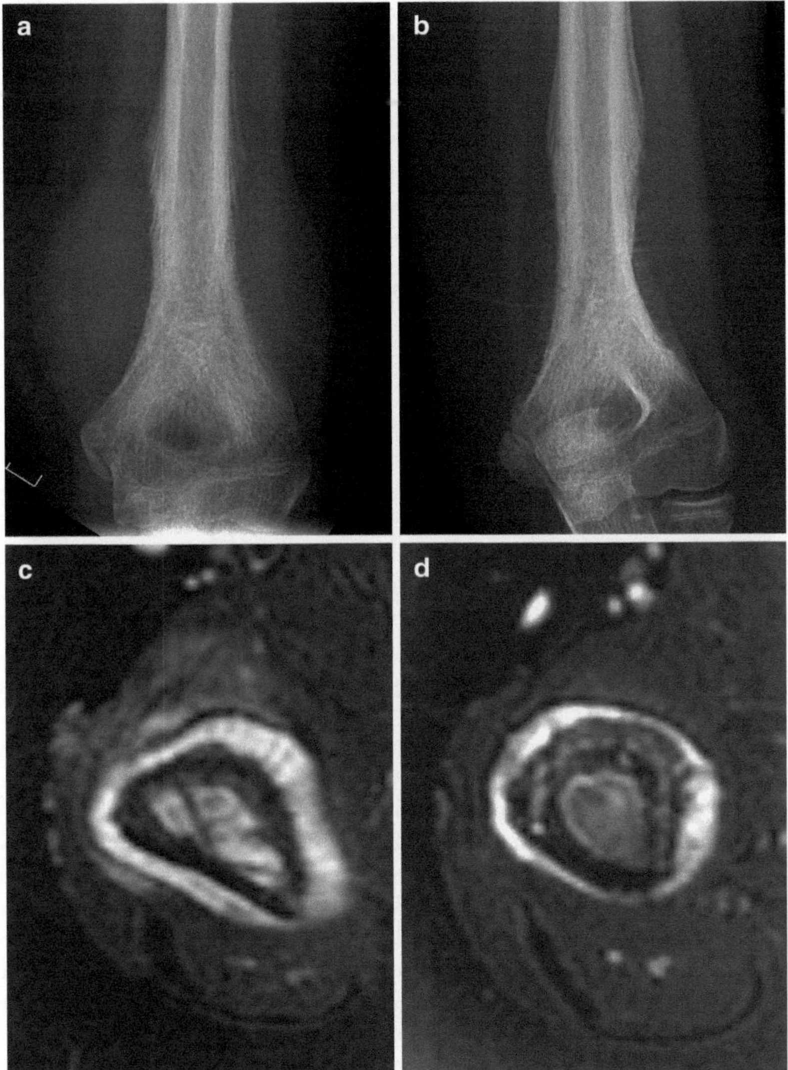

Fig. 2.9 Ewing sarcoma in a distal humerus. (**a**) Radiography shows a large soft tissue mass, periosteal reactions (spiculated, lamellated, and interrupted), Codman angle, and osteolysis (permeative and moth-eaten). (**b**) Radiography taken 7 weeks later shows a posttreatment partial response. Seen are a resolving soft tissue mass and progressive mineralization (maturation) of periosteal reactions, along with some sclerosis and redefinition of the cortex. (**c** and **d**) MRI (T2-weighted, fat-saturated) taken at the same time as (**b**) also shows tumor improvement in the soft tissue and subperiosteal tumor, periosteal reaction, and marrow.

in comparison with fat. After the administration of intravenous gadolinium contrast, bone sarcomas typically demonstrate a variable degree of internal enhancement. Areas that lack enhancement are typically representative of necrosis, hemorrhage, or mineralization within the tumor. At our institution, intravenous contrast is routinely administered initially on pretherapeutic baseline MRI studies. After the administration of intravenous contrast, MRI can be used to guide biopsy to the enhancing, vascularized portions of a tumor and help avoid necrotic, nonenhancing tissue, which may not be diagnostic. Intravenous contrast is also used on subsequent preoperative MRI studies for evaluation of the tumor response to therapy (discussed later in this chapter). Finally, intravenous contrast is given for postoperative MRI scans to increase the conspicuity of residual or recurrent tumor (see Chap. 14, "Follow-up Evaluation and Surveillance After Treatment of Bone Sarcomas," for further discussion of magnetic resonance [MR] pulse sequences and the rationale for their use).

Computed Tomography

In essence, CT can be described as sophisticated, cross-sectional, computer-enhanced radiography. Like conventional radiographs, CT images basically distinguish between air, fat, water, and mineral, but with CT, many more shades of gray or density are detected by computer enhancement. These images provide exquisite detail of bone anatomy, including cortical continuity or disruption of cancellous bone, and evaluation of periosteal reactions. CT excellently demonstrates tumor matrix mineralization inside and outside the bone. Because it is a cross-sectional imaging technique, CT can simplify the appearance of complex anatomy in areas such as the joints, pelvis, and spine, where there may be too many curving and overlapping surfaces to allow complete anatomic evaluation by conventional radiography. As CT scanners have improved over the past decade or so, reconstruction techniques and volumetric scanning have allowed CT to compete with MRI's ability to provide multiple imaging planes. Reformatted images in the sagittal and coronal planes are very useful, and at MD Anderson, we routinely acquire them in almost all cases in which CT is performed for skeletal disease. Images in the oblique and nonconventional planes may also be obtained. Three-dimensional and volumetric CT images can assist in preoperative planning. Plastic models made from the three-dimensional CT images are also useful in the design and manufacture of customized prostheses with an accurate fit. When there is a contraindication to MRI, CT with contrast media may be used in its place for evaluation of the extent of bone disease.

Skeletal Scintigraphy

Like MRI, skeletal scintigraphy is a highly sensitive but nonspecific imaging modality for detection of bone lesions; however, unlike regional MRI, it provides a global picture of the entire skeleton. Radionuclide bone scans using 99m technetium methylenediphosphonate (99mTc-MDP) are routinely obtained during the workup of patients with bone sarcoma. The bone scan not only shows the primary bone sarcoma and its specific location but also reveals remote metastases elsewhere in the skeleton, which might otherwise remain undetected at baseline. This modality is also useful in demonstrating "skip metastases" that may occur separately from the primary sarcoma in the same bone. Skeletal scintigraphy remains the imaging technique of choice for screening for bone-to-bone metastases. Such metastases are relatively uncommon among bone sarcomas and most often seen in patients with osteosarcoma or Ewing sarcoma. Because multiplicity is more common in bone metastases from nonbone primary solid-organ or soft tissue tumors, myeloma, or lymphoma, these diagnoses should be excluded if multiple bone lesions are discovered by scintigraphy.

Other Modalities

PET imaging using [^{18}F]fluorodeoxyglucose (^{18}F-FDG) is currently being used in patients with bone sarcomas. It is a functional imaging modality that detects the accumulation of radiolabeled glucose in tissues with high metabolic activity (seen in numerous malignancies) and is used in the form of fused PET/CT in modern imaging practices. Like skeletal scintigraphy, PET/CT provides whole-body imaging. An advantage of PET/CT over skeletal scintigraphy is that it can reveal metastases in soft tissues as well as bone.

Fluoroscopy or ultrasonography, in addition to CT or MRI, can be used to guide needles for biopsy of a bone sarcoma for diagnosis.

Assessment of Tumor Extent

After diagnosis, the local extent of the bone tumor and its distant spread in the body are determined for staging. The local extent of a bone sarcoma can be identified as intramedullary (one anatomic compartment) or extramedullary (two or more compartments). Determining the intramedullary extent involves assessment of the longitudinal medullary length, the presence of epiphyseal involvement, and the presence of skip metastases. These factors determine the level of subsequent local bone resection, if needed. Extramedullary extension is defined by cortical breakthrough and involvement of the adjacent soft tissues, specific muscle groups, major neurovascular bundles, and the adjoining growth plate or joint. Accurate, detailed evaluation of extramedullary extension is required for deciding whether to perform limb-salvage surgery. The distant extent of a bone sarcoma involves the presence of regional metastases (other than skip metastases) and distant metastases, which most commonly occur in the lung.

Plain radiography can demonstrate gross local extension by showing cortical breakthrough and extraosseous mineralized matrix, if present. However, it is MRI that is the most comprehensive imaging modality for determining the local extent. CT can also demonstrate cortical breakthrough, and the mineralized extraosseous components of a bone sarcoma are easily seen on noncontrasted scans; however, like plain radiography, CT has a limited role for the purpose of staging because of a lack of soft tissue contrast resolution.

Both regional and distant metastasis can occur with bone sarcomas. Skeletal scintigraphy can demonstrate intracompartmental skip metastases, but if they are too close to the primary tumor, they may be obscured by the extended field of radioactive uptake exhibited by the tumor. The technique provides a global picture of the entire skeleton and is highly sensitive but nonspecific. Although most active osteoblastic metastases yield positive findings on a radionuclide bone scan, up to 5% of osteolytic metastases can be missed. At times, skeletal scintigraphy may even show mineralizing lung metastases in patients with osteosarcoma. Nevertheless, MRI is superior to skeletal scintigraphy in detection of bony metastases, and whole-body MRI has been shown to be more sensitive than skeletal scintigraphy for the detection of bony metastases (Eustace et al. 1997). However, whole-body MRI is not widely used at the time of this publication, and conventional MRI is only utilized for regional scanning.

For detection of lung metastases, CT is the optimal imaging technique. Nodal metastases, although rarely seen with bone sarcomas, can be demonstrated with CT or MRI. Ultrasonography has a limited role in the assessment of spread of bone sarcomas but may be helpful in distinguishing reactive lymph nodes from metastatic disease, detecting local recurrence, and guiding biopsy in these circumstances.

Magnetic Resonance Imaging

MRI produces soft tissue contrast superior to that of other imaging modalities, making it the ideal noninvasive method of evaluating the local extent of bone tumors (Aisen et al. 1986). The relationship of the tumor to vital structures, such as nerves, vessels, muscles, fascial planes, growth plates, and articular surfaces, is best demonstrated with MRI, allowing accurate preoperative planning for en bloc resection and use of metallic prostheses, bone allografts, or autografts. Flap placement after surgery at the operative site can also be anticipated and planned using MRI.

MRI allows simultaneous assessment of the intramedullary and soft tissue extent of bone sarcomas. It reveals the length of tumor involvement in the medullary cavity, the size of the associated soft tissue masses, and the degree of enhancement, which is indicative of tumor viability and vascularity. Essential information obtained with MRI also includes the relationship of soft tissue extension to the surrounding structures, such as nerves, vessels (abutted or encased), muscles, other bones, and visceral organs, and the extension of the tumor across the fascial planes (Fig. 2.10). As noted above, bone sarcomas rarely metastasize to lymph nodes, but enlarged lymph nodes, when present, are often easily detected with MRI.

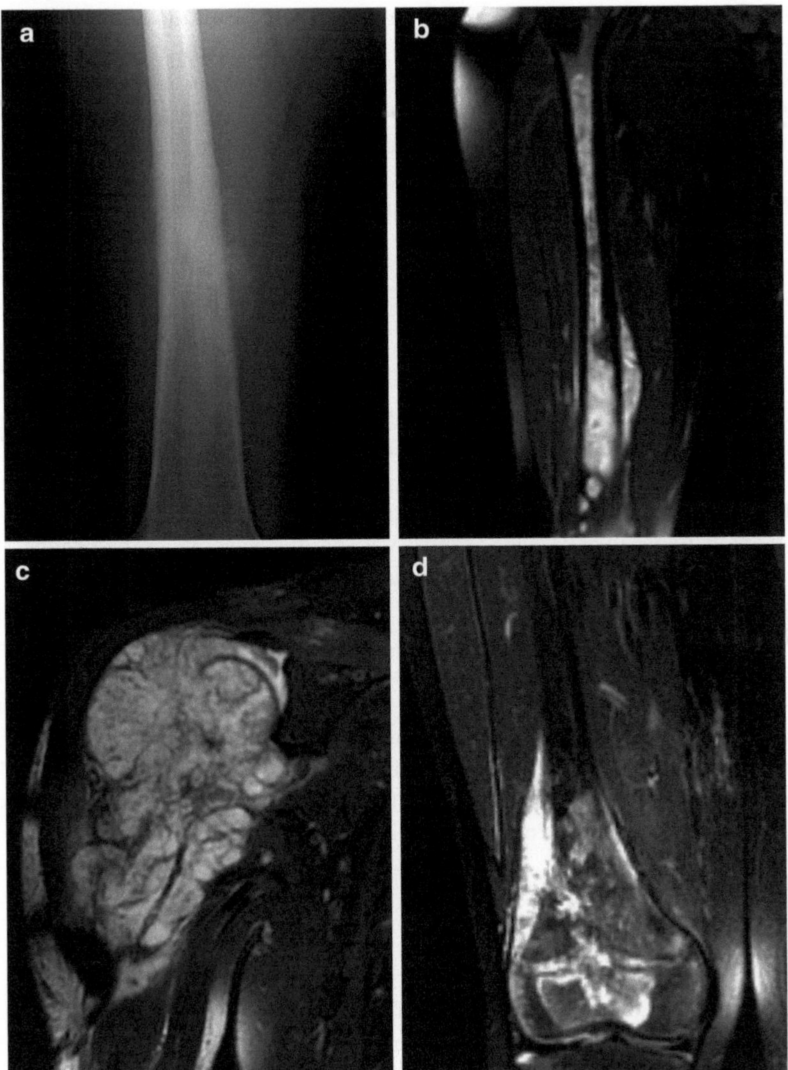

Fig. 2.10 A spectrum of extent of disease. (**a**) A radiograph and (**b**) coronal T2-weighted MRI scan of a femur osteosarcoma with a predominant diaphyseal location and osteoid matrix inside and outside the bone. MRI demonstrates extensive intramarrow extension, skip metastases, and an extraosseous mass corresponding to, but with much greater involvement than, what is seen using radiography. (**c**) An osteosarcoma in a proximal humerus with extensive soft tissue disease extending superiorly into the shoulder joint. (**d**) An osteosarcoma in a distal femur with extension through the growth plate into the epiphysis and down to the subarticular bone.

Evaluation of a bone sarcoma requires examination of the marrow cavity of the entire bone in order to exclude the possibility of skip metastases, the presence of which indicates a worse prognosis. At our institution, if a bone sarcoma is suspected, the entire bone is evaluated in the coronal plane using fast spin echo T1-weighted and fat-saturated fast spin echo T2-weighted images. Inversion recovery sequences are prescribed as an alternative to the fat-saturated images, especially in the presence of significant metal (see Chap. 14). Specific surface coils, such as an extremity or long-bone coil, are utilized to enhance image quality and spatial resolution. Additional pulse sequences are obtained in the axial plane, including fast spin echo T1-weighted images, fat-saturated fast spin echo T2-weighted images, and fat-saturated fast spin echo T1-weighted images after administration of intravenous gadolinium.

Computed Tomography

Although CT can be useful in diagnosis of a malignant bone tumor, its use in assessment of the local extent of the tumor is very limited. MRI provides superior contrast resolution between the tumor and surrounding normal tissue and is, consequently, the first-line method for determining local extent in the extremities. In patients who cannot safely undergo MRI, such as those with cardiac pacemakers and defibrillators, both CT and ultrasonography may play a useful role in determination of the local extent of the tumor.

In the chest, abdomen, and pelvis, CT is the primary cross-sectional method of diagnosis for nonmusculoskeletal disease. MR sequences, even short ones, take at least a minute or two to acquire, increasing the likelihood of significant motion artifact. The normal physiologic motion of the heart, lungs, and intestines and the transmitted motion that affects such internal organs as the liver and kidneys decrease the quality of the MR images. CT scans, on the other hand, now take mere seconds and can be performed in 1 breath hold, essentially eliminating motion artifact.

Chest CT

When a patient is diagnosed with a sarcoma, a conventional radiograph and a CT scan of the chest are obtained to evaluate for metastatic disease. If there is no sign of metastases in the chest or in the included portion of the upper abdomen and if there are no factors, such as elevated levels of liver enzymes, to suggest other disease, no additional CT scans are typically performed. Often, however, particularly in older patients, the chest radiograph and CT scan will not be pristinely normal. Many people harbor small pulmonary nodules, the majority of which, particularly in patients without known cancer, are benign. In patients with bone sarcoma, the likelihood of metastatic nodules increases when these small nodules are present, and follow-up to determine biologic activity or growth may be necessary.

A single pulmonary nodule with spiculated borders stands a reasonable chance of representing a primary lung cancer, particularly in older patients or those who smoke. A patient with such a nodule should be evaluated with a biopsy. Smoother, multiple nodules are more typical of metastatic disease. Smooth, multiple nodules are atypically granulomas, such as histoplasmomas. If the pulmonary nodule is large enough, PET scanning or a biopsy may be useful. For smaller nodules, follow-up CT scans are often performed. Metastatic nodules may be expected to grow or even shrink after chemotherapy, whereas granulomas often remain stable. Other intrinsic pulmonary diseases may also be discovered incidentally with chest CT.

Skeletal Scintigraphy

Skeletal scintigraphy with 99mTc-MDP provides a global view of the skeleton and is routinely used in assessment of tumor spread to detect remote bony metastases. Mineralizing lung metastases from osteosarcoma may be seen on radionuclide bone scans. The technique is highly sensitive but nonspecific; lesions that appear "hot" on bone scans must be studied on plain radiographs of the bones to exclude the possibility of benign bone lesions such as fractures.

Evaluation of Response to Treatment

After chemotherapy, radiation, or both, patients with bone sarcomas undergo routine follow-up with plain radiographs and MRI scans to assess response. In patients who undergo surgery, such imaging techniques are used to assess the presence of residual or recurrent tumor or metastases and to detect hardware complications (see also Chap. 14).

Radiography is useful for demonstrating shrinkage and ossification of a bone tumor, which are both favorable signs in osteosarcoma and Ewing sarcoma. Radiography can also detect hardware failure, due to either mechanical factors or osteomyelitis, after limb-salvage surgery. Recurrent tumor may also be demonstrated as an osteolytic lesion or as increased mineralization. However, as described above, plain radiography is a screening imaging modality with inherent limitations.

MRI has a major role in the evaluation of response of bone sarcomas to therapy. A posttherapeutic decrease in the degree of internal contrast enhancement and/or shrinkage of the tumor is considered a positive response to therapy. At times, a sarcoma may become larger after treatment yet still have responded favorably to therapy if the enlargement coincides with decreasing enhancement. The enlarging portion of the tumor in this scenario represents therapy-induced cell death and necrosis. Increased tumor contrast enhancement (typically accompanied by an increase in the size or nodularity of all or part of the tumor) constitutes a potential failed therapeutic response and requires reevaluation of the patient's therapeutic regimen. Changes in MR enhancement reflect general trends in the degree of tumor necrosis but, at the time of this publication, do not replace the accuracy of histologic evaluation. Although research efforts have assessed tumor response through methods such as dynamic MRI (Choyke et al. 2003), MR-coupled molecular imaging

(Pathak 2005), and diffusion-weighted imaging (Uhl et al. 2006), all imaging studies remain preoperative adjuncts to histopathologic examination in determining the percentage of tumor necrosis. MRI is also effective for detection of tumor recurrence locally and regionally.

PET scanning using ^{18}F-FDG has been found useful in evaluating therapeutic response in patients with bone sarcoma. FDG PET/CT has been shown to be capable of providing prognostic information in patients with osteosarcoma. Costelloe et al. (2009) studied 31 patients with FDG PET/CT before and after the administration of chemotherapy, prior to surgical resection. The investigators found that a high maximum standardized uptake value (SUV_{max}) using lean body mass before and after chemotherapy indicated worse progression-free survival, while a high SUV_{max} value after chemotherapy indicated worse overall survival. Although PET/CT may or may not be performed with intravenous contrast and does not image the lungs as well as diagnostic chest CT, this fused imaging modality provides functional and anatomic information of the entire body in a single imaging session and may become standard practice in the evaluation of bone sarcomas.

Key Practice Points

- Radiography is fundamental to the initial characterization and diagnosis of a bone tumor and is the first imaging study that should be performed.
- Aggressive benign bone lesions may mimic malignant bone lesions on radiographs and other imaging studies.
- Because of its many excellent imaging properties, MRI is the optimal imaging modality for simultaneous evaluation of the intraosseous and soft tissue extent of bone sarcomas, including their relationship to adjacent vital structures.
- Because of its sectional display of osseous anatomy, CT can be more helpful than plain radiography in complex anatomic areas such as the spine and pelvis or when bony detail is critical to assessment.
- Skeletal scintigraphy should be routinely performed to detect remote bone metastases.
- MRI is useful for assessing tumor response to therapy through change in size and/or contrast enhancement.

Suggested Readings

Aisen AM, Martel W, Braunstein EM, et al. MRI and CT evaluation of primary bone and soft-tissue tumors. Am J Roentgenol. 1986;146:749–56.
Choyke PL, Dwyer AJ, Knopp MV. Functional tumor imaging with dynamic contrast-enhanced magnetic resonance imaging. J Magn Reson Imaging. 2003;17:509–20.

Costelloe CM, Macapinlac HA, Madewell JE, et al. ^{18}F-FDG PET/CT as an indicator of progression-free and overall survival in osteosarcoma. J Nucl Med. 2009;50:340–7.

Enneking WF. A system of staging musculoskeletal neoplasms. Clin Orthop Relat Res. 1986;(204):9–24.

Eustace S, Tello R, DeCarvalho V, et al. A comparison of whole-body turboSTIR MR imaging and planar ^{99m}Tc-methylene diphosphonate scintigraphy in the examination of patients with suspected skeletal metastases. Am J Roentgenol. 1997;169:1655–61.

Johnson LC. A general theory of bone tumors. Bull N Y Acad Med. 1953;29:164–71.

Kransdorf MJ, Jelinek JS, Moser Jr RP, et al. Soft-tissue masses: diagnosis using MR imaging. Am J Roentgenol. 1989;153:541–7.

Lodwick GS, Wilson AJ, Farrell C, et al. Determining growth rates of focal lesions of bone from radiographs. Radiology. 1980;134:577–83.

Madewell JE, Ragsdale BD, Sweet DE. Radiologic and pathologic analysis of solitary bone lesions. Part I: internal margins. Radiol Clin North Am. 1981;19:715–48.

Morrison WB, Dalinka MK, Daffner RH. Bone tumors. ACR appropriateness criteria. Reston: American College of Radiology; 2005. p. 1–5.

Murphy Jr WA. Imaging bone tumors in the 1990s. Cancer. 1991;67:1169–76.

Nomikos GC, Murphey MD, Kransdorf MJ, et al. Primary bone tumors of the lower extremities. Radiol Clin North Am. 2002;40:971–90.

Oudenhoven LF, Dhondt E, Kahn S, et al. Accuracy of radiography in grading and tissue-specific diagnosis—a study of 200 consecutive bone tumors of the hand. Skeletal Radiol. 2006;35: 78–87.

Pathak AP. Magnetic resonance imaging of tumor physiology. Methods Mol Med. 2005;124: 279–97.

Ragsdale BD, Madewell JE, Sweet DE. Radiologic and pathologic analysis of solitary bone lesions. Part II: periosteal reactions. Radiol Clin North Am. 1981;19:749–83.

Stacy GS, Mahal RS, Peabody TD. Staging of bone tumors: a review with illustrative examples. Am J Roentgenol. 2006;186:967–76.

Sweet DE, Madewell JE, Ragsdale BD. Radiologic and pathologic analysis of solitary bone lesions. Part III: matrix patterns. Radiol Clin North Am. 1981;19:785–814.

Tehranzadeh J, Mnaymneh W, Ghavam C, et al. Comparison of CT and MR imaging in musculoskeletal neoplasms. J Comput Assist Tomogr. 1989;13:466–72.

Uhl M, Saueressig U, van Buiren M, et al. Osteosarcoma: preliminary results of *in vivo* assessment of tumor necrosis after chemotherapy with diffusion- and perfusion-weighted magnetic resonance imaging. Invest Radiol. 2006;41:618–23.

Chapter 3
Percutaneous Image-Guided Biopsy for Diagnosis of Bone Sarcomas

Kamran Ahrar

Contents

Chapter Overview Percutaneous image-guided biopsy plays an essential role in diagnosis and management of all cancer patients, including those with primary bone tumors. For the biopsy procedure to be successful in characterizing bone tumors, appropriate planning is of utmost importance. This planning starts with review of both plain radiographs and cross-sectional imaging studies. The interventional radiologist should select an appropriate imaging modality to guide the biopsy and carefully plan the biopsy to minimize the risk for any neurovascular complications. For patients who will undergo limb-salvage operations, careful attention should be given to the biopsy approach such that the orthopedic surgeon will be able to resect the biopsy track using the standard approach for the selected operation. Both fine-needle aspiration and core biopsy are used for sampling of bone tumors; the two techniques are often complementary. Nearly all image-guided bone biopsies can be performed under moderate intravenous sedation in an outpatient setting. These procedures are safe, complications are rare, and the recovery is

K. Ahrar (✉)
Section of Interventional Radiology, Department of Diagnostic Radiology, Unit 1471,
Division of Diagnostic Imaging, The University of Texas MD Anderson Cancer Center,
1515 Holcombe Boulevard, Houston, TX 77030, USA
e-mail: kahrar@mdanderson.org

P.P. Lin and S. Patel (eds.), *Bone Sarcoma*, MD Anderson Cancer Care Series,
DOI 10.1007/978-1-4614-5194-5_3,
© The University of Texas M. D. Anderson Cancer Center 2013

negligible. The expedited diagnosis and short recovery possible with percutaneous biopsy, in contrast with open surgical biopsy, allow for immediate institution of the appropriate therapy.

Introduction

Radiographic characterization of a bone lesion, together with the medical history and physical examination, often helps narrow the differential diagnosis to a short list of possibilities. However, to establish the definitive diagnosis, a biopsy is usually necessary. For malignant lesions, it is especially important to confirm the exact diagnosis before initiating neoadjuvant chemotherapy, radiation therapy, and surgical resection. The biopsy should provide adequate material so that an unequivocal pathologic diagnosis can be established.

At MD Anderson Cancer Center, percutaneous biopsy is generally the preferred procedure for obtaining diagnostic tissue from primary bone tumors. In this chapter, we describe our rationale for and approach to performing percutaneous image-guided biopsies. These procedures are performed in the Interventional Radiology Suites. The facilities dedicated to this operation include clinic space for patient consultation, a preprocedure patient preparation area, state-of-the-art imaging equipment, and a postprocedure recovery area.

Percutaneous Versus Open Biopsy

When compared with open surgical biopsy, percutaneous image-guided biopsy of primary bone tumors has several advantages. Whereas open surgical biopsies often require general anesthesia and sometimes hospitalization, percutaneous procedures are typically performed on an outpatient basis with intravenous conscious sedation. Neoadjuvant chemotherapy or radiation therapy is delayed for 10 days to 3 weeks after open biopsy to allow for wound healing, but these therapies can be initiated immediately after percutaneous biopsy. Open biopsies may cause gross tumor contamination of the field, tumor cell dissemination from oozing vessels after tour- niquet release, hemorrhage, and hematoma formation. However, complications are exceedingly rare after percutaneous bone biopsies. Percutaneous image-guided biopsy allows sampling of various tumor quadrants and immediate assessment of tissue viability. And finally, percutaneous biopsies are more cost-effective than are open surgical biopsies.

With careful patient selection and planning, percutaneous bone biopsy is a highly effective method of establishing a diagnosis for a variety of bone tumors and tumorlike lesions. Nondiagnostic biopsies, or samples that do not yield a specific pathologic diagnosis, are rare. In our experience, a nondiagnostic biopsy usually does not result from an inadequate quantity of sample material. Suboptimal prebiopsy imaging and characterization of the tumor are potential causes of a biopsy result being nondiagnostic. Another contributor is indiscriminate use of biopsy for any lesion, irrespective of its radiographic features, size, or location.

In a study of 110 patients who underwent percutaneous biopsy, the diagnostic accuracy rates were 98% for correct determination of benign versus malignant tumors and 88% for correct histologic diagnosis (Jelinek et al. 2002). In that study, high diagnostic accuracy was achieved for biopsies in both sclerotic and solid, nonsclerotic lesions. Biopsies in tumors that were predominantly cystic, as determined by computed tomography (CT) or magnetic resonance imaging (MRI), resulted in several nondiagnostic samples.

When percutaneous biopsy samples are nondiagnostic, an open surgical biopsy may be warranted. In a study of 141 patients with suspected primary musculoskeletal neoplasms, 25 (18%) required open biopsies because of inconclusive results of percutaneous core biopsies (Yao et al. 1999). However, diagnostic dilemmas after percutaneous biopsy may not always be resolved with open surgical biopsy. This situation is particularly the case when a patient does not have cancer but exhibits a radiographic abnormality that is suggestive of malignancy. In the study by Yao et al., only 72% of the subsequent open biopsies yielded a specific diagnosis, and the remaining 28% were inconclusive.

Assessment of the Patient

At MD Anderson, all patients who undergo percutaneous biopsy in Interventional Radiology first have a consultation to assess their suitability for safely undergoing the procedure. During the consultation, a patient's age, cardiopulmonary status, body size, weight, and level of existing pain are considered to determine an appropriate sedation method. Most percutaneous biopsies are performed with local anesthesia and moderate intravenous sedation consisting of small doses of anxiolytic drugs (e.g., midazolam hydrochloride) and analgesic agents (e.g., fentanyl citrate). Young children, patients with borderline cardiopulmonary function, patients who are morbidly obese, and patients with severe cancer-related pain may require higher levels of sedation or anesthesia, i.e., deep intravenous sedation or general anesthesia administered by an anesthesiologist. In addition to determination of sedation method, the prebiopsy consultation includes a review of the patient's clinical history, which should consider any tumor-related symptoms, such as neurovascular compromise. A focused physical exam is performed to document any sensory, motor, or pulse deficit.

Prebiopsy adjustments to patients' medications may be needed. Long-acting anticoagulants (e.g., warfarin) should be switched to short-acting agents (e.g., enoxaparin) that can be discontinued 12 h before the biopsy and restarted shortly after the biopsy. Antiplatelet agents (e.g., aspirin or clopidogrel) should be discontinued for an appropriate amount of time to allow recovery of platelet function; we recommend discontinuation of aspirin for 3–7 days prior to the biopsy and of clopidogrel for 3–5 days prior. Laboratory evaluation of patients who undergo bone biopsy should include assessment of coagulation pathways. At minimum, a platelet count of 50,000/μL is required. The international normalized ratio (INR) should not exceed 1.6. A low platelet count or abnormal INR should be corrected prior to biopsy.

During the consultation, the risks and benefits of percutaneous biopsy are discussed with the patients and their families. Informed consent is obtained at the time of consultation. A prebiopsy consultation helps detect unanticipated problems in advance and prevents delays and cancellations of procedures. The results are improved quality of care and patient satisfaction.

Prebiopsy Planning

One of the most important predictors of outcome in establishing the diagnosis of any bone tumor is the thoroughness of both prebiopsy evaluation and planning of the procedure. This process begins with the review of appropriate imaging studies. In our practice, these studies often include plain radiography and MRI of the affected bone (Figs. 3.1 and 3.2). In the workup for suspected bone sarcomas, MRI should include images taken before and after administration of intravenous contrast material (Figs. 3.1b and 3.2b). MRI scans help guide the biopsy by outlining the extent of bone marrow involvement, identifying any soft tissue components, and detecting any areas of cystic degeneration or necrosis. Plain radiographs add to this evaluation by localizing areas of cortical breakdown or sclerosis that may not be well depicted by MRI.

Based on careful evaluation of images, an area within the tumor that is most likely to yield a diagnostic sample is selected for biopsy. In selecting this site, the soft tissue component is preferred over the dense sclerotic portion of the tumor. Furthermore, cystic or necrotic areas are avoided. Once the target area is selected, a route is prescribed to provide a short path from the puncture site at the skin surface to the target. More important than the length of the path, the trajectory of the needle should be free of any vital structures, such as neurovascular bundles in the appendicular skeleton and visceral organs in the chest, abdomen, or pelvis. Also, consideration is given to including the biopsy site in the future surgical resection field. Track seeding from needle biopsy is exceedingly rare, and despite anecdotal reports (Davies et al. 1993), it has not been shown to be a major cause of morbidity in patients with bone sarcomas (Ahrar et al. 2004). Nevertheless, when limb-salvage surgery is contemplated for primary bone tumors, anatomically based guidelines should be followed such that the surgeon could resect the biopsy track using a standard incision, without the need for additional soft tissue resection (Liu et al. 2007).

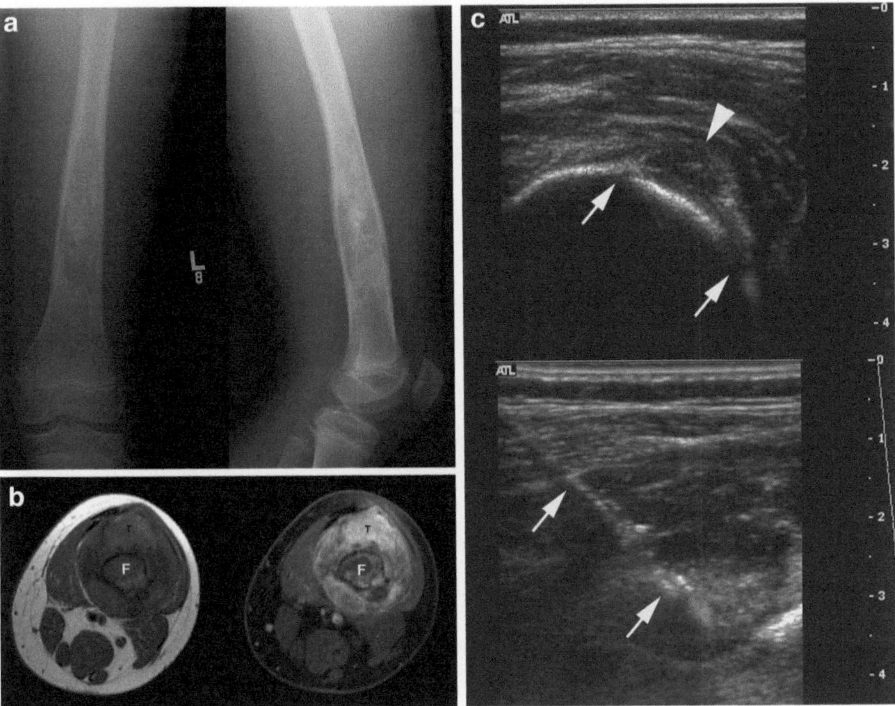

Fig. 3.1 Evaluation of an 11-year-old boy who presented with pain involving his left thigh. (**a**) Anteroposterior and lateral radiographs of the left femur demonstrate an aggressive, sclerotic lesion with expansion of the distal left femur. (**b**) Precontrast axial T1-weighted (*left*) and postcontrast, fat-suppressed axial T1-weighted (*right*) MRI scans of the distal femur demonstrate heterogeneous enhancement of the femur (F) and a circumferential soft tissue mass surrounding the bone. The maximum enhancement is seen in the anterior aspect of the tumor (T). (**c**) A transverse ultrasound image (*top*) of the distal left thigh demonstrates a soft tissue mass (*arrowhead*) and breaks in the cortex of the femur (*arrows*). A longitudinal ultrasound image (*bottom*) of the same lesion shows the entire length of the biopsy needle (*arrows*) placed within the tumor. A pathologic diagnosis of high-grade osteoblastic osteosarcoma was made on the basis of 14-gauge core biopsy samples. This diagnosis was later confirmed after resection of the tumor. Images © 2013, Kamran Ahrar.

Imaging Modalities

MD Anderson's Interventional Radiology Suites contain ultrasonography, fluoroscopy, CT, MRI, and angiography equipment. One or more of these imaging modalities is selected to guide needle placement and tissue sampling. Each modality has certain advantages and disadvantages.

Ultrasonography provides real-time imaging and is capable of depicting the entire needle as it advances from the puncture site at the skin surface to the target (Saifuddin et al. 2000). Duplex Doppler ultrasonography allows detection of

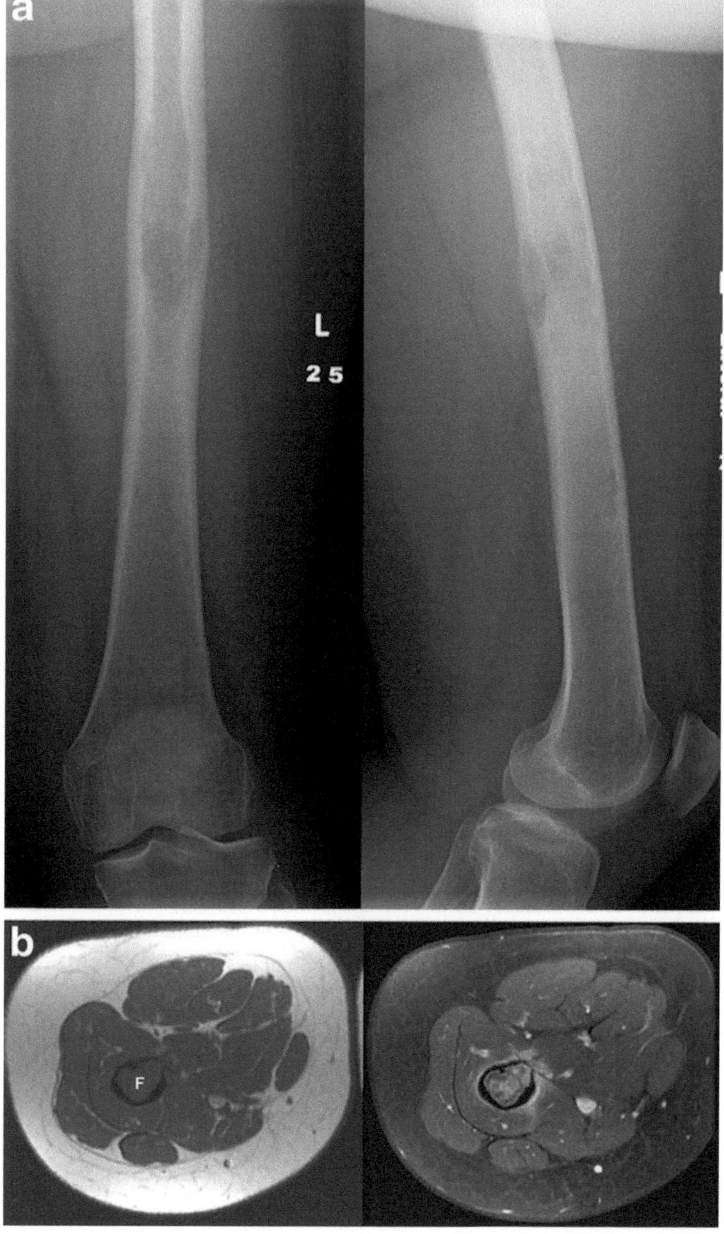

Fig. 3.2 Evaluation of a 55-year-old woman who presented with left thigh pain. (**a**) Anteroposterior and lateral radiographs of the left femur demonstrate an aggressive, expansile lesion involving the midshaft of the left femur. Observed are endosteal scalloping, lytic destructive changes, and faint calcifications. (**b**) With the patient in prone position, precontrast axial T1-weighted (*left*) and post-contrast, fat-suppressed axial T1-weighted (*right*) MRI scans of the distal femur demonstrate heterogeneous enhancement of the femur (F) with extension of the tumor through the posterior femoral cortex. A scant soft tissue component is associated with this tumor. (**c**) An axial CT image of both thighs demonstrates the abnormal expansion of the left femur (F) with punctate areas of calcification. (**d**) Axial CT images with the patient in prone position demonstrate placement of the biopsy needle within the target area for sampling of the tumor. This track was chosen so that it can be incorporated into the resected specimen at the time of surgery. A pathologic diagnosis of chondrosarcoma was established based on evaluation of 14-gauge core biopsy samples. Images © 2013, Kamran Ahrar.

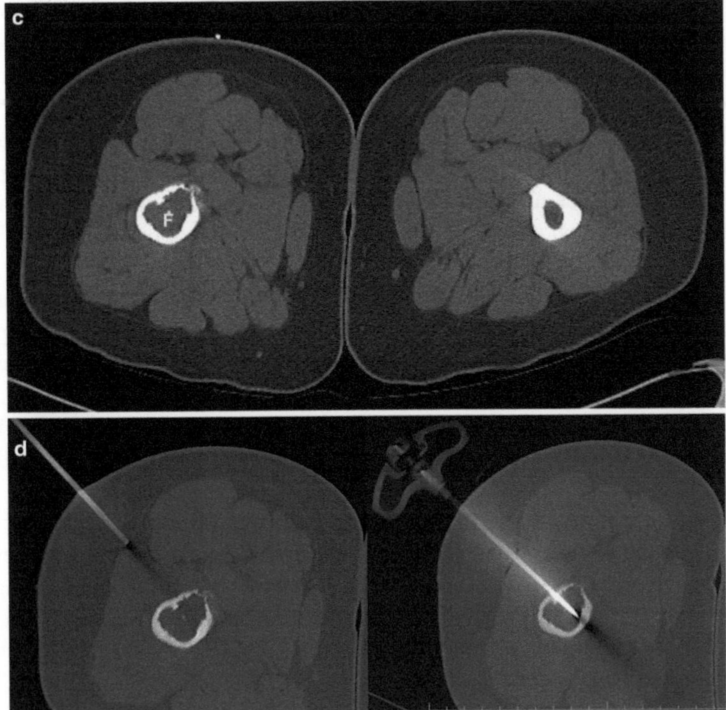

Fig. 3.2 (continued)

arteries and veins in and around the tumor. Interrogation of the needle path with duplex Doppler ultrasonography prevents inadvertent injury to blood vessels and hemorrhagic complications. Ultrasonography is ideal for targeting the extraosseous soft tissue components of bone tumors (Fig. 3.1c). At MD Anderson, we have used ultrasonography successfully for performing percutaneous biopsies in patients with osteosarcoma when prebiopsy MRI demonstrated the presence of a soft tissue component (Ahrar et al. 2004). On the other hand, ultrasonography cannot be used for targeting sclerotic tumors or lesions deep to the cortical bone.

Fluoroscopy alone can be used to target bone lesions that are visualized using plain radiography, including lytic, sclerotic, or marrow-infiltrating tumors (Murphy et al. 1981). We often use duplex Doppler ultrasonography in conjunction with fluoroscopy to help select a safe path for needle placement that is free of vascular structures.

CT provides excellent cross-sectional imaging (Fig. 3.2c) for targeting and sampling bone tumors (Leffler and Chew 1999). In addition to depicting the tumor, CT provides high-resolution images of the visceral organs in the chest, abdomen, and pelvis, enabling safe placement of the biopsy needle in almost any part of the axial skeleton. There are only a few disadvantages to the use of CT in diagnostic biopsies of bone sarcomas. When compared with MRI or ultrasound imaging, noncontrast CT is less optimal for characterizing the soft tissue component of tumors in the appendicular skeleton. Unlike ultrasonography, which provides real-time continuous imaging, ordinary CT guidance does not provide real-time imaging; rather, imaging is performed intermittently.

CT fluoroscopy allows real-time, continuous CT imaging of the needle during the biopsy. The only disadvantage of CT fluoroscopy is that the physician performing the biopsy receives an additional radiation dose. We utilize this technique for more complex biopsies, including cases in which the target is small or the lesion is in the head, neck, or spine.

In selected cases, we use MRI for targeting small tumors or lesions that are not visualized with CT, ultrasonography, or fluoroscopy. MRI-guided biopsies require special equipment, including titanium needles and nonferromagnetic patient-monitoring devices.

In the era of modern cross-sectional imaging, diagnostic angiography is not used often for assessment of tumors. However, assessment of vascularity can still be useful in certain cases. For example, we perform diagnostic angiography in patients with parosteal osteosarcoma so that we can localize and sample the hypervascular component of the tumor, which tends to correspond to an area of dedifferentiation. Establishing this diagnosis is important because it affects the clinical management of the patient. With multidetector CT scanners that are now available for clinical practice, CT angiography can provide the same information and preclude the need for conventional angiography.

Biopsy Techniques

On the day of biopsy, patients are asked to arrive shortly before the procedure. They are prepared in the preprocedure area with assessment of their vital signs and establishment of intravenous access for administration of agents for sedation. Patients are then transferred to one of the Interventional Radiology Suites for the appropriate procedure (decided on previously). The patient is assisted with placement on the procedure table in a position (supine, prone, or decubitus) that provides optimal access to the biopsy site. During the procedure, the patient's cardiopulmonary status is continuously monitored and recorded by the Interventional Radiology nursing staff.

Initial imaging is performed to confirm appropriate positioning of the patient and to mark the puncture site on the skin surface. Moderate sedation is commenced at that time. The patient is then prepared using usual sterile technique, and the puncture site and the needle track are infiltrated with a local anesthetic (e.g., lidocaine). A small stab incision is created at the biopsy site, and the needle is placed into the incision and directed toward the lesion (Fig. 3.2d).

Most biopsies are performed in a "coaxial" fashion (White et al. 1996). With this technique, a guide needle is placed into the target lesion. A smaller-gauge needle is then inserted through the guide needle into the lesion, allowing the interventional radiologist to sample the tumor multiple times with multiple biopsy needles through a single track. In fine-needle aspiration (FNA), the simplest form of biopsy, individual tumor cells are aspirated through a small needle. FNA samples require careful evaluation for cellular atypia by an experienced cytopathologist. Cytospin preparations and cell blocks can be obtained from FNA biopsy samples for further evaluation. On the other hand, the tissue core biopsy technique yields fragments of tumor that can be processed for histologic assessment. Core biopsy samples enable evaluation of tissue architecture in addition to cellular atypia. FNA and core biopsy samples are often complementary for successful diagnostic biopsy.

There are numerous commercially available biopsy needles, but with respect to bone biopsies, they can be classified into three types:

1. We use simple biopsy needles (e.g., Chiba type, 18–12 gauge, Cook, Bloomington, IN) as guide needles. Similar needles (slightly smaller in diameter, 22–14 gauge) are used to obtain FNA biopsy samples in coaxial fashion.
2. Spring-loaded, cutting-type needles (20–14 gauge, Cook) are used to obtain core biopsy samples from the soft tissue component of bone tumors. These needles can be used alone or through a guide needle in coaxial fashion.
3. Finally, trephine biopsy needles (e.g., Elson/Ackermann, 14 gauge, Cook; or Core-Assure, 11 gauge, Parallax, Sunnyvale, CA) are used to sample sclerotic bone tumors.

The type and size of the needle used for biopsy are initially determined based on the imaging characteristics of the bone tumor and the differential diagnosis. In general, a bone biopsy will start with FNA of the most appropriate area within the tumor. Once the biopsy is started, immediate assessment of the initial FNA sample by a cytopathologist determines the course of the rest of the procedure, i.e., the number and type of samples collected for various laboratory assessments. At MD Anderson, the cytopathology service, consisting of a technologist, laboratory facilities, and a board-certified cytopathologist, is always available; this service is located immediately adjacent to the Interventional Radiology Suite for prompt assessment of every biopsy specimen.

In the initial FNA sample, the cytopathologist confirms tissue viability and lack of necrosis. Experienced cytopathologists are often capable of making a preliminary diagnosis based on their initial evaluation of FNA samples; for example, spindle cell proliferations are suggestive of osteosarcoma; hyaline cartilage proliferation is suggestive of chondrosarcoma; and small, blue, round tumor cells are suggestive of Ewing sarcoma. In cases of suspected osteosarcoma, large (e.g., 14-gauge) core biopsy samples should be obtained with cutting-type needles; at least 4 of these high-quality samples are required for accurate diagnosis and possible subtyping of the tumor. On the other hand, Ewing sarcoma can be diagnosed largely on the basis of cytologic features, and a core biopsy may not be necessary. In fact, for Ewing sarcoma, rather than a core biopsy, additional FNA samples are often recommended for cytogenetic and electron microscopy evaluation. Furthermore, unlike osteosarcoma, Ewing sarcoma lacks a substantial matrix, and attempted core biopsy with a large needle may yield fragmented tumor tissue.

Close collaboration and direct communication between the interventional radiologist and cytopathologist enable collection of the appropriate type and amount of samples and help accurate and efficient determination of the diagnosis. In this way, the number of nondiagnostic samples and the need for repeat biopsy are minimized.

Postbiopsy Care

As the biopsy proceeds, once the cytopathologist confirms that adequate material has been obtained, the needles are removed. Hemostasis is achieved by manual compression of the puncture site for a short period of time (1–3 min). A sterile dressing is applied to the biopsy site; it can be removed in 24 h. The patient is then transferred to the Interventional Radiology recovery area for observation and recovery from sedation (a minimum of 1 h). Prior to discharge from the department, the patient's pain is assessed, and when needed, appropriate analgesics are prescribed. Discharge instructions cover care of the biopsy site, including keeping the site dry for 24 h, and observation for unexpected developments, such as redness, swelling, or bleeding; contact information for Interventional Radiology and the Emergency Center is provided.

Potential Complications

We always inform patients of potential complications of percutaneous biopsy. The risks include hemorrhage, infection, damage to adjacent structures, pneumothorax, and track seeding. In reality, complications are exceedingly rare. In 7 reported series of percutaneous musculoskeletal biopsies involving a total of 714 patients, 5 (0.7%) complications were reported, 1 (0.1%) of which required treatment (Table 3.1).

Table 3.1 Reported complications of percutaneous biopsy

Author (year)	No. of patients	Complications		
		No.	Type	Treatment
Murphy et al. (1981)	169	2	Pneumothorax	Chest tube (1)
Yao et al. (1999)	141	0		
Leffler and Chew (1999)	43	0		
Jelinek et al. (2002)	110	1	Hematoma	None
Ahrar et al. (2004)	35	0		
Puri et al. (2006)	121	2	Transient neurologic	None
Krause et al. (2008)	95	0		

Key Practice Points

- Optimal prebiopsy characterization of suspected tumors with plain radiography and cross-sectional imaging is essential for successful patient selection and tissue sampling.
- The biopsy site, approach, and guiding imaging modality are chosen based on prebiopsy diagnostic studies.
- Immediate assessment of the FNA specimen by a cytopathologist determines appropriate sampling of the tumor.
- Soft tissue tumors are best sampled by large (14-gauge) cutting-type needles.
- Sclerotic bone tumors are best sampled by trephine biopsy needles.
- FNA biopsy samples are useful in tumors that lack a well-formed matrix.
- For any bone biopsy prior to limb-salvage surgery, anatomically based guidelines should be followed such that the surgeon can resect the biopsy track using a standard incision, without the need for additional soft tissue resection.

Suggested Readings

Ahrar K, Himmerich JU, Herzog CE, et al. Percutaneous ultrasound-guided biopsy in the definitive diagnosis of osteosarcoma. J Vasc Interv Radiol. 2004;15:1329–33.

Davies NM, Livesley PJ, Cannon SR. Recurrence of an osteosarcoma in a needle biopsy track. J Bone Joint Surg Br. 1993;75:977–8.

Jelinek JS, Murphey MD, Welker JA, et al. Diagnosis of primary bone tumors with image-guided percutaneous biopsy: experience with 110 tumors. Radiology. 2002;223:731–7.

Krause ND, Hddad ZK, Winalski CS, Ready JE, Nawfel RD, Carrino JA. Musculoskeletal biopsies using computed tomography fluoroscopy. J Comput Assist Tomogr. 2008;32:458–62.

Leffler SG, Chew FS. CT-guided percutaneous biopsy of sclerotic bone lesions: diagnostic yield and accuracy. Am J Roentgenol. 1999;172:1389–92.

Liu PT, Valadez SD, Chivers FS, et al. Anatomically based guidelines for core needle biopsy of bone tumors: implications for limb-sparing surgery. Radiographics. 2007;27:189–206.

Murphy WA, Destouet JM, Gilula LA. Percutaneous skeletal biopsy 1981: a procedure for radiologists – results, review, and recommendations. Radiology. 1981;139:545–9.

Puri A, Shingdale VU, Agarwal MG, et al. CT-guided percutaneous core needle biopsy in deep seated musculoskeletal lesions: a prospective study of 128 cases. Skeletal Radiol. 2006;35:138–43.

Saifuddin A, Mitchell R, Burnett SJ, et al. Ultrasound-guided needle biopsy of primary bone tumours. J Bone Joint Surg Br. 2000;82:50–4.

White LM, Schweitzer ME, Deely DM. Coaxial percutaneous needle biopsy of osteolytic lesions with intact cortical bone. Am J Roentgenol. 1996;166:143–4.

Yao L, Nelson SD, Seeger LL, et al. Primary musculoskeletal neoplasms: effectiveness of core-needle biopsy. Radiology. 1999;212:682–6.

Chapter 4
Orthopedic Oncologic Surgical Specimen Management and Surgical Pathology

A. Kevin Raymond and Alexander J. Lazar

Contents

A.K. Raymond (✉)
178 Drakes Landing, Brunswick, GA 31523, USA (retired from Section of Orthopaedic
Pathology, Department of Pathology, Division of Pathology and Laboratory Medicine,
The University of Texas MD Anderson Cancer Center, Houston, TX, USA)
e-mail: kraymond1950@yahoo.com

A.J. Lazar (✉)
Department of Pathology, Division of Pathology and Laboratory Medicine,
The University of Texas MD Anderson Cancer Center, Houston, TX, USA

Department of Dermatology, Division of Internal Medicine,
The University of Texas MD Anderson Cancer Center, Houston, TX, USA
e-mail: alazar@mdanderson.org

P.P. Lin and S. Patel (eds.), *Bone Sarcoma*, MD Anderson Cancer Care Series,
DOI 10.1007/978-1-4614-5194-5_4,
© The University of Texas M. D. Anderson Cancer Center 2013

Chapter Overview The pathologist is an integral member of the multidisciplinary team central to the successful treatment of bone tumors. The role of the pathologist is to provide morphology-derived information pertaining to diagnosis and status of disease. Communication between all members of this team is vital at all junctures of workup and treatment. During the evaluation of biopsies, critical information from the history, physical examination, and imaging studies should be taken into account and integrated with histological observations to ensure a correct diagnosis. Later on during the course of treatment, the pathologist is called upon to advise the surgeon as to the status of resection margins and adequacy of surgery. And later still, the pathologist provides the medical oncologist with an assessment of the response to preoperative chemotherapy. In each case, the evaluation of bone specimens requires a systematic approach to specimen preparation and analysis. Mineralization is intrinsic to the structure and function of bone. However, it adds a significant degree of difficulty to bone specimen management; osseous tissues are not easily dissected or cut using traditional techniques. Special methods are required for analyzing bone specimens and sarcomas of bone. Although complex and time consuming, the procedures, when carried out correctly, will reward the pathologist and clinician with accurate, reliable information that provides insight into diagnosis, classification, staging, and treatment efficacy.

Introduction

Historically, the primary role of the pathologist in the evaluation of the bone-tumor patient has been to provide an accurate morphology-based diagnosis that will allow the initiation of appropriate therapy. The pathologist has also been expected to provide information about tumor stage: the extent of disease within the primary site, including adjacent structures (e.g., bone and immediately overlying connective tissues), the involvement of regional structures (e.g., blood vessels and lymph nodes), and the status of the resection margins. In addition, with the advent of multidisciplinary therapy, particularly the use of preoperative therapy (e.g., chemotherapy, radiation therapy, biological modifiers), the pathologist is now expected to provide both qualitative and *quantitative* assessment of the tumor's response to preoperative therapy. Because the latter has been found to be a singular prognostic indicator, it has assumed a central position in postchemotherapy surgical specimen analysis. The response is used to determine the form of postoperative chemotherapy: responders receive the same form of chemotherapy that was given preoperatively, while nonresponders are given an alternative chemotherapy regimen. This chapter will focus on the techniques applicable to the preparation and analysis of specimens from bone-tumor patients. Specific tumor types will be addressed in subsequent chapters.

The Sarcoma Group at MD Anderson Cancer Center favors a multidisciplinary approach to the morphological analysis of bone tumors. Although bone-tumor symptomatology is typically nonspecific, clinical information—in particular, demographics—may nevertheless prove pivotal in the analysis of potential bone tumors. Although the tendencies are statistical, bone tumors are associated with unique demographic properties; each type of tumor has a relatively strong tendency to occur within certain age groups and in one sex more frequently than the other. Furthermore, each bone tumor tends to occur with unique frequency in specific bones, in specific aspects of those bones (i.e., surface vs medullary cavity), and, when intramedullary, within specific compartments (i.e., epiphysis, diaphysis, or metaphysis) of those bones. Although histological analysis is the final arbiter, clinical information provides a context within which to apply histological criteria while assessing diagnostic probabilities. In light of this interdependence of clinical and pathological diagnostic criteria, clear lines of communication between the treatment and diagnostic arms of the multidisciplinary team are vital.

The review of imaging studies should be considered an integral part of histological analysis and diagnosis in skeletal pathology. If the pathologist cannot interpret the imaging studies, he or she should review them with a radiologist, preferably one with an interest in musculoskeletal disease. Just as each type of bone tumor is associated with unique demographic characteristics, each tumor type also has a relatively well-defined spectrum of radiographic changes that is exhibited in most cases. The contribution of imaging studies to the diagnostic evaluation of bone tumors cannot be overestimated nor overstated.

In summary, although some espouse a philosophy of reviewing histological slides in the absence of clinical information, we are committed to a multidisciplinary approach: viewing each case as a *patient* rather than a *specimen*. It is our opinion that for each patient, all available clinical, radiology, and pathology information should be incorporated into the diagnostic process; the potential consequences of not doing so are far too serious to consider otherwise.

Surgical Pathology Specimens

Although there appears to be an endless range of specimens resulting from orthopedic surgery, they can be grouped into a limited number of specimen types: biopsies, frozen sections, curettage specimens, and "definitive" (i.e., resection, ablation) surgical specimens.

Biopsy Specimens

Diagnostic biopsies are generally done in one of two forms: percutaneous image-guided needle biopsy or open surgical biopsy. Each technique has advantages and disadvantages. As described in the previous chapter, percutaneous needle biopsy is the standard technique employed for most diagnostic procedures at MD Anderson. In almost all cases at our institution, the biopsy is done by specially trained radiologists and performed under imaging guidance (see Chap. 3, "Percutaneous Image-Guided Biopsy for Diagnosis of Bone Sarcomas"). The needle biopsy has a number of advantages over other techniques. Its minimal/absent contamination of normal tissues and the fact that it can be repeated or supplemented by open biopsy if results are nondiagnostic are compelling reasons for accepting its use in orthopedic oncology.

In most cases, cytopathological evaluation acts as an adjunct to histopathological evaluation for gauging the adequacy of a percutaneous core biopsy. In this scenario, the core biopsy is rolled across a slide. The slide is then stained and reviewed under the microscope *at the time of biopsy.* Experience has shown that if the core is adequate, the number of cells that exfoliate on the slide will be sufficient to allow a tentative statement as to possible diagnosis. If the cytology is considered insufficient for diagnosis, additional cores can be obtained during the same procedure. In general, cytopathological evaluation enables an estimation of specimen adequacy, whereas histological evaluation yields the final diagnosis; rather than being competitive, the roles of the two techniques are complementary.

Frozen Sections

With the emergence of the needle biopsy as a reliable diagnostic tool, the *need* for frozen-section diagnosis has sharply declined. For evaluating potential bone tumors, diagnostic frozen sections are largely confined to one of two scenarios: an emergent clinical situation (e.g., pathologic fracture) or adding an element of confidence in the face of an equivocal biopsy-based diagnosis. The questions posed to the surgical pathologist are generally focused to establish or confirm a diagnosis or assess the status of resection margins.

The presence of mineralized tissue offers a challenge to the pathology laboratory when faced with bone specimens. It is frequently said that frozen-section techniques cannot be employed with bone tumors: "You can't freeze bone." However, in most cases, careful examination of the specimen will allow the identification of areas of the specimen that are sufficiently soft to allow frozen-section analysis of a technical quality that will enable confident diagnosis. In addition, the use of disposable knives has decreased the impact of the consequences (e.g., knife chipping) of cutting mineralized tissue. We add to the probability of diagnostic accuracy by performing touch imprint cytologic analysis in conjunction with frozen-section analysis.

In general, we attempt to utilize only a portion of the available tissue for frozen section while preserving part for "permanent sections" (or "permanents") and special studies. However, there are times when it may be necessary to submit all available tissue for frozen-section analysis. In such cases, we request additional tissue for permanents. All frozen blocks are subsequently melted and submitted for formalin fixation, decalcification, paraffin embedding, and slide preparation to create permanent sections.

For evaluating potential hematologic neoplasia involving bone, we do not recommend frozen section as the routine method because of the potential introduction of significant artifacts. However, there are circumstances in which intraoperative examination becomes a necessary option, for example, cases in which other biopsy techniques have failed to yield diagnostic tissue and time-critical clinical situations mandating immediate surgical intervention. In both situations, frozen-section analysis serves as a guide to finding suitable tissue for successful diagnostic evaluation.

If the differential diagnosis of a lesion has been narrowed to metastasis versus hematologic malignancy, we generally perform frozen-section analysis to initiate disease-specific special studies. If frozen section suggests that the lesion is a hematologic malignancy, an established protocol of tests (i.e., immunohistochemical analysis, flow cytometry, and cytogenetic testing) is performed, and the remainder of the tissue is submitted for histological analysis using formalin-fixed, paraffin-embedded tissue. If the frozen section shows metastatic carcinoma, the subsequent workup is a function of the suspected primary tumor type. Usually, histological analysis of one or two permanent sections is sufficient to corroborate the frozen-section impressions. However, additional studies are frequently required to clarify the tumor site of origin and/or to assess prognostic markers (e.g., estrogen and progesterone receptors and HER-2/Neu in breast cancer).

Curettage Specimens

Occasionally, primary malignant bone tumors are not excised en bloc but removed in piecemeal fashion by curettage or other means. In certain areas, such as the spine, this approach may be the only means of removing the tumor. In other situations, an unresectable tumor may be "debulked" for the purpose of temporary palliation. In these cases, the submission of two or three blocks of tissue is generally sufficient to confirm the diagnosis. Additional sampling can be done as a matter of interest or for more detailed or specific clinicopathological correlation.

From the perspective of the pathologist, an "open biopsy" and a "curettage" are effectively the same procedure, differing only in the amount of tissue submitted and the intent for which the procedure was undertaken: diagnosis or treatment assessment. In each case, the specimen consists of intermixed fragments of tumor, bone, and connective tissue.

If the lesion is a primary bone lesion and the diagnosis is known or strongly suspected, we submit four or five sections and then follow the principle of "representative sections." This principle, discussed further later in this chapter, holds that by subjecting a specimen to gross examination, we can select limited portions of tissue for histological analysis that are representative of the entire disease process. For lesions treated with curettage, the exceptions to this rule are cases of suspected aneurysmal bone cysts and nonossifying fibroma. Such lesions can manifest as either true diagnostic entities or degenerative "patterns" that appear within other primary bone tumors. If the histological findings together with the demographics and imaging findings are "classic" for these entities, analysis of representative sections can yield a diagnosis. However, if there are atypical features, histological analysis of all submitted tissue may be required for diagnostic resolution. Aneurysmal bone cyst and nonossifying fibroma represent diagnoses of exclusion. The most feared misdiagnosis is osteosarcoma, which can be mistaken for either of these two entities.

Definitive Surgical Specimens

The products of definitive orthopedic surgical procedures fall into a limited number of categories:

1. Curettage, or so-called intralesional excision: removal of tumor in one or more pieces without surrounding normal tissue and without consideration of resection margin status.
2. "Simple" or "marginal" excision: removal of an intact tumor with minimal surrounding normal tissue.
3. "Wide" or "en bloc" resection: removal of tumor with a larger quantity of normal tissue to provide a wide margin.
4. Amputation/ablation: removal of the extremity or region containing a tumor.

It should be noted that whereas advanced tumors are frequently removed by amputation, such procedures do not always produce wide margins, particularly when central locations, such as the shoulder and pelvic girdles, are involved. Operations such as amputations are not "radical" simply because an extreme amount of tissue is being sacrificed. Rather, in musculoskeletal oncology, the term *radical* specifically refers to the removal of the entire tumor-bearing anatomic compartment.

When working with the definitive surgical specimen, the primary issues of specimen management are diagnosis, classification, determination of extent of disease, evaluation of resection margin status, and, when applicable, assessment of response to preoperative therapy. The "final diagnosis" may have been established prior to definitive surgery. However, with the use of limited biopsy specimens (e.g., needle biopsy), the diagnosis is frequently sufficient to initiate therapy but incomplete in detail, that is, a "working diagnosis." Questions pertaining to precise tumor classification and subclassification may still need to be answered. On the other hand, although the diagnosis may be established prior to surgery, analysis of factors pertaining to staging and response to therapy remains the domain of the definitive surgical specimen. The techniques for addressing these issues follow.

Preparation of Osseous Tissues by the Surgical Pathologist

The preparation and analysis of definitive surgical specimens can be quite laborious and time consuming. The specimen must be carefully inspected, dissected, and cut into pieces small enough to be assessed using routine processing equipment. The adequacy of surgical margins must be assessed. Bones must be decalcified prior to cutting tissue for histological slides. In many cases, the response to preoperative therapy (i.e., amount of tumor necrosis) must be determined quantitatively. The approach to each of these processes in individual cases is a function of the type of specimen and the intent of the procedure.

Specimen Dissection

Pathologists generally view their specimen dissection as a personal accomplishment, and therefore, there are probably as many dissection strategies as there are pathologists implementing them. At MD Anderson, we assign responsibility for gross examination and selection of tissues to be processed to a physician—occasionally a trainee, but usually a staff pathologist with experience in bone pathology. Specifically, we do not assign this work to pathologist assistants, histotechnologists, or histotechnicians. We summarize here the dissection techniques routinely employed at MD Anderson.

Dissection techniques for bone are both similar and dissimilar to those employed in nonskeletal disciplines of pathology. Soft tissues can be readily addressed with use of the familiar scalpel, forceps, and scissors. However, the presence of mineralized tissue adds aspects of dissection virtually unique to bone pathology.

Small Specimens

Unhindered by significant amounts of adherent normal tissue, needle biopsies, open biopsies, curettage specimens, and material submitted for frozen section require little if any dissection. Individual pieces are either submitted in their entirety or cut to fit processing vehicles (e.g., cassettes, slides). When working with curettage specimens, the tissue fragments seldom require anything more than washing and separating the submitted pieces or cutting them to fit processing cassettes.

Large Specimens

With respect to dissection, "large specimens" can be roughly divided into two groups: resections and ablative specimens. In addition to containing tumor-bearing tissue and the parent bone, each of these specimen types contains larger amounts of normal tissue than are seen in small specimens, which must be addressed.

Resection specimens generally include a segment of the tumor-containing bone and small amounts of attached overlying soft tissue, which may or may not contain tumor secondary to direct extension from the primary site. Depending on anatomic location, the specimen may include a portion of adjacent bone and intervening joint structures that have been removed because of functional considerations, for example, the resection of distal femur for tumor involving the distal metaphysis and epiphysis frequently includes the adjacent normal knee joint components and a segment of proximal tibia. Dissection of these specimens requires removal of tumor-free normal tissues followed by bone cutting. Because normal soft tissues cannot be cut on a bone saw, they must be removed or incised; unaltered soft tissues will catch on the saw teeth, resulting in damage to the tissues and a dangerous situation for the prosector due to potential loss of control of the specimen while it is running through the saw. On occasion, photographic considerations may dictate leaving the bone-joint-bone components or bone with soft tissue intact during the initial longitudinal sectioning of the bone specimen. Special care must be taken with these specimens so that the soft tissues do not catch in the bone saw blade and drag the prosector's hands into the blade. Although illogical, many of us appear to have a natural tendency to protect the specimen rather than ourselves. This possibility should be considered ahead of time and a conscious decision made as to what the response will be should specimen drag occur. Although somewhat obsessive, this preemptive way of thinking has saved the author's fingers on several occasions.

Ablative specimens include those resulting from a transmedullary or transarticular amputation, for example, above-knee amputation, disarticulation, hemipelvectomy (hindquarter amputation), forequarter amputation, and hemicorpectomy. Each of these specimens includes large amounts of normal tissue in continuity with the tumor-containing bone and the tumor itself. In each case, dissection is a two-step procedure in which the surgical specimen is first reduced to the tumor and parent tumor-containing bone, in essence, reducing the *surgical* specimen to a *pathology* specimen. Following removal of the attached normal tissues, dissection of the tumor-containing bone is performed by cutting the bone on a bone saw. Removal of the soft tissues is generally accomplished by one of two approaches: removing the tumor-containing bone from the specimen or removing the skin and soft tissues from the surface of the tumor and tumor-containing bone.

In the first of these choices, the skin and soft tissues overlying the tumor-containing bone are incised to the level of the tumor and parent bone. The incision is then extended around the tumor-containing bone. The skin and soft tissues overlying the major joint compartment are frequently incised to the level of the major neurovascular bundle, allowing examination of the major vessels for evidence of tumor involvement. Next, the intact tumor-containing bone is removed from the attached normal tissues. The margins and soft tissues may be examined for evidence of locoregional involvement. Finally, the bone is submitted for band-saw sectioning. This technique is limited by its requirement to perform largely "blind" dissection through a narrow, constricted, and limited incision.

An alternative approach is to first remove the bulk of the skin and subcutaneous tissue from the specimen. Although "skinning" the specimen is a somewhat grotesque prospect, the resulting complete 360° tissue accessibility yields a specimen that is much easier to work with. The first step is to retain the needle or open biopsy site, including skin and underlying connective tissue, in continuity with the underlying tumor-distorted bone so that the biopsy site and track are available for histological analysis. This can be accomplished by first incising an ellipse around the skin and soft tissue of the biopsy site, which is generally overlying the aspect of the tumor closest to the skin. Retaining the biopsy site is followed by circumferentially incising the skin through underlying subcutaneous fat to the level of skeletal muscle/fascia at the distal extreme of the specimen (e.g., wrist, ankle). This circumferential "limiting incision" is followed by a perpendicular, longitudinal incision running the length of the specimen (from the circumferential limiting incision to the biopsy-site-including ellipse overlying the tumor) and then continuing on to the specimen resection margin. The skin and subcutaneous tissues are then removed via a combination of sharp and blunt dissection. This procedure leaves a bone specimen that is covered by muscle, fascia, joint, and neurovascular structures, all of which are now visible in a form resembling the pictures and diagrams in anatomy textbooks. The major vasculature can then be examined for tumor contamination. After this, the soft tissues are removed in a logical, controlled, layer-by-layer manner. The resulting tumor and parent bone are then cut on a band saw. With a little practice, this technique will only add 5 or 10 min to the overall dissection but will make all other aspects of dissection much easier.

With removal of the skin and soft tissue from the tumor-containing bone, the full circumference of the bone is available for sectioning. A decision as to the plane of section is a function of desired end results and should be made in consultation with the multidisciplinary treatment team members. In general, long bones are cut in a sagittal, coronal, or oblique longitudinal plane, effectively "bivalving" the tumor-containing bone. In contrast, flat bones are frequently cut in a serial fashion in the sagittal plane. These planes generally fulfill the needs of most clinical/radiologic/pathological correlations. However, each case should be individualized with a goal of directing the dissection toward resolving clinical questions. In the absence of such clinicopathological issues, photography needs may be given voice.

Although some pathologists fix and decalcify the definitive specimen when it is intact or after bivalving, we do not favor this practice. We have had better success by taking the initial fresh or formalin-fixed, band-saw-cut specimen and, while it is still mineralized, cutting it into pieces that fit standard processing cassettes. We then place these smaller, thinner pieces of tissue into cassettes and submit them for fixation, decalcification, and further processing. We find that this approach results in more thorough tissue processing.

Cutting bone is a compromise between dissection and distortion of the involved tissues. Potential distortions include deposition on and impregnation of bone by bone dust and thermal/heat/burn effects. We recommend the use of a heavy-duty band saw with a half-inch blade for making the larger cuts (e.g., bivalving a bone or cutting a bone into multiple serial planes). Although this type of saw is a powerful instrument, we find the added stability provided by the wide blade provides a degree of safety not afforded by thinner blades, which may bend, break, or dislodge. The cutting action of a traditional saw, such as the band saw, results in the production of significant amounts of bone dust that are invariably forced into the interstices of both cancellous and lamellar bone. Thus, the cut surface of the specimen must be thoroughly washed with water immediately after cutting to minimize bone-dust contamination; a surgical brush is very effective for such cleaning. The resulting cut specimen is then further cut into pieces that will be accommodated by standard processing cassettes.

In our experience, the best results for cutting major bone specimens into cassette-sized pieces (length, width, *and thickness*) are obtained using an IsoMet® (Buehler Ltd., Lake Bluff, Ill). The IsoMet is a geology saw used for cutting rocks (Fig. 4.1). It has a diamond-impregnated circular metal blade that passes through a water bath. The advantages of this saw are several. It cuts with a very narrow blade, resulting in minimal tissue loss. It cuts with a grinding action that provides minimal

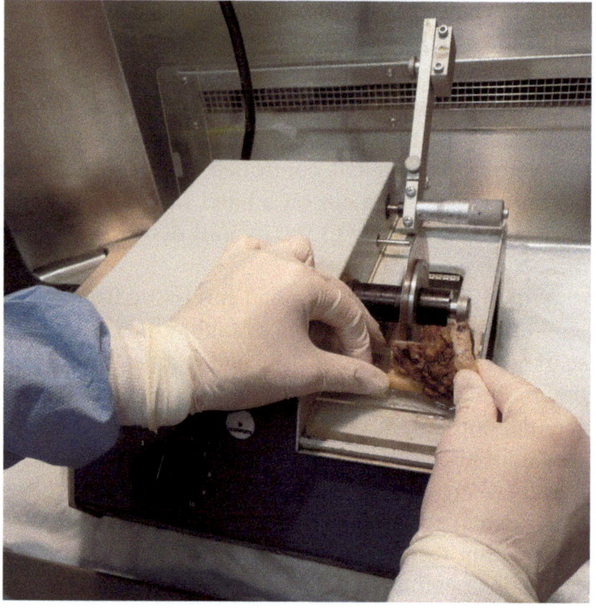

Fig. 4.1 A Buehler IsoMet saw. This low-speed saw is used for sectioning hard specimens. It allows precise cuts with minimal distortion of tissues.

mechanical and thermal tissue distortion. At the same time, the presence of the water bath minimizes impregnation of bone dust into the specimen cut surface. As a result, when compared with other saws, use of the IsoMet results in fewer artifacts in the dissected tissue.

Although we have tried a variety of smaller saws (e.g., jigsaw, table saw, and vibrating saw), we have found them inferior to the combination of the band saw and IsoMet saw. Each of the others has problems with cutting accuracy and control, the production of significant bone-dust artifacts, and/or an inability to cut sections thin enough to be directly placed into cassettes.

Unmodified, the practice of freezing intact, whole specimens and then cutting them on a band saw is discouraged. This technique furnishes specimens that result in unparalleled, magnificent gross photographs since both osseous and nonosseous tissues are intact and retain their normal anatomic relationships. However, freezing frequently and unpredictably ruins tissue for histological analysis (i.e., causes "frozen-section artifact"). With a little planning and thought, this technique can be modified to provide raw material that allows an excellent histological outcome, as well as spectacular photography. If the specimen is to be frozen, then clinical information and imaging studies need to be studied and integrated with the specimen *immediately*. In doing so, the plane that will fulfill photographic needs, and therefore the plane in which the specimen is ultimately to be cut, can be established. Then the tumor can be incised in a plane parallel to the ultimate cut surface, and tumor tissues obtained for histological analysis. The removed tissues are immediately placed in appropriate fixatives and submitted for study. Only after tissue has been obtained for histological assessment and other potential studies is the specimen frozen. Thorough freezing usually takes at least 24 h. The specimen is then cut on a band saw and photographed. It is our opinion that, because of the potential for irreparable tissue damage, whole-specimen freezing should be done with great care and reserved for selected specimens.

Fixation and Decalcification

In our practice, we have verbalized a working philosophy that "there is no such thing as a soft bone specimen." Admittedly somewhat of an overstatement, it serves to emphasize the fact that virtually all bone specimens should be decalcified prior to paraffin embedding and microtome cutting. Although we allow exceptions to this rule, it is with the knowledge that we are taking risks. The potential for information gain and the necessity of proceeding without decalcification must be balanced with the potential consequences of cutting mineralized tissue, up to and including complete specimen loss. In truth, the unavoidable position of intentionally cutting undecalcified (i.e., mineralized) tissue is largely limited to the performance of intra-operative frozen-section histological analysis.

There is some tendency to view small specimens such as biopsies, curettage specimens, and lung metastases as having insufficient mineralization to warrant decalcification. This perception is absolutely not true. The presence of even microscopic amounts of mineralized tissue can be enough to preclude the preparation of technically excellent histological slides and thereby impede or even negate diagnosis. Biopsies and curettage specimens may contain mineralized tumor or fragments of cancellous and/or cortical bone. The presence of these mineralized tissues will result in a variety of artifacts, including chips or linear defects in the tissue, chatter, tissue compression, and shattering, or the inability to fully process the tissue. Lung metastases are frequently and erroneously processed without decalcification, resulting in any or all of the above-listed artifacts. On occasion, mineralized tissue may even pop out of the block upon impact of the microtome on the tissue.

Decalcification requires complete tissue fixation. Decalcification without fixation results in a variety of artifacts, for example, the release of gas bubbles into the tissue and the formation of what might be referred to as "pseudophysaliferous cells." We fix all tissue in 10% neutral buffered formalin. The length of time necessary for fixation is proportional to the volume and thickness of the tissue. Bone needle biopsies need the least fixation and decalcification, but both processes are required. As a rule of thumb, we will not process on the day of biopsy any needle biopsy that has not been placed in formalin before 3 p.m. With our tissue-processing schedule, this policy allows a minimum of 6 h of fixation before decalcification and subsequent processing.

In most cases, the decision to proceed with, or refrain from, decalcification appears fairly straightforward; tissue mineralization is often grossly evident. However, it should be kept in mind that there are limits to our ability to detect mineralization through visual inspection and palpation. As a result, we obtain plain-film specimen X-rays of all tissue blocks after fixation. For those blocks without unequivocal, gross evidence of mineralization, this initial examination will determine whether any calcium is present and whether decalcification is necessary. At the same time, the initial specimen X-rays set a pre-decalcification mineralization baseline for all blocks undergoing decalcification.

In many laboratories, the endpoint of decalcification is determined by the "crunch" technique. That is, tissue is placed in solution for decalcification for a predetermined length of time. Periodically, the tissue is removed and tested by finger compression. If the tissue "crunches," it needs more decalcification; if no crunch is felt or heard, the tissue is deemed decalcified and submitted for processing. This technique is somewhat imprecise and may result in a wealth of artifacts.

We have chosen an alternative method. All tissue samples with evidence of calcium are submitted for X-ray-monitored decalcification. We use a 5% solution of formic acid for decalcification; it is somewhat slower than other techniques but results in the production of slides with excellent histological detail while retaining tissue antigenicity for potential immunohistochemical analysis. After fixation and X-ray, the tissue cassettes are placed on a perforated ceramic platform within a covered glass container, filled with dilute formic acid solution, under which a magnetic stir bar spins. The cassettes are removed each morning and X-rayed. If there is residual calcium, the cassette is returned to decalcify further; this process is repeated for up to 7 days. If a small amount of residual calcium remains at 7 days, the specimen may continue processing at the discretion of the pathologist. When there is no X-ray evidence of calcium, the remainder of processing is the same as for nonmineralized tissue; that is, the cassette is submerged in 10% neutral buffered formalin and then transferred to an automated tissue processor. The tissue is then embedded in paraffin, cut on a microtome, mounted on glass slides, stained, and cover-slipped.

A word of warning must be given: not all that is hard is mineralized. Dense unmineralized collagen can be as difficult to cut as mineralized tissue. This problem is frequently encountered with certain bone-producing tumors, that is, certain forms of osteosarcoma, including osteoblastic osteosarcoma, parosteal osteosarcoma, well-differentiated intramedullary osteosarcoma, and osteosarcoma that has been treated with chemotherapy. Despite apparently adequate decalcification, the tissues remain difficult to cut, and no amount of time in decalcification will help since the problem is not calcium but dense collagen.

It should be kept in mind that the decision of whether to decalcify a specimen is essentially irrevocable. Should a mineralized specimen be processed without decalcification, processing can be rerun in reverse and the specimen subsequently submitted for decalcification. However, this process is extremely destructive, and the resulting histological materials have extreme distortion and are seldom more than barely interpretable. On the other hand, when done properly, contemporary decalcification has minimal impact on our ability to produce technically excellent histological slides while at the same time preserving the properties inherent to other formalin-fixed, paraffin-embedded tissue. In short, when in doubt, submit the tissue for decalcification; the minimal resulting delay is a small price to pay.

Tissue Submission

As with all surgical specimens, questions concerning the amount of tissue to be submitted for histological examination from bone cases are difficult to answer objectively. As pathologists, we are torn in two directions: academic curiosity, which inspires submission of massive amounts of tissue, versus economy and efficiency, which favors submission of the minimum amount of tissue that will allow appropriate analysis of the case.

We tend to submit a greater proportion of tissue for histological analysis in cases in which the procedure is performed for diagnosis; the less certain the diagnosis, the greater the proportion of tissue that is submitted.

Entire Specimen

Since diagnostic features may be confined to small portions of the specimen, we find it effective and efficient to submit large amounts of tissue when managing *diagnostic* biopsies. In the case of needle core biopsies, we always submit the entire specimen. When there are multiple cores, we place each core, or core fragment, in its own individual cassette. Placing multiple pieces of tissue in a single cassette might seem to be an efficient method of handling tissue, but it is frequently disappointing; it can cause problems in the three-dimensional orientation of those pieces during paraffin embedding. Improper placement results in the tissue being oriented "obliquely" across multiple planes and in each piece being oriented differently. Such misorientation results in an inability to obtain complete tissue surfaces for histological examination of each core or core fragment. As a result, multiple levels must be cut so that all surfaces can be seen. In turn, this results in the waste of large amounts of tissue in the pursuit of complete analysis. If special procedures are to be performed, this unnecessary tissue depletion may be a critical problem. By submitting one core per cassette and cutting a single surface cut for hematoxylin and eosin (H&E) staining from each of the resulting paraffin blocks, we are able to achieve multiple goals: review the maximum amount of tissue available, selectively perform special studies on limited tissue with the highest probability of diagnostic results, and preserve tissue for future diagnostic or investigational use. An exception to this rule of one fragment per cassette may be in the case of an open biopsy, where tissue is more abundant; for such specimens, we allow multiple pieces per cassette.

As alluded to earlier, aneurysmal bone cyst and nonossifying fibroma present potential management problems. The histological features in these conditions are relatively nonspecific and may represent either a specific entity or a reactive/degenerative pattern seen as secondary processes in a wide variety of primary bone tumors. As a result, when the entire clinical/radiologic/histological picture supports a diagnosis of aneurysmal bone cyst or nonossifying fibroma, submission of a small amount of tissue has a high probability of allowing accurate diagnosis. However, if there are atypical clinical or radiologic features, then large amounts of tissue, up to and including entire biopsy or curettage specimens, may have to be reviewed to exclude elements of the differential diagnosis and achieve confident diagnostic specificity.

Representative Sections

Submitting specimens in their entirety is both logistically and economically impractical in the vast majority of cases. Therefore, the standard method of selecting tissue for histological analysis is governed by the principle of *representative sections*. The essence of this concept resides in the ability of the pathologist to examine gross specimens and submit a limited amount of tissue for histological analysis, with confidence that this limited tissue will be "representative" of the entire disease process. This process assumes that the reviewer is familiar with the diversity and subtleties of gross bone pathology and is therefore in a position to decide which portions of the tumor to sample for histological examination. However, because bone tumors are rare and tend to be referred to a limited number of specialty hospitals, few pathologists see sufficient numbers of bone tumor specimens to become comfortable or experienced in their gross analysis and management.

As in other areas of pathology, we translate the concept of representative sections into a system of standardized tissue submission, and this method has been largely adopted in sarcoma pathology. In cases in which all of the submitted tissue fits in five or fewer cassettes, we submit the tissue in its entirety. In cases in which the pathological condition is unknown and the specimen is no more than 10 cm in greatest dimension, we submit ten sections from tumor areas that appear similar. If the specimen is larger than 10 cm, we then submit one additional block of tissue per centimeter of the tumor's greatest dimension from areas that are similar. We also submit additional sections from areas whose gross appearance differs from the dominant gross appearance.

Evaluation of Surgical Margins

Unlike the spread of epithelial malignancies, direct extension of primary bone tumors into normal soft tissues tends to be a process that can be appreciated at the gross level. Sarcomas do not tend to insidiously microscopically infiltrate normal tissues any significant distance from the parent tumor. Therefore, careful gross examination is generally adequate for assessing soft tissue margins. If the external surface of the specimen is free of gross tumor and there is freely mobile overlying normal soft tissue or the tumor-bearing compartment is removed intact with a layer of normal boundary tissue (e.g., an intact fascial plane) overlying the tumor, we accept gross examination as sufficient for margin evaluation. On the other hand, we do submit tissue from any area in which the soft tissue margin is nonmobile or fixed to the underlying tumor. If there are doubts concerning any of these parameters, tissue is submitted for histological analysis.

Examination of the medullary cavity margin is approached somewhat differently for several reasons. Primary bone tumors can insidiously infiltrate normal bone, track along intraosseous blood vessels, and have areas of tumor discontinuity (i.e., so-called skip metastasis). At the same time, the physical realities of orthopedic surgery introduce an element of uncertainty concerning the correlation between radiology-defined tumor limits and the surgically established margins; the extent of bone surgery must be assessed through soft tissue and abstracted from X-ray-established measurements. If margin evaluation by pathology-based gross or histological analysis is necessary, it should be done at the time of surgery. The appropriate imaging studies should be correlated with the specimen and the specimen dissected and cut on the band saw at this time. This approach allows direct inspection of the tumor and establishment of its relationship to the resection margins at a time when additional intervention is easily initiated. As a routine, we also perform frozen-section analysis on the medullary cavity contents obtained from the portion of the bone remaining in the patient. To avoid any misunderstandings, gross margin review is almost always done with the operating surgeon in attendance.

We liberally use colored inks to designate specimen margins and discriminate among multiple margins when necessary. After initial application, the specimen is daubed with clean, dry 4×4 cotton gauze pads to remove excess ink. After a brief period of air drying, a dilute acid is sprayed on the ink to complete drying.

Gross Description

Providing accurate and meaningful gross descriptions of bone specimens can be challenging. The length and detail of the gross description are largely a function of the size, type, and intent of the specimen.

Biopsy Specimens

Although limited, there is potential information to be gained from the gross description of small specimens (e.g., needle biopsy, open biopsy, curettage, frozen section). In general, reproducible qualities (e.g., color, consistency, texture), together with a quantitative estimate (e.g., focal vs diffuse) of these factors, are included. Bone-producing tumors tend to be yellow to yellow-white and have a texture that is generally sclerotic or granular. In contrast, cartilaginous tumors tend to be blue to blue-gray and semitranslucent. Small cell tumors are characteristically white or beige and fleshy. Many tumors may be tan, brown, or red-black and hemorrhagic; such features may be intrinsic to the tumor or a function of secondary changes. The color of formalin-fixed tissue is almost always "gray-tan," except in areas of hemorrhage, where it is "brown-black."

In addition, the size and shape of small specimens are included in the gross description. The latter should also be included in the "section code" for clinical/pathological correlation and documentation. After tissue processing and embedding, small specimens have few characteristics other than number, size, and shape that can be used to arbitrate specimen management problems, for example, specimen confusion, mix-up, or loss.

Gross evaluation of curettage specimens is hampered by the fact that most such specimens are generally covered by, and immersed in, large amounts of blood, which obscure the true gross appearance of the underlying pathological process. Thus, curettage specimens must be washed before gross inspection. This washing can be accomplished in a number of ways. We place the tissue in a covered container with either water or formalin and then shake it. We then pour the contents through a strainer and examine the resulting "washed" specimens on a paper towel.

Definitive Specimens

The gross description of larger bone specimens can be somewhat problematic. A working knowledge of skeletal anatomy is a prerequisite for this task. In addition, an organized approach to the collection of information is important for thoroughness and completeness. We have developed and adopted a standard format for gross descriptions that achieves consistency while minimizing the length by eliminating extraneous information and verbiage. The essence of this system is the division of the gross description into sections defined by paragraphs of predetermined content. This system is meant to be flexible, with the precise content, order, and number of paragraphs dictated by the needs of the individual institution. We structure our reports as follows:

1. The first paragraph serves to list the specimen components with their sizes. If a structure is normal, a statement is made to that effect (e.g., "… the articular cartilage is unremarkable"), and no further description is given.
2. The second paragraph is dedicated to the primary pathological findings: the tumor's location with reference to relationships to normal structures, its size in three dimensions, and its physical attributes (e.g., color, texture, and consistency). When working with most nonskeletal specimens, documentation of tumor location is at best an estimate since once the specimen leaves the patient, points of orientation become vague and are at best an approximation. In these cases, tumor location is generally described in terms of reference to a resection margin or other nonspecific but constant anatomic landmark. Therefore, tumor location, size, and qualitative description are included in a single paragraph. In contrast, in bone specimens, the intrinsic anatomic features present allow specific reference points and orientation, thereby allowing precise reproducible localization of the tumor and enabling accurate clinical/pathological correlation. In light of this, some of us have divided this section into two paragraphs. The first paragraph

includes all tumor measurements (size and location) in reference to anatomic compartment and structures. The second paragraph describes the physical characteristics of the tumor.

3. The next paragraph is intended for description of any predisposing or "accessory" pathological findings (e.g., enchondroma, nonossifying fibroma).

4. The next paragraph is used to summarize any inking code that might be employed for specimen orientation. In general, it is helpful to first give the ink color, followed by a brief description of the tissue designation; the information is given left to right, as it would be read.

5. The final paragraph is used to indicate the section code. If margins are included within a tissue block, their form (i.e., perpendicular vs *en face*) should be noted. Because of our left-to-right written language, we find it useful to give the alpha-numeric section code first, followed by the tissue designation.

The well-defined nature of skeletal anatomy allows precise designation of tumor location. Tumors arise either within the bone's medullary cavity or on the periosteal cortical surface. If in the medullary cavity, the tumor will have arisen within a given compartment: epiphysis, metaphysis, or diaphysis. Larger tumors may arise in one skeletal compartment and extend into another or through the cortex to involve soft tissues.

When reporting morphological features, we try to be as direct and specific as possible rather than including long descriptive statements. For example, matrix is either present or absent, and if present, it is either bone or cartilage and specifically stated as such. At the same time, each particular matrix has a specific color, texture, and consistency, and those are described.

The use of preoperative chemotherapy adds another layer of complexity to the visual examination of bone specimens. The gross appearance of treated tumors depends upon a combination of factors: the original appearance of the tumor, together with the superimposition of secondary and degenerative processes. The histological hallmark of response to chemotherapy is tumor cell dropout. This finding may be accompanied by inflammation, granulation tissue, fibrosis, bone healing, cyst formation, hemorrhage, and/or pathologic fracture. The gross features of most of these secondary changes may be self-evident. However, gross discrimination between viable and nonviable tumor is less obvious. Viable tumor tissue tends to have vibrant colors, significant luster, and an overall "wet" appearance. In contrast, nonviable tumor tissue *tends* to have subdued, bland colors and to lack luster; furthermore, after several minutes of exposure to air, nonviable tumor tissue tends to appear "dry" or dehydrated. Unfortunately, like viable tumor, various reactive processes (e.g., granulation tissue) also tend to retain luster, making retention of color and luster an observation of limited specificity and reliability. In contrast, a dull, dehydrated appearance is a *relatively* reliable indicator of tumor necrosis but does not discriminate between spontaneous necrosis and response to preoperative therapy.

As a final note, a comment on the timing of specimen dictation may be helpful. In practice, we urge prosectors not to describe specimens while they dissect, but rather after dissection is completed. We have found that dictating the gross description after dissection decreases unnecessary description as the specimen is "revealed" to the prosector during dissection. It also serves to eliminate the inclusion of dissection techniques from the gross description; such information is generally unnecessary but is frequently included in pathology reports as a matter of convention. We have adopted the position that other than the plane in which a bone has been cut, only unusual dissection techniques are included in our reports; the usual techniques are assumed.

Mapping of Postchemotherapy Specimens

With the development of effective drugs, chemotherapy assumed a central role in the multidisciplinary treatment of a number of primary malignant bone tumors, for example, osteosarcoma and Ewing sarcoma. It subsequently became evident that preoperative chemotherapy could be used to assess the effectiveness of a particular drug or combination of drugs in the treatment of a specific tumor within the idiosyncratic physiologic milieu of an individual patient. Furthermore, it became apparent that there is a relationship between the *amount* of therapy effect and the subsequent response to postoperative chemotherapy and even ultimate patient survival. Response to preoperative therapy is a prognostic factor. In fact, when looking at prognostic factors (e.g., tumor size and location, patient age and sex), response to preoperative therapy is the most powerful one for osteosarcoma.

The finding of this therapy–survival relationship mandated the development of techniques that would enable the *quantitative* evaluation of response to therapy. At the same time, the recognition that bone sarcomas have imaging characteristics (seen on plain films, computed tomography [CT], magnetic resonance imaging [MRI], and positron emission tomography [PET]) that change following therapy necessitated the development of techniques for radiology and pathology documentation and correlation. Unlike the response in other solid tumors, response to therapy in bone tumors is not necessarily accompanied by a decrease in tumor size; tumor cells may be eliminated by chemotherapy, but tumor-produced matrix remains largely intact. However, bone tumors develop qualitative morphological changes in response to therapy that may be reflected in imaging changes.

The technique of "specimen mapping" was developed to address the issues of quantitative analysis of response to therapy while enabling detailed correlation between clinical, radiologic, gross, and histological findings. Mapping was designed to allow the examination of large amounts of tumor while introducing an element of consistency and reproducibility to specimen management and quantitative response-to-therapy analysis.

Intrinsic to mapping is the construction of a pictorial record of the specimen sampling. We use specimen X-rays in mapping, but a number of other visual techniques for record keeping are available, including specimen photograph, specimen sketch, and specimen photocopy. Specimen X-rays can be done in one of two ways. In the first, a specimen X-ray is prepared using the intact bivalved bone that will be the subject of analysis. After the surface of the specimen has been cut and pieces placed in cassettes, a record of the bone-cutting schema is drawn on the X-ray using lead or wax pencil; pencil has the advantage of being potentially not visible when photographed. In the second method, the entire specimen surface is cut into tissue block–sized pieces, reassembled, and submitted for X-ray. The pieces are then placed in numbered processing cassettes and the numbers transposed, in pencil, onto the X-ray. We have tried both of these techniques and prefer the latter.

Details of the mapping procedure are as follows. The specimen is cut in a coronal, sagittal, or oblique longitudinal plane that is designed to maximally demonstrate the presence of posttherapy viable tumor. Discussion with the surgeon and review of the preoperative imaging studies help to establish the optimal plane for cutting the tumor-containing bone. Historically, the arteriogram was an important study for guiding the selection of the plane, but now such data are generally available only when the preoperative chemotherapy includes intra-arterial chemotherapy (e.g., cisplatin). Most high-grade malignant tumors have hypervascular profiles on arteriograms prior to therapy. With successful treatment, this hypervascularity resolves in areas of tumor necrosis; conversely, residual hypervascularity corresponds to residual viable tumor. When using arteriograms as a guide, the bone is cut in the plane that will demonstrate the largest amount of hypervascular tumor.

After the plane of section is chosen, the bone is cut on a band saw, photographed, X-rayed, and submerged in 10% neutral buffered formalin. The surface resulting from this plane of section is further cut in a gridlike pattern into small pieces that fit standard processing cassettes. Additional sections of tumor are cut from other areas that are suggestive of residual viable tumor and not represented in the single longitudinal plane. After cutting, the pieces are reassembled into the proper anatomic relationship and resubmitted for specimen X-ray (Fig. 4.2). The resulting X-ray and cassettes are labeled with matching section codes, and the cassettes are then submitted for additional fixation, decalcification, final processing, and slide preparation. Although a number of alternatives are possible, we find that the combination of X-ray and histological analysis allows closer comparison with preoperative findings. At the same time, we submit additional sections of tumor from parts of the tumor outside the initial cut surface. Although a written record of the site of origin of these sections is kept, these are sections for which there is no mapping representation; the number of these so-called random sections is equal to the number of mapped sections.

For the final analysis, a physical, pictorial "map" of the specimen can be constructed to depict a record of the histological analysis. This map establishes the presence or absence of viable and nonviable tumor within the specimen and its precise relationship to normal structures. Other findings (e.g., hemorrhage, cyst formation) can be indicated on the map as needed. The map can then be correlated with other preoperative studies, such as MRI and PET scans, to evaluate tumor response. However, accurate, detailed pictorial tumor mapping is an extremely time-consuming endeavor: 2–4 h for small, noncomplex specimens and 4–20 h for large, complex cases. We no longer routinely construct pictorial maps for each posttherapy specimen; the decision of whether to employ formal pictorial mapping is a case-by-case determination.

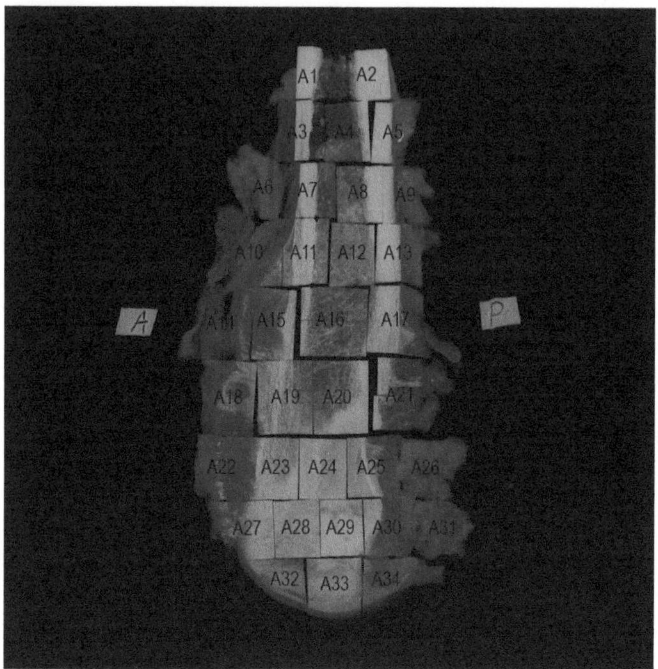

Fig. 4.2 Mapping of a tumor specimen. An osteosarcoma of the distal femur is shown after it has been cut into a grid and reassembled. Each sector of the grid has a specific label. Radiography of the mapped specimen enables subsequent correlation of the microscopic findings for each cassette to the findings for the larger specimen.

Histological estimation of response to therapy is time consuming and complex (Fig. 4.3). A familiarity with the appearance of untreated tumor is a prerequisite. The basis of this examination is an estimation of how much tumor is present and how much of that tumor is still viable. The hallmark of successful response to therapy is dropout or disappearance of the neoplastic cells from the tumor-involved area. Although referred to in terms of "tumor necrosis," the process of cell death probably reflects therapy-induced tumor cell *apoptosis.* Any tumor cell with an intact, nonapoptotic nucleus is interpreted as viable. For purposes of analysis, it is assumed that all spaces between or within the tumor-produced matrix were occupied by viable neoplastic cells prior to preoperative therapy. An estimate is made as to the percentage of tumor that is viable versus tumor that is nonviable. For reporting purposes, this estimate is expressed in terms of "percentage tumor necrosis."

A number of approaches have been used in the quantitative analysis of response to therapy. Currently, two methods of tumor necrosis calculation are employed at MD Anderson. One is based on a slide-by-slide determination of percentage of tumor necrosis per slide and then a mathematical calculation for the entire case.

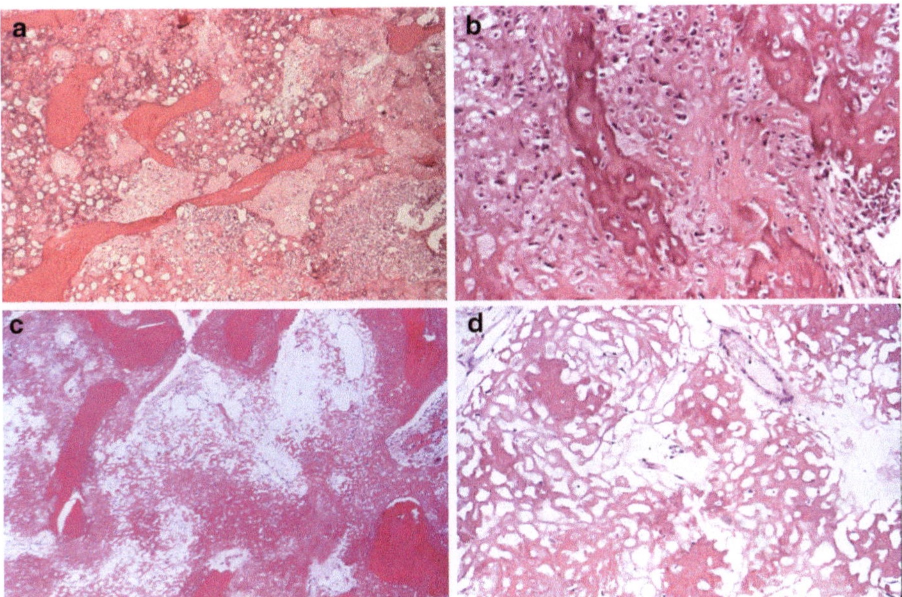

Fig. 4.3 An osteoblastic osteosarcoma before and after chemotherapy. Before chemotherapy (**a**, **b**), the tumor is seen to have pleomorphic spindle-shaped cells producing abundant osteoid. After chemotherapy (**c**, **d**), evidence of necrosis is seen: the tumor is largely devoid of cells, and empty spaces are observed in the osteoid matrix.

Alternatively, the analysis consists of a postreview overall impression of the case. For those who are new to this procedure, we recommend the slide-by-slide approach. In reporting the results of response-to-therapy analysis, we do not limit this part of the pathology report to a simple statement of percentage of tumor necrosis. In addition to the amount of nonviable tumor, we add descriptive comments as to the form, pattern, size, and location of viable tumor. From a practical point of view, it is rare to see any significant areas of viable tumor (i.e., >1.0 cm) in a neoplasm that has responded well to preoperative therapy. Historically, the clinical interpretation of response to preoperative chemotherapy has been viewed as a "threshold phenomenon"; patients with 90% or greater tumor necrosis are considered to have had a good response to therapy, while patients with less than 90% tumor necrosis are considered to have had a poor response. Although at the time of this writing, "threshold necrosis" is used to make decisions about therapy, most investigators believe that the relationship between response to preoperative therapy and survival is more complex than a simple numerical threshold above which patients survive and below which patients do not—a reminder that medicine is not a science, but a finely practiced art.

Pathology Report

The final pathology report contains the results of gross and histological analysis, together with the findings of any special studies and morphology-based clinico-pathological correlation. The need for prolonged decalcification results in a delay of specimen availability for histological analysis and thus a delay in the ability to construct and issue a final pathology report. Although understood in theory, this is frequently a source of friction between pathologist and clinician. In light of this, we encourage a close working relationship between pathologist and clinician in the form of conversations, telephone calls, e-mails, and preliminary reports to transmit information as it becomes available and thus fill the void caused by delayed final reports.

The form of the pathology report has become a contentious issue. It is our opinion that the final pathology report is the domain of the individual surgical pathologist. However, considering the magnitude of its impact, and the changing needs of the clinical arm, it is not unreasonable that input pertaining to content of the pathology report should be sought from all report recipients.

At this time, the issue of *narrative* versus *synoptic* reporting remains unresolved. Standardized synoptic reports have the advantages of easy reading, thoroughness, and consistency; an example is shown in Fig. 4.4. However, many pathologists are more comfortable with the traditional narrative report. We have mixed opinions concerning this issue, and the choice of reporting style may be best left up to the individual pathologist. Recommended reporting elements and a suggested format have been produced by the College of American Pathologists under the Cancer Protocols program (Rubin et al. 2011; http://www.cap.org/apps/docs/committees/cancer/cancer_protocols/2011/Bone_11protocol.pdf).

Complete reports should be the end result of all pathology studies. However, the rarity of bone tumors makes it difficult to gather significant amounts of meaningful data concerning bone tumors. In light of this, bone tumor pathology reports should be as detailed and complete as possible, although some might consider this over-reporting. There should be detailed and precise information regarding all aspects of the tumor: location, classification, extent of disease, resection margins, and where applicable, evaluation of response to preoperative therapy.

Photography

A detailed discussion concerning the principles of medical specimen photography is beyond the scope of this work. However, considering the volume of work that we do, we would like to share a few practices that we have found useful and enhance photographs without adding significant effort.

a

SARCOMA INVOLVING BONE:

Classification:	[generic tumor type]
Group:	conventional/variant
Type:	[specific type; see Dahlin and Unni, 1977]
Major component:	[type], _%
Minor component(s):	[type], _%
Site:	
Side:	right/left
Bone:	[bone]
End:	proximal/mid/distal
Compartment:	medullary cavity / surface
Part:	epiphysis/metaphysis/diaphysis
Invasion:	yes/no
Cortex:	yes/no
Overlying soft tissue:	yes/no, distance
Blood vessel:	yes/no
Metastases:	yes/no
Skip mets:	yes/no
Other:	yes/no
Regional involvement:	yes/no, what
Resection margins:	[involved?] yes/no
Distance from tumor	
Status post-chemotherapy:	yes/no
Amount therapy effect:	_%
Other:	

Comment:

b

POST-TREATMENT OSTEOSARCOMA INVOLVING BONE, MARGINS FREE:

Classification:	osteosarcoma
Group:	conventional
Type:	osteoblastic osteosarcoma
Major component:	osteoblastic 60%
Minor component(s):	fibroblastic 25%
	chondroblastic 15%
Site:	bone
Side:	right
Bone:	femur
End:	distal
Compartment:	medullary cavity
Part:	metaphysis
Extension:	into diaphysis
	focal invasion of epiphysis
Invasion:	yes
Cortex:	yes
Overlying soft tissue:	3 cm into true soft tissue
Blood vessel:	no
Metastases:	yes
Skip mets:	yes
	2 cm diameter
	2.6 cm proximal to primary
Other:	no
Regional involvement:	no
Resection margins:	free of tumor
Distance from tumor:	tumor 2.6 cm from proximal resection margin
Status post-chemotherapy:	yes
Amount therapy effect:	80%
Other:	

Comment: Viable tumor is largely present as scattered atypical cells singly and in small aggregates. However, there are several 1.0–2.0-cm foci of viable fibroblastic osteosarcoma present both within the medullary cavity and more frequently in the subperiosteal, extraosseous soft tissue.

Fig. 4.4 A sample synoptic pathology report. (**a**) General information contained in the report. (**b**) A specific example of a completed report.

Appropriate lighting: Careful lighting is crucial. The basket-weave architecture of mineralized bone matrix, with the retraction of intervening nonmineralized tissue, imparts a unique three-dimensional architecture to bone and bone-tumor surfaces. In turn, this can lead to extensive shadows when a single light is used during photography. Therefore, we routinely employ at least two lights and two reflectors, resulting in evenly lighted surfaces.

Background: This is a much underappreciated consideration. An even, flat, clean background is necessary to prevent viewer distractions. Colored backgrounds are popular with some investigators. However, this practice ignores the problem of "optical color bleed." There are no "pure" colors in nature. Rather, all biological colors are actually a liberal mixture of many colors, a feature largely unappreciated or overlooked. When an artificial colored background is employed, there will be colors common to both the monochromic background and polychromatic specimen. As a result, the colors of the specimen and background will merge at the interface, resulting in a loss of definition of the specimen edge; the interface may not be sharp or well defined. In contrast, black is the absence of color, and no such merging occurs, resulting in a sharp specimen/background interface. We find that a sheet of developed X-ray film results in a consistent, matte, black surface that, when covered by nonreflective glass, results in an ideal background upon which specimens can be positioned for photography.

Clean: Nothing can be more distracting or unsightly than a poorly cleaned specimen. When necessary, needle biopsy specimens can be rinsed with water or formalin. As previously discussed, curettage specimens are usually saturated in blood and can be rinsed with water or formalin. Larger surgical specimens pose a greater challenge as a result of bone saw artifacts: bone dust and scorching. Areas of medullary cavity cancellous bone should be thoroughly rinsed with water and generally must be lightly scrubbed with a brush. Surgical brushes do an excellent job, and they are generally readily available. In addition, as a result of the high-speed cutting action of a bone saw and its interaction with cortex, bone dust frequently becomes scorched, resulting in brown-green material adherent to cortical bone. The side of a scalpel blade can be used to scrape this material off the cortex.

Cut surface: Although there are exceptions, bone photography is largely limited to the cut surface of the tumor-containing bone. For convenience and cost-effectiveness, it is tempting to put both sides of a bivalved specimen in a single view; however, doing so is counterproductive if the images will be presented or published. When such images are projected, audience members usually assume that when two structures are shown, they must be different. As a result, they will look back and forth searching for differences ("the Wimbledon perspective") rather than listening to a speaker. Therefore, photograph each side separately; the tighter view also results in a better quality photograph.

Crop: The specimen should occupy the largest possible area within the photographic field. Remember that current digital projection only allows a horizontal plane. If you photograph in a vertical plane to increase the size of the image, the computer will automatically reorient the image sideways. You can increase pixel density using vertical photography, but you must remember to crop and reorient the photograph, or it will be projected sideways.

Couple of views: Film and computer memory are cheap; bone specimens are rare. Thus, multiple views are suggested. In particular, remember to shoot close-ups so that features of interest can be readily seen. We suggest a low-power view encompassing the entire bone, followed by a view limited to the entire tumor (i.e., cropping out normal bone), and then close-ups of the tumor surface so that tissue variation between tumor and normal tissue, together with other aspects of tumor color and texture, can be appreciated.

Dry: Remember to dry the specimen. This will remove remnants of blood and debris. At the same time, it will remove fluids that otherwise provide unwanted reflective surfaces.

Recolorization: A final comment on "the one that got away": There are circumstances in which a specimen is dissected and cut but must be formalin fixed before photography can be accomplished. The fixed specimen can be photographed, but, other than in cartilage-containing tumors, the results are generally unsatisfactory. However, there is a technique that will regenerate specimen color: "recolorization." The fixed specimen is submerged in 80% ethanol for a period of time and then photographed. It should be kept in mind that this technique is far from perfect and has a number of limitations. The "color" resulting from this practice is at some variance from natural colors, but it is generally better than no color. The length of time it takes to recolorize a specimen is a direct function of the amount of time the specimen has been in formalin. We find that 4–6 h of alcohol processing is required for specimens with 24–48 h of formalin fixation. The time for recolorization increases with longer periods of fixation. We have not tried this technique in specimens with greater than 7 days fixation. The recolorization process is temporary, and the color begins to fade as soon as the specimen is removed from alcohol. Therefore, the specimen must remain in alcohol until photography; literally, the specimen should be transferred from the alcohol to the photography surface for immediate photography. In our experience, recolorization is a one-time opportunity. That is, once recolorization is performed, the color quickly retreats to the "gray-tan" of formalin-fixed tissue; the process cannot be repeated.

Special Studies

In specific clinical scenarios or pathological findings, the use of special diagnostic procedures—electron microscopy, immunohistochemistry, and molecular studies—may be indicated.

Electron Microscopy

In the past, samples of all bone specimens were submitted for electron microscopy. However, that was at a time when electron microscopy was largely supported by external funding. Today, tissues from suspected small cell tumors and those in which prior biopsy materials have yielded nonspecific results are the only tissues routinely submitted for electron microscopy. We use glutaraldehyde for fixation and embed all materials within 24 h. The final decision to use electron microscopy is delayed until the light microscopy results for a specimen have been reviewed and a clear need for the test is evident.

Immunohistochemistry

Our current methods of fixation and decalcification allow the production of material in which antigenicity appears to remain intact, and immunohistochemical studies are routinely performed. In cases in which there is significant suggestion of a specific differential diagnosis (e.g., small cell tumor) through initial screening techniques (e.g., frozen-section or cytologic analysis at the time of a procedure), unstained slides are prepared along with the initial H&E-stained slides. This approach allows the block to be cut for multiple purposes at once, enabling efficient use of tissue while maximally preserving it for future studies and decreasing turnaround time. The tissue is cut in a "sandwich" fashion in which a predetermined number of sections are cut and mounted on slides for immunohistochemical analysis. The first and last slides are stained with H&E and reviewed. If a pathological process is present in the first and last slides, it is presumed that it is present in the intervening slides, which are then available for special studies.

Molecular Studies

Some sarcomas of both bone and soft tissue are associated with recurrent unique chromosomal translocations, usually balanced or reciprocal, that result in the fusion of one gene from each chromosome to produce a unique chimeric gene. These translocations are generally specific for a particular sarcoma, but identical transcripts have been described in differing histological types, such as clear cell sarcoma and angiomatoid fibrous histiocytoma (Hallor et al. 2006). A fusion gene transcript often encodes a unique and inappropriately regulated transcription factor that promotes transcription of genes important to neoplastic growth and perhaps malignant transformation in these rare tumors (Lazar et al. 2006).

Ewing sarcoma was the first sarcoma recognized to have a recurrent chromosomal translocation. The characteristic translocation involves a reciprocal exchange of the long arms of chromosomes 11 and 22 and is designated t(11;22)(q24;q12) (Fig. 4.5a, b). On chromosome 11q24 resides the *FLI1* gene, which is a member of the ETS family of genes and functions as a transcription factor (Fig. 4.5b–e). The *EWSR1* gene resides on chromosome 22q12 and has an RNA-binding domain and an activation domain (Fig. 4.5e). The fusion gene contains the activation domain (exons 1–7) of the *EWSR1* gene fused to the DNA-binding domain of the *FLI1* gene, which creates a novel transcription factor that aberrantly regulates the transcription of genes believed important in the biology of this tumor (Delattre et al. 1992). The active fusion gene is formed on the derivative chromosome 22, while the affected chromosome 11 does not result in a functional chimeric gene and thus contains what is termed a "silent breakpoint." Together, the many types of *EWSR1-FLI1* chimeric fusion transcripts involving various combinations of exons from these two genes are estimated to be present in greater than 90% of Ewing sarcoma cases. At least six other members of the ETS gene family residing on different chromosomes can be involved as alternative sites of translocations. The most common of these is *ERG* on 21q22, which is present in approximately 5% of cases; the remaining fusion partners are very rarely encountered and are present in less than 1% of all cases in aggregate, though this percentage could increase as testing for these less common fusion transcripts becomes more routine (Romeo and Dei Tos 2010).

It is now widely recognized that ancillary cytogenetic and molecular techniques are critical for the diagnosis of Ewing sarcoma, and genetic confirmation is evolving as the standard of care for making this diagnosis (Folpe et al. 2005). Genetic confirmation is particularly critical when unusual clinical or histological presentations are encountered. While positive immunohistochemical stains for markers such as CD99 (O13) and FLI-1 are helpful in combination with negative results for other pertinent immunostains, these methods often lack the sensitivity and specificity to reliably deliver a definitive diagnosis.

The historical gold standard for demonstrating a translocation is chromosomal karyotyping (Fig. 4.5a) when fresh material is available for the cytogenetics laboratory from a surgical or needle biopsy. This technique offers the advantage of being open ended; thus, it will demonstrate any cytogenetic event present. Only small amounts of pure and viable tumor are required. The disadvantages of the technique are that tumors are often difficult to grow in culture, definitive results are often not available for more than a week, and, because MD Anderson is a referral center, often only formalin-fixed, paraffin-embedded material is available with the patient referral for verification of the diagnosis. The karyotypes can be very complex, and translocations can be small and cryptic, but methods such as spectral karyotyping (SKY) and fluorescence in situ hybridization (FISH) can help clarify the chromosomal status.

FISH with formalin-fixed, paraffin-embedded samples is the most common modality at MD Anderson for cytogenetic testing for Ewing sarcoma (Fig. 4.5c). This method involves the use of highly specific hybridizing DNA probes that flank the *EWSR1* locus. We use the commercially available probe set produced by Vysis/Abbott Molecular (Des Plaines, IL). Each probe is labeled with a different

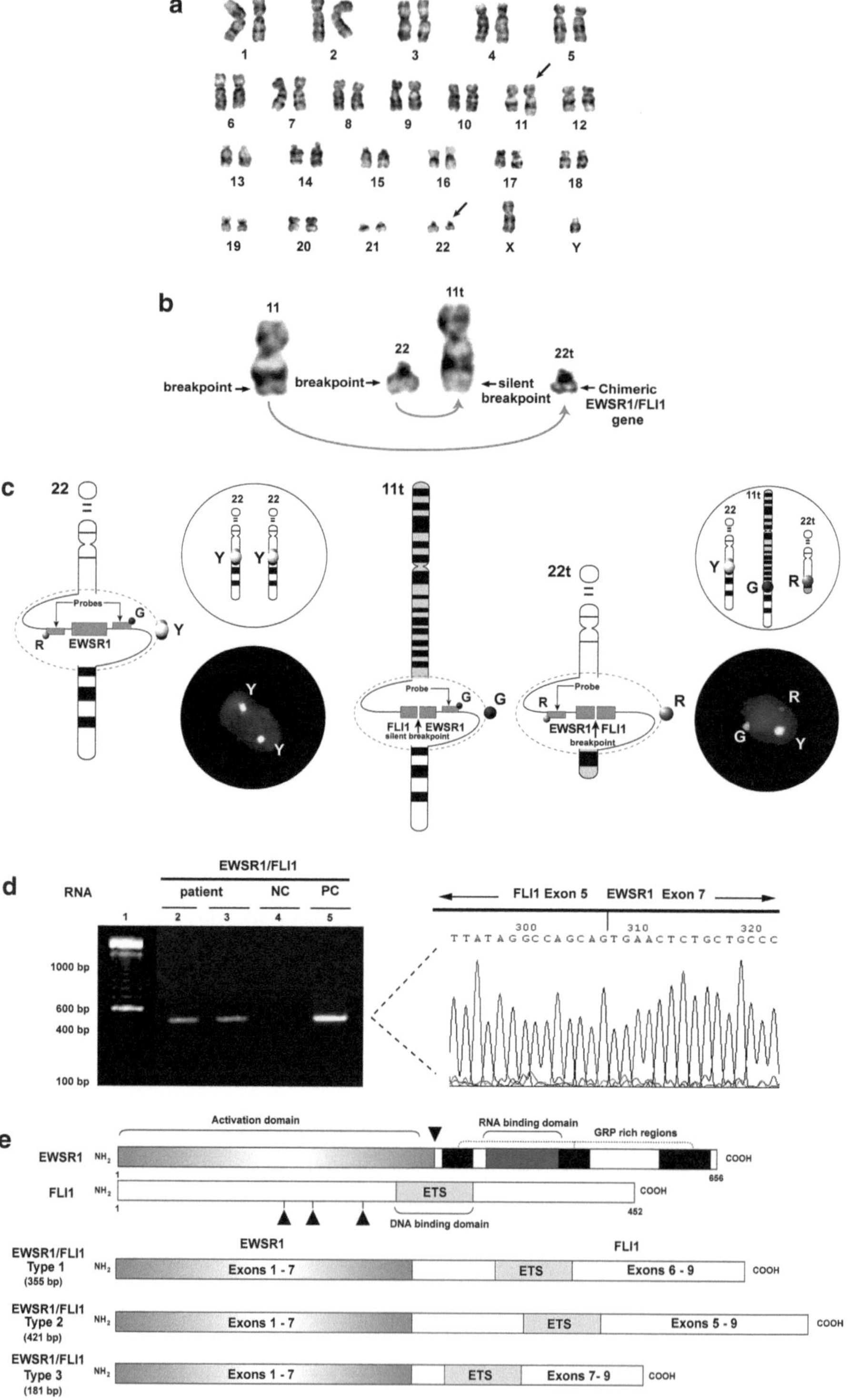

a
1 2 3 4 5
6 7 8 9 10 11 12
13 14 15 16 17 18
19 20 21 22 X Y

b
11 22 11t 22t
breakpoint breakpoint silent breakpoint Chimeric EWSR1/FLI1 gene

c
22
Probes
R EWSR1 G Y
22 22
Y Y
Y Y

11t
Probe
FLI1 EWSR1 G G
silent breakpoint

22t
Probe
EWSR1 FLI1 R R
breakpoint
22 11t 22t
Y G R
R G Y

d
RNA
EWSR1/FLI1
patient NC PC
1 2 3 4 5
1000 bp
600 bp
400 bp
100 bp

FLI1 Exon 5 EWSR1 Exon 7
300 310 320
T T A T A G G C C A G C A G T G A A C T C T G C T G C C C

e
Activation domain
RNA binding domain
GRP rich regions
EWSR1 NH2 COOH
656
FLI1 NH2 ETS COOH
1 452
DNA binding domain

EWSR1/FLI1 Type 1 (355 bp)
EWSR1 FLI1
NH2 Exons 1 - 7 ETS Exons 6 - 9 COOH

EWSR1/FLI1 Type 2 (421 bp)
NH2 Exons 1 - 7 ETS Exons 5 - 9 COOH

EWSR1/FLI1 Type 3 (181 bp)
NH2 Exons 1 - 7 ETS Exons 7 - 9 COOH

fluorescent chromophore; a red-labeled probe hybridizes to the centromeric side of the *EWSR1* locus and a green-labeled probe to the telomeric side. When the probes hybridize to an intact *EWSR1* locus, they are in extremely close proximity, and their overlapping spectra produce a single yellow signal. Thus, a cell lacking a rearrangement at *EWSR1* has two yellow signals—one for each of the chromosome 22 pair. When one of the two *EWSR1* loci is rearranged, the green and red signals no longer segregate together to produce a yellow signal, and thus three signals (red, green, and yellow) are noted. This process is illustrated in Fig. 4.5c, in which representative nuclei with intact and rearranged signals are also shown. The advantage of this method is that it is robust and will detect all rearrangements of the *EWSR1* locus regardless of the ETS family member involved, and thus one probe set can be used for all cases. Only in exceptional, rare cases of Ewing sarcoma is the *EWSR1* locus not involved; for instance, there are a few reports that a homolog of this gene, *TLS/FUS* (16p11), can substitute for *EWSR1*. The FISH method can be used for paraffin sections, cytologic smears, and touch preps and to confirm findings in the metaphase spreads used to produce traditional karyotypes. The disadvantage of the method is that no information is given regarding the identity of the fusion partner. At least five other types of

Fig. 4.5 The chromosomal translocation of Ewing sarcoma. (**a**) This conventional karyotype shows a balanced reciprocal translocation between chromosomes 11 and 22 (depicted by *black arrows*). (**b**) Enlarged images of chromosomes 11 and 22 illustrate the breakpoints, including the silent breakpoint on the derivative chromosome 11 and the active site that produces the functional chimeric gene on the derivative chromosome 22. (**c**) Fluorescence in situ hybridization (FISH) relies on two unique DNA probes that hybridize to the centromeric (R, a red-labeled probe) and telomeric (G, a green-labeled probe) flanking regions of the *EWSR1* locus. The spectral overlap of these two probes produces a *yellow* (Y) signal when they co-localize, and thus two *yellow* signals are present in the normal intact interphase nucleus (with a 4′,6-diamidino-2-phenylindole [DAPI]—counterstained nucleus). In Ewing sarcoma, the telomeric probe (*green*) is most commonly transferred to the *FLI1* locus on chromosome 11. The centromeric (*red*) probe remains on the derivative chromosome 22. Since the two derivative chromosomes (11 and 22) segregate independently, nuclei with one *red*, one *green*, and one *yellow* signal (representing the translocated chromosome 22, the translocated chromosome 11, and the unaffected chromosome 22, respectively) are detected. (**d**) The EWS-FLI1 fusion transcript can also be detected by the RT-PCR technique from RNA extracted from tumor cells. Two independent samples from a patient (lanes 2 and 3) show a type 2 EWS-FLI1 fusion transcript combining exon 5 of *FLI1* in frame with exon 7 of *EWSR1* (confirmed by DNA sequencing of the amplicon). Testing with negative and positive controls (indicated here by "NC" and "PC") is routinely performed. (**e**) The *EWSR1* gene encodes a protein with an activation domain and an RNA-binding domain, and the *FLI1* gene is a member of the ETS family of transcription factors and has a DNA-binding domain. Among the numerous variant chimeric gene combinations are types 1–3, and each combines the activation domain of *EWSR1* (N-terminal) and the DNA-binding domain of *FLI1* (C-terminal), creating a novel transcription factor. The type 1 fusion transcript is most common and represents more than 50% of all fusion transcripts. (Portions of this figure are courtesy of Lynne V. Abruzzo, Kimberly J. Hayes, Bogdan A. Czerniak, Dolores Lopez-Terrada, and Kim Vu [MD Anderson Cancer Center and Texas Children's Hospital, Houston, TX].)

sarcoma—desmoplastic small round cell tumor, extraskeletal myxoid chondrosarcoma, clear cell sarcoma, and subsets of both myxoid liposarcoma and angiomatoid fibrous histiocytoma—can also contain rearrangements at the *EWSR1* locus but do not involve an ETS family member (Romeo and Dei Tos 2010). Fortunately, the clinical, histological, and immunophenotypic features of these other lesions are usually readily distinguished from Ewing sarcoma, so the nonspecific results are not often a problem in the practical application of this methodology; however, they can be an issue in small or poorly preserved biopsy specimens. Molecular diagnostic results should never be acted upon in the absence of a sound clinico-pathological characterization of a tumor and patient.

Finally, polymerase chain reaction (PCR) methods in which cDNA is reverse transcribed from RNA extracted from fresh, frozen, or formalin-fixed, paraffin-embedded tumor specimens can be used to elucidate the precise fusion transcript. The disadvantages of this method are that high-quality RNA can be very difficult to extract from formalin-fixed tissue, and multiple sets of PCRs and primers are necessary to reliably detect all of the variant translocations. In our experience, it is increasingly difficult to extract high-quality RNA from paraffin blocks that have been fixed for more than 5 years. It is vitally important to sequence the DNA of the PCR amplicon to confirm its identity, as illustrated in Fig. 4.5d. This method is employed at MD Anderson. Usually, only FISH or only reverse transcription (RT)-PCR is employed, as both methods provide molecular diagnostic confirmation. In practice, results can often be obtained faster with RT-PCR than with FISH, but RT-PCR may fail to detect unusual fusion genes if probes for such genes are not included in the test. Another caveat is that FISH is more likely than RT-PCR to provide interpretable results in decalcified specimens, and so the type of fixation and processing of the specimen can also be important in selecting the molecular diagnostic approach.

There is preliminary evidence that the identity of the fusion partner of *EWSR1* and the breakpoints of the *FLI1* and *EWSR1* genes may impart prognostic information (de Alva et al. 1998), though more recent large prospective studies of pediatric cohorts have not reproduced this finding (van Doorninck et al. 2010). The detection of fusion transcripts in peripheral blood or bone marrow in patients with primary Ewing sarcoma after treatment is associated with relapse (Avigad et al. 2006). While these results are intriguing, they must be considered preliminary at present because they are based on relatively small retrospective studies and need corroboration with further study. Nevertheless, it has become clear that the information imparted by FISH, RT-PCR, and other genetic tests will become increasingly important in the future for Ewing sarcoma and other diseases.

Key Practice Points

- Correlation between clinical, radiographic, and histological findings is mandatory.
- The principle of representative sections, which enables a reliable histological analysis of the tumor specimen to be made on the basis of limited samples, requires the pathologist to be familiar with the gross appearance of bone tumors in order to be able to select the essential areas for study.
- All bone tumor specimens require decalcification unless there are compelling reasons in a specific case to forgo this procedure.
- The hallmark of response to preoperative chemotherapy is cell dropout (i.e., apoptosis [often called "tumor necrosis"]).
- Gross criteria might give a qualitative sense of the degree of tumor necrosis but are not adequate means of quantitatively judging the response to preoperative therapy.
- Detailed mapping of postchemotherapy specimens is the only reliable method of deriving an accurate measure of percentage of tumor necrosis.
- Molecular confirmation of the diagnosis by FISH or RT-PCR, in correlation with appropriate clinical, radiographic, and histological data, is the gold standard for diagnosis of Ewing sarcoma.

Suggested Readings

Avigad S, Cohen IJ, Zilberstein J, et al. The predictive potential of molecular detection in nonmetastatic Ewing family of tumors. Cancer. 2006;100:1053–8.

Ayala AG, Raymond AK, Ro JY, Carrasco CH, Fanning CV, Murray JA. Needle biopsy of primary bone lesions. M.D. Anderson experience. Pathol Annu 1989;24:219–51.

Bjonsson J, McCleod RA, Unni KK, Ilstrup DM, Pritchard DJ. Primary chondrosarcoma of long bones and limb girdles. Cancer. 1998;83:2105–19.

Dahlin DC, Unni KK. Osteosarcoma of bone and its important recognizable varieties. Am J Surg Pathol. 1977;1:61–72.

Dahlin DC, Coventry MB, Scanlon PW. Ewing's sarcoma: a critical analysis of 165 cases. J Bone Joint Surg Am. 1961;43:185–92.

Dayton AS, Ro JY, Schwartz MR, Ayala AG, Raymond AK. Raymond's paragraph system: an alternative format for the organization of gross pathology reports and its implementation in an academic teaching hospital. Arch Pathol Lab Med. 2009;133:298–302.

de Alva E, Kawai A, Healey JH, et al. *EWS-FLI1* fusion transcript is an independent determinant of prognosis in Ewing's sarcoma. J Clin Oncol. 1998;16:1248–55.

Delattre O, Zucman J, Plougastel B, et al. Gene fusion with an ETS DNA-binding domain caused by chromosome translocation in human tumours. Nature. 1992;359:162–5.

Dorfman H, Czerniak BA (1998) Bone tumors. Mosby, Saint Louis

Evans HL, Ayala AG, Romsdahl MM. Prognostic factors in chondrosarcoma of bone: a clinicopathologic analysis with emphasis on histologic grading. Cancer. 197740:818–31.

Fletcher CDM, Unni KK, Mertens F (eds). World Health Organization classification of tumours. Tumours of soft tissue and bone. Pathology & genetics. IARC Press, Lyon: 2002.

Folpe AL, Goldblum JR, Rubin BP, et al. Morphologic and immunophenotypic diversity in Ewing family tumors: a study of 66 genetically confirmed cases. Am J Surg Pathol. 2005;29: 1025–33.

Hallor KH, Micci F, Meis-Kindblom JM, et al. Fusion genes in angiomatoid fibrous histiocytoma. Cancer Lett. 2006;251:158–63.

Jaffe HL, Lichtenstein L. Benign chondroblastoma of bone: a reinterpretation of the so-called calcifying or chondromatous giant cell tumor of bone. Am J Pathol. 1942;18:969–91.

Lazar A, Abruzzo LV, Lee S, Pollock RE, Czerniak BA. Molecular diagnosis of sarcomas: chromosomal translocations in sarcomas. Arch Pathol Lab Med. 2006;130:1199–207.

Lewis MM, Kenan S, Yabut SM, Norman A, Steiner G. Periosteal chondroma. A report of ten cases and review of the literature. Clin Orthop. 1990;256:185–92.

Lichtenstein L, Jaffe HL. Chondrosarcoma of bone. Am J Pathol. 1943;19:553–89.

Nakashima Y, Unni KK, Shives TC, Swee RG, Dahlin DC. Mesenchymal chondrosarcoma of bone and soft tissue: a review of 111 cases. Cancer. 1986;57:2444–53.

Raymond AK, Ayala AG. Specimen management after osteosarcoma chemotherapy. Contemp Issues Surg Pathol. 1988;11:157–83.

Raymond AK, Chawla SP, Carrasco CH, et al. Osteosarcoma chemotherapy effect: a prognostic factor. Semin Diagn Pathol. 1987;4:212–36.

Romeo S, Dei Tos AP. Soft tissue tumors associated with EWSR1 translocation. Virchows Arch. 2010;456:219–34.

Rubin BP, Antonescu CR, Gannon FH, et al. Protocol for the examination of specimens from patients with tumors of bone. Washington DC: College of American Pathologists; 2011. Available at http://www.cap.org/apps/docs/committees/cancer/cancer_protocols/2011/ Bone_11protocol.pdf. Accessed 19 Jun 2012.

Subbiah V, Anderson P, Lazar AJ, Burdett E, Raymond K, Ludwig JA. Ewing sarcoma: standard and experimental treatment options. Curr Treat Options Oncol. 2009;10:126–40.

Toomey EC, Schiffman JD, Lessnick SL. Recent advances in the molecular pathogenesis of Ewing sarcoma. Oncogene. 2010;29:4504–16.

Turcotte RE, Kurt AM, Sim FH, Unni KK, McLeod RA. Chondroblastoma. Hum Pathol 1993;24:944–9.

Unni KK, Inwards CY. Dahlin's bone tumors: general aspects and data on 10,165 Cases, 6th edn. Wolters Kluwer/Lippincott, Williams & Wilkins, Philadelphia: 2009.

Unni KK, Inwards CY, Bridge JA, Kindblom LG, Wold LE. Tumors of the bones and joints. AFIP atlas of tumor pathology. Series 4; Fascicle 2. ARP Press, Silver Spring: 2005.

van Doorninck JA, Ji L, Schaub B, et al. Current treatment protocols have eliminated the prognostic advantage of type 1 fusions in Ewing sarcoma: a report from the Children's Oncology Group. J Clin Oncol. 2010;28:1989–94.

Chapter 5
Osteosarcoma

Patrick P. Lin and Shreyaskumar Patel

Contents

Chapter Overview The treatment of osteosarcoma forms the basis of therapy for most other sarcomas. The concepts that were developed originally for the staging, pathologic analysis, chemotherapy, and surgical management of osteosarcoma have now been applied to many other diseases. Most cases of osteosarcoma are classified as conventional osteosarcoma, which is a high-grade tumor arising typically in an adolescent patient or young adult. For these patients, the standard treatment consists

P.P. Lin (✉)
Department of Orthopaedic Oncology, Unit 1448, Division of Surgery,
The University of Texas MD Anderson Cancer Center,
P.O. Box 301402, Houston, TX 77230, USA
e-mail: plin@mdanderson.org

S. Patel
Department of Sarcoma Medical Oncology, Unit 450, Division of Cancer Medicine,
The University of Texas MD Anderson Cancer Center, 1400 Holcombe Boulevard,
Houston, TX 77030, USA
e-mail: spatel@mdanderson.org

P.P. Lin and S. Patel (eds.), *Bone Sarcoma*, MD Anderson Cancer Care Series,
DOI 10.1007/978-1-4614-5194-5_5,
© The University of Texas M. D. Anderson Cancer Center 2013

of preoperative chemotherapy, wide surgical excision, careful pathologic mapping of the resected tumor, and postoperative chemotherapy based upon the percentage of necrosis of the tumor. There are many uncommon variants of osteosarcoma that behave differently than conventional osteosarcoma. Osteosarcoma of the craniofacial bones resembles conventional osteosarcoma histologically, but its prognosis is different since metastasis is uncommon. Other variants discussed in this chapter have distinctive radiographic, histologic, or demographic characteristics. Secondary osteosarcoma, which arises in a preexisting bone lesion, has a markedly worse prognosis than other forms of osteosarcoma.

Introduction

Osteosarcoma is the most common primary sarcoma of bone. Nevertheless, it is, like all sarcomas, a rare disease. Approximately 1,000 new cases arise in the United States each year. Most of these occur in young patients, with a peak age of incidence in the second decade. Cases of primary conventional osteosarcoma may arise in older patients, but as age increases, secondary osteosarcoma is more likely. Such tumors develop in patients who have had a preexisting lesion or disease in the bone, such as Paget disease. The diagnosis of secondary osteosarcoma carries significance in terms of prognosis and expected response to treatment; secondary osteosarcoma does not respond well to chemotherapy and has a worse outcome than that of primary conventional osteosarcoma.

The term *osteosarcoma* usually carries the connotation of a high-grade, bone-forming sarcoma that has occurred in a young person. In essence, this description characterizes *conventional osteosarcoma*, which is the proper name for such disease. Conventional, or classic, osteosarcoma accounts for most cases of osteosarcoma, but there also exist many other, rarer variants of osteosarcoma that have different clinical characteristics, prognoses, and treatment approaches. Thus, a clear distinction should be made as to which type of osteosarcoma is meant when the disease is discussed.

The management of conventional osteosarcoma represents the model of multidisciplinary treatment that is the foundation of therapy for other sarcomas. The management of certain rare sarcomas, such as dedifferentiated chondrosarcoma, is based on the protocols used for conventional osteosarcoma. The hope is that sarcomas that are currently considered resistant to therapy might one day be treated successfully with a similar strategy, if newer, more effective agents can be identified in the future.

It should be recognized that certain other tumors are now believed to be closely related to osteosarcoma. In particular, malignant fibrous histiocytoma (MFH) of bone, which is discussed in Chap. 8 ("Rare Bone Sarcomas"), may be a variant of osteosarcoma. Although MFH of bone may be nearly identical in histologic appearance to MFH of soft tissue, the behavior of MFH of bone and its response to treatment are more akin to those of conventional osteosarcoma.

Table 5.1 Classification of osteosarcomas

Conventional (classic) osteosarcoma
Osteoblastic osteosarcoma
Chondroblastic osteosarcoma
Fibroblastic osteosarcoma
Rare variants of high-grade osteosarcoma
Telangiectatic osteosarcoma
Small cell osteosarcoma
Epithelioid osteosarcoma
Giant cell–rich osteosarcoma
Osteosarcoma of the craniofacial bones
Well-differentiated intramedullary osteosarcoma
Parosteal osteosarcoma
Periosteal osteosarcoma
High-grade surface osteosarcoma
Secondary osteosarcoma

This chapter discusses the staging and diagnostic workup of suspected cases of osteosarcoma, as well as the management of conventional osteosarcoma and its variants. The classification of osteosarcoma is shown in Table 5.1, which is based on the World Health Organization (WHO) classification of bone-forming tumors (Schajowicz 1993), with a few modifications. In particular, several clinical variants that are recognized in Table 5.1 are not part of the original WHO classification. Osteosarcoma of the craniofacial bones and secondary osteosarcoma are two important entities with characteristics that clearly set them apart from conventional osteosarcoma. These diseases are discussed in separate sections below. In addition, several rare histologic variants are noted. These include telangiectatic, small cell, epithelioid, and giant cell-rich osteosarcoma. Emphasis in this chapter will be placed upon variants that are unique in their clinical presentation, prognosis, or treatment. Other variants may be distinctive in terms of their histologic appearance but have the same treatment and prognosis as those of conventional osteosarcoma and will therefore be mentioned only briefly.

Diagnostic Workup and Staging

The workup of osteosarcoma includes a detailed history taking and physical examination. The presenting symptoms typically include deep-seated, constant, gnawing pain and swelling at the affected site. Pain in multiple areas may portend skeletal metastasis and should be investigated appropriately. The family history is important, as there may be clues to inherited familial disorders such as retinoblastoma and Li–Fraumeni syndrome (*TP53* gene mutation), both of which give rise to osteosarcoma. Beyond the history and examination, the standard studies for evaluation of potential osteosarcoma are laboratory tests, an X-ray of the entire affected

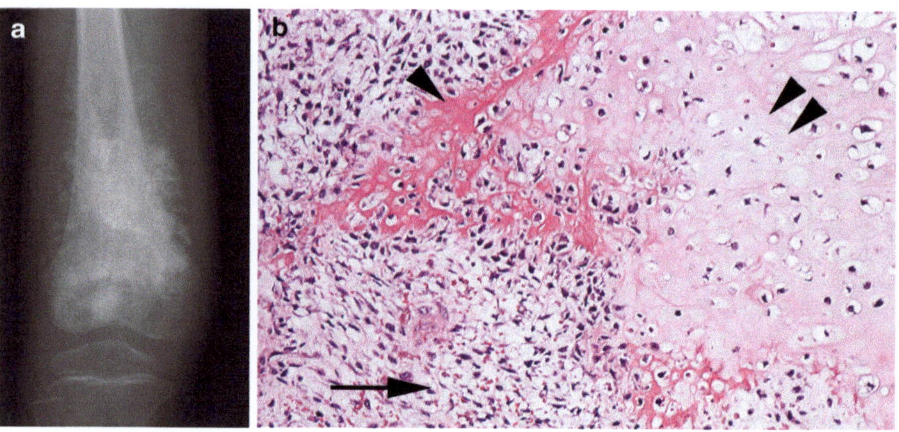

Fig. 5.1 Radiographic and histologic hallmarks of osteosarcoma. (**a**) Osteosarcoma classically presents in the distal femur of a skeletally immature patient or young adult. Fluffy ossification is present in the soft tissues, while the bone shows mixed sclerotic and lytic areas. (**b**) Histologically, areas of osteoblastic (*single arrowhead*), chondroblastic (*double arrowhead*), and fibroblastic (*single arrow*) differentiation may be visible in the same tumor to varying degrees. The presence of osteoid formation by malignant spindle cells is the essential diagnostic criterion for osteosarcoma. Image © 2013, A. Kevin Raymond, used with permission.

bone, a magnetic resonance imaging (MRI) scan of the entire affected bone, a chest X-ray, a chest computed tomography (CT) scan, a whole-body technetium bone scan, and a percutaneous image-guided biopsy.

Laboratory tests should include a complete blood count; measurement of serum electrolytes, blood urea nitrogen, creatinine, calcium, phosphate, and magnesium; and liver function tests. High levels of the enzymes alkaline phosphatase and lactic dehydrogenase, which offer a rough measure of overall tumor burden, have been correlated with worse prognosis by some authors (Meyers et al. 1992).

An X-ray of the affected bone is an important test since it provides diagnostic information and offers a measure by which response to treatment can be judged qualitatively. For diagnostic purposes, the entire bone must be included to evaluate for skip metastases, which are discontinuous tumors in the primary bone site. The presence of fluffy, cloudlike ossification in the soft tissues combined with a permeative, destructive lesion of bone is the classic presentation of osteosarcoma (Fig. 5.1). The amount of ossification can be quite variable, and initially there may not be much ossification, particularly with telangiectatic osteosarcomas, which are almost purely osteolytic lesions. With a positive response to treatment, the extraosseous tumor ossifies and becomes more radiodense. Development of a very clear, mature edge of ossification delineating the border of the tumor portends an excellent response to systemic therapy.

Cross-sectional and multiplanar imaging is obtained with MRI, which provides detailed anatomic information about the extent of disease in the extraosseous soft tissues and the bone marrow. Again, the entire bone should be included. A chest

Table 5.2 Musculoskeletal Tumor Society staging system

Stage	Grade	Tumor	Metastasis
IA	G1	T1	M0
IB	G1	T2	M0
IIA	G2	T1	M0
IIB	G2	T2	M0
III	Any	Any	M1

Abbreviations: G1, any low-grade tumor; G2, any high-grade tumor; T1, intracompartmental tumor location (confined to bone); T2, extracompartmental tumor location; M0, no metastases; M1, any metastases (regional or distant metastasis, including lymph nodes). Adapted with permission from Enneking WF, Spanier SS, Goodman MA. A system for the surgical staging of musculoskeletal sarcoma. *Clin Orthop Relat Res* 1980;(153):106–120.

X-ray and chest CT scan are important to screen for pulmonary metastases. A whole-body technetium Tc 99m bone scan is obtained to evaluate possible skeletal metastasis. Occasionally, a bone scan shows activity in pulmonary lesions, which may help to determine whether the lesions represent metastatic disease.

Beyond these standard studies, another imaging study, ^{18}F-labeled fluorodeoxyglucose (^{18}F-FDG) positron emission tomography (PET) with CT, is often performed at presentation. Although it is still not widely accepted as the standard of care, the test is attractive to clinicians because of its potential use for screening for occult metastases and, more importantly, for monitoring response to treatment. Improvements in the specificity and sensitivity of the scan may enable the test to be used as a surrogate measure of chemotherapy response before resection of the tumor. Such use may have important therapeutic implications for both medical oncologists and orthopedic surgeons.

Like the PET/CT scan, an arteriogram of the tumor is not a standard test, but it is vital to intra-arterial therapy. The arteriogram offers an excellent means of monitoring the effectiveness of treatment. A marked decrease in the hypervascular blush associated with radiocontrast dye uptake indicates a positive response to chemotherapy.

The diagnosis of osteosarcoma still must be verified by histopathologic examination of biopsy tissue. At MD Anderson Cancer Center, needle biopsy has traditionally been favored over open biopsy. Biopsy techniques are discussed in detail in Chap. 3, "Percutaneous Image-Guided Biopsy for Diagnosis of Bone Sarcomas." In the rare instance in which diagnostic tissue is not obtained by needle biopsy, a small open biopsy should be performed by an experienced orthopedic oncologist. Placement of the biopsy incision in line with the future incision for tumor resection is important since the biopsy track must be subsequently resected.

The Musculoskeletal Tumor Society (MSTS) staging system (Table 5.2) has traditionally been used for staging purposes. Using this system, nonmetastatic conventional osteosarcoma is typically staged as IIB. Stage IIA applies in the rare instance in which the tumor is purely intramedullary without extraosseous growth.

Table 5.3 American Joint Committee on Cancer staging system for bone tumors

Stage	Tumor	Nodes	Metastasis	Grade
IA	T1	N0	M0	G1, 2 low grade, GX
IB	T2	N0	M0	G1, 2 low grade, GX
	T3	N0	M0	G1, 2 low grade, GX
IIA	T1	N0	M0	G3, 4 high grade
IIB	T2	N0	M0	G3, 4 high grade
III	T3	N0	M0	G3, 4
IVA	Any T	N0	M1a	Any G
IVB	Any T	N1	Any M	Any G
	Any T	Any N	M1b	Any G

Definitions: T1, tumor 8 cm or less in greatest dimension; T2, tumor more than 8 cm in greatest dimension; T3, discontinuous tumors in the primary bone site; N0, no regional lymph node metastasis; N1, regional lymph node metastasis; M0, no distant metastasis; M1a, lung; M1b, other distant sites; G1, well differentiated—low-grade; G2, moderately differentiated—low-grade; G3, poorly differentiated; G4, undifferentiated; GX, grade cannot be assessed. Reprinted with permission of the American Joint Committee on Cancer (AJCC), Chicago, Illinois. The original source for this material is the *AJCC Cancer Staging Manual,* 7th edition (2010), published by Springer Science and Business Media LLC, www.springer.com.

Stage III applies if metastasis is present, regardless of where it occurs. Most commonly, metastasis occurs in the lungs through hematogenous spread. The second most common site is the skeleton. Lymph node involvement is rare and generally occurs late in the course of disease.

The MSTS-based system is still widely used and is currently favored at MD Anderson. However, one of the criticisms of this staging system is that it does not stratify patients with conventional osteosarcoma except on the basis of metastasis. Conventional osteosarcoma, by definition, is a high-grade tumor and therefore is considered a minimum of stage II, not stage I. The distinction between intra- and extraosseous tumor (stage IIA vs IIB) does not separate patients in a manner that carries much prognostic significance.

The more recent version (seventh edition) of the American Joint Committee on Cancer (AJCC) staging system (Edge et al. 2010) incorporates into the system the size of the tumor and the presence of skip metastases (Table 5.3). Once again, stage I disease represents low-grade tumor, while stage II disease is characterized by high-grade tumor. The designations A and B are determined by tumor size, with 8 cm being the cutoff point. Stage III represents cases with skip metastases, and the new stage IV is characterized by metastatic disease. At the time of this writing, this staging system has not yet gained widespread acceptance or usage. The 8-cm cutoff is not universally accepted as the most appropriate way of distinguishing large versus small tumors. It is unknown whether the staging system will be modified further in future editions or retained in its present form as the standard. Given the ongoing advances in the understanding of the basic biology of the disease, it is likely that the staging of the future will incorporate more molecular-based parameters.

Conventional Osteosarcoma

Clinical Features

Conventional osteosarcoma is primarily a disease of young people; the peak age of incidence is in the second to third decade. This disease is rare in the elderly and, curiously, the very young. It has a slight predominance in males. The most common site of occurrence is around the knee: foremost the distal femoral metaphysis, followed by the proximal tibial metaphysis. Together, these sites account for nearly half of all cases. The proximal femoral and proximal humeral metaphyses are the next most common sites. Occurrence in the pelvis and spine is rarer, which is fortunate because in these areas the surgical difficulties are greater and the rates of recurrence correspondingly higher.

Conventional osteosarcoma has three histologic subtypes: *fibroblastic*, *chondroblastic*, and *osteoblastic* osteosarcoma. In all three subtypes, there is production of osteoid (immature bone matrix) by malignant spindle-shaped sarcoma cells. The presence of osteoid, in essence, defines osteosarcoma. Typically, in any given tumor, all three subtypes may be found to varying degrees; a tumor's designation as a particular subtype simply refers to the predominant subtype of the tumor. Fibroblastic osteosarcoma has a greater proportion of fibroblastic spindle cells relative to the amount of osteoid. Chondroblastic osteosarcoma has a greater proportion of chondrocytes and cartilaginous matrix relative to the amount of osteoid. Osteoblastic osteosarcoma is composed chiefly of osteoblasts and dense, abundant osteoid.

Primary Treatment

Approach and Rationale

The treatment regimen for conventional osteosarcoma at MD Anderson is unique. Although similar to that of other centers in that it involves systemic chemotherapy and surgery, it is distinguished by the tailoring of postoperative chemotherapy and the use of intra-arterial preoperative chemotherapy. As we describe below, the rationale for this approach is based on both theoretical grounds and experience at MD Anderson.

Many articles have been published on different chemotherapeutic regimens for conventional osteosarcoma. Comparison across different trials is difficult, and it is hazardous to ascribe superiority to one therapeutic strategy over another. Although various protocols employ similar chemotherapeutic agents, differences in dosing and scheduling can affect the comparability of the results.

A number of principles emerge from the published experience with the disease. First, successful treatment requires both systemic chemotherapy and surgical resection of disease. The chances of cure with either alone are quite low, although not zero. Before the era of effective chemotherapy, the rate of cure for patients who underwent immediate amputation was approximately 15–20%. That low rate indicates that in most patients, microscopic metastatic disease is present at the time of presentation. As with surgery alone, the chances of long-term disease control with chemotherapy alone are poor. The experience at MD Anderson has shown that patients who were treated aggressively with chemotherapy alone and had durable remissions eventually developed relapses (Jaffe et al. 2002).

Another principle that has emerged from the published experience is that a combination of active agents is necessary to achieve optimal results. The most active agents currently include doxorubicin, cisplatin, ifosfamide, and methotrexate. Historically, methotrexate was one of the first agents identified as being effective for osteosarcoma, but as a single agent, it results in a somewhat lower rate of response compared with the other drugs. Doxorubicin and cisplatin have higher rates of response and are therefore now the frontline agents. Ifosfamide and methotrexate are the next most active agents. The combination of gemcitabine and docetaxel (Taxotere) has been shown recently to have some activity against the disease and may be considered a reasonable alternative second-line regimen. Older drugs with weaker activity include dactinomycin, bleomycin, and cyclophosphamide.

Several key questions regarding chemotherapy remain unanswered at this time. There continues to be debate over what constitutes the optimal combination of chemotherapeutic agents. Should two, three, four, or more agents be employed? Addition of more agents is not wholly beneficial because it may compromise the dose intensity of the most effective agents. There is also debate over whether the strategy of "tailoring" chemotherapy has merit. This concept involves changing the postoperative chemotherapeutic agents for patients who have not responded well to the initial agents. Finally, there is controversy over the utility of intra-arterial versus intravenous therapy.

To make some sense of the controversy over these issues, it is useful to bear in mind that there are inherent differences among tumors, and all tumors are not created equal. Some respond well to chemotherapy, and some do not. More importantly, some tumors respond well to certain agents but not others. These differences are simply a manifestation of the genetic heterogeneity of tumors.

When viewed in this context, the rationale of the MD Anderson approach to chemotherapy becomes clearer. Rather than relying on a uniform combination of agents to treat all tumors, we build flexibility into the treatment scheme. The two drugs that are given preoperatively, doxorubicin and cisplatin, are the ones that have induced greatest responsiveness in previous trials. They are ideal candidates for combination in full doses because of their nonoverlapping mechanisms of action and toxicity profiles. This combination gives patients the highest probability of achieving a response to the initial therapy. After four cycles of preoperative treatment, patients undergo surgical resection of the primary tumor. If the percentage of tumor necrosis is not outstanding (i.e., if it is less than 95%), then postoperatively patients are switched to the next two most active agents, ifosfamide and methotrexate. These drugs are given at high doses to maximize their effectiveness.

The concept of tailoring chemotherapy based on patients' therapeutic response has existed for some time. In a study by Meyers et al. (1992) from Memorial Sloan-Kettering Cancer Center, tailoring chemotherapy was attempted, but no significant improvement in survival was found. It should be noted, however, that in this and other studies, many agents were included in the preoperative regimen, and it was impossible for the clinician to know which of the agents were active or inactive. The T12 protocol at Memorial Sloan-Kettering included methotrexate, doxorubicin, cisplatin, bleomycin, cyclophosphamide, and dactinomycin before surgery.

MD Anderson's approach to tailoring chemotherapy represents a clear departure from previous attempts. Only two agents, doxorubicin and cisplatin, are given before surgery. If the tumor response is inadequate, it seems logical to switch to alternative agents rather than to persevere with inactive agents. Indeed, review of data at MD Anderson has shown that the survival rate of patients who have poor responses to the frontline regimen can be significantly improved by switching to high-dose ifosfamide and methotrexate. Between 1980 and 1992, 123 patients age 16 years and over were treated for conventional osteosarcoma of the extremities. Throughout this period, patients received doxorubicin and cisplatin as the primary agents, and these were the exclusive agents in the early years. During the latter part of the study period, between 1989 and 1992, high-dose ifosfamide and methotrexate were given to patients who had had poor responses (less than 90% tumor necrosis) after the frontline regimen. The 5-year continuous disease-free survival rate was 67% for these patients, a significant improvement over the 24% rate for poor-responding patients who did not receive ifosfamide and methotrexate after surgery ($P=0.015$, Benjamin et al. 1995). Of note, patients who received methotrexate alone did not fare as well as did patients who received both ifosfamide and methotrexate. Nevertheless, even with the use of postoperative tailoring with ifosfamide and methotrexate, the survival rates were significantly worse than those for patients who had had a good response (at least 90% necrosis) after preoperative therapy; at 10 years, the latter group's continuous disease-free survival and overall survival rates were 74% and 76%, respectively.

It is likely that the tailoring of chemotherapy is still in its infancy. At present, our ability to characterize tumors on a molecular level is still at a primitive state. There may one day be a means to determine at the time of diagnosis whether a patient's tumor carries the biological targets for specific agents. As our ability to characterize tumors in molecular terms improves, it is conceivable that the choice of postoperative chemotherapy will be guided by biological targets within the resistant clones of tumor cells.

One of the benefits of tailoring chemotherapy is that patients are not uniformly subjected to the harsh toxic effects of chemotherapy. All of the agents mentioned above can have serious long-term deleterious effects. Maximizing dose intensity of chemotherapy for all patients indiscriminately subjects many patients to complications that seriously detract from their overall quality of life and functional outcomes. Identification of patients who need only a moderate course of postoperative chemotherapy should be an important aspect of future efforts to improve treatment.

Apart from tailoring chemotherapy, the other unique aspect of the chemotherapy approach at MD Anderson is the intra-arterial administration of cisplatin, when feasible, before surgery. The conceptual basis for this strategy is that it delivers a higher dose of chemotherapy to the primary site compared with other means of administration. Data from the Rizzoli Institute have shown that the percentage of patients who have a good response to initial chemotherapy is higher for patients who receive intra-arterial, as opposed to intravenous, cisplatin (Bacci et al. 1992). Furthermore, data at MD Anderson clearly indicate that the rate of local recurrence is directly related to patients' responses to chemotherapy. Patients who have excellent responses to induction chemotherapy have significantly lower rates of local recurrence. By enhancing the chemotherapeutic effect at the primary site, quick palliation of symptoms is achieved. Furthermore, limb-salvage surgery is facilitated, and a greater percentage of patients have successful preservation of the extremity.

Chemotherapy Schedule

Our standard treatment protocol is shown in Fig. 5.2. To summarize, patients receive four cycles of intravenous doxorubicin (90 mg/m^2) and intra-arterial cisplatin (120 mg/m^2) before surgery. The percentage of tumor necrosis is determined by careful pathologic mapping of the resection specimen. Our current practice is to separate optimal from suboptimal necrosis based on a cutoff of 95%, instead of the 90% cutoff used in MD Anderson's published data (described above). This practice is based on a separate analysis of our data set evaluating the effect of necrosis in increments of 5% instead of 10%, which suggested that the continuous disease-free survival rate of patients with 85–90% tumor necrosis was superior to that of patients with 91–95% necrosis. One possible explanation for this finding could be that the group of patients with 85–90% necrosis was switched to ifosfamide and methotrexate, while the 91–95% group did not receive this intensified postoperative therapy. So, currently, patients who have excellent responses (at least 95% tumor necrosis) receive an abbreviated postoperative regimen: four cycles of doxorubicin (75 mg/m^2) and ifosfamide (10 g/m^2). Although cisplatin has also been used instead of ifosfamide for good responders, the preference at MD Anderson is for ifosfamide in the postoperative setting. Patients who have less-than-excellent responses (less than 95% tumor necrosis) are switched to a regimen of ifosfamide (14 g/m^2) and methotrexate (10–12 g/m^2). Depending on tolerance, patients are given up to six cycles of high-dose ifosfamide at 3- to 4-week intervals and six cycles of high-dose methotrexate at 2-week intervals, alternating the drugs every three cycles.

Several points regarding the delivery of drugs are worth noting. The cardiotoxicity of doxorubicin is lessened by administering it using a continuous infusion, which is given over 72–96 h. Intra-arterial cisplatin (120 mg/m^2) may be given concurrently with doxorubicin intravenously via central venous access. Pretreatment hydration with 5% dextrose (D5) half-normal saline and posttreatment hydration with intravenous mannitol solution are important to decrease the nephrotoxic effects of cisplatin.

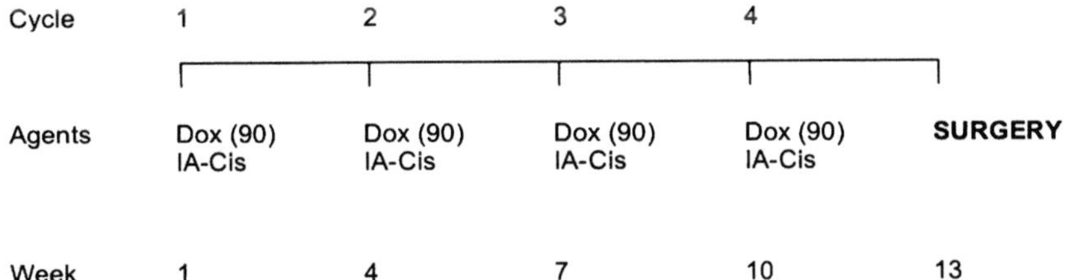

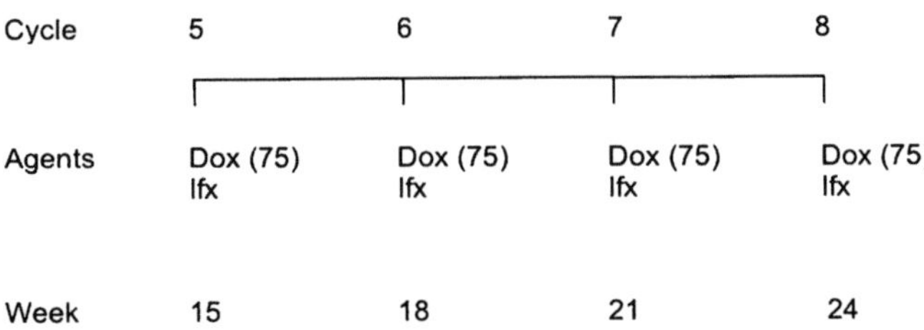

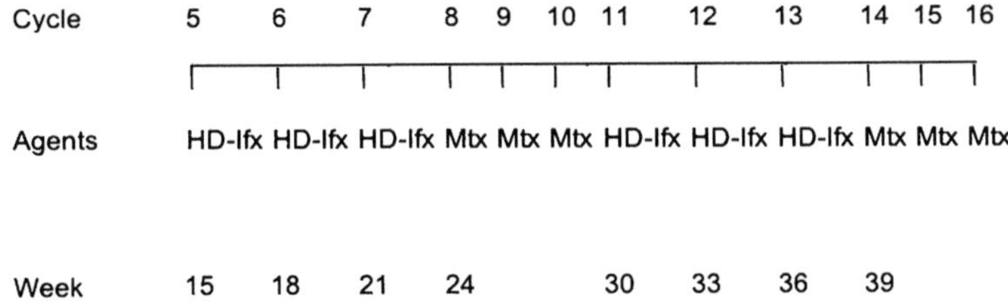

Fig. 5.2 A schematic diagram of the schedule for standard chemotherapy for conventional osteosarcoma at MD Anderson. All patients receive the same preoperative chemotherapy. Postoperative chemotherapy is based on the response to preoperative chemotherapy, as determined by the percentage of tumor necrosis in the resected specimen. Historically, patients were considered "good responders" if at least 90% necrosis was observed. Currently, the preferred cutoff for "excellent responders" at MD Anderson is 95% necrosis. Patients achieving this tumor response are treated with a shorter course of postoperative chemotherapy. Conversely, patients who do not have an excellent response are treated postoperatively with ifosfamide and methotrexate (six cycles each, depending on tolerance). *Dox* doxorubicin (90 or 75 mg/m^2), *IA-Cis* intra-arterial cisplatin, *Ifx* ifosfamide, *HD-Ifx* high-dose ifosfamide, *Mtx* methotrexate.

Surgery

Definitive management of osteosarcoma requires surgical resection of the primary site of disease with wide, negative margins. In the past, various authors recommended a bone margin of 3–7 cm, but most of these recommendations were made before the advent of MRI scans. Smaller margins are acceptable now that MRI enables visualization of the tumor border. Whenever feasible, a 1- to 3-cm margin is advisable, particularly for diaphyseal osteotomies, in which the removal of an extra centimeter of bone usually carries no functional consequence. However, for epiphyseal-sparing resections and other difficult situations, a 1-cm (or less) margin may be acceptable if the preoperative MRI shows clear delineation of the tumor border. Careful intraoperative inspection of a close margin with the pathologist is important to minimize the chance of recurrence at that location.

An adequate soft tissue margin is more difficult to define. Data from the surgical experience at MD Anderson indicate that the risk of local recurrence largely depends on the response to chemotherapy. Patients with 99–100% tumor necrosis have a 1% local recurrence rate. This finding has relevance for the debate regarding surgical margins. Assignment of an arbitrary numeric distance as being an "adequate" margin for all cases is simplistic and not especially helpful. The current challenge is to determine before surgery how well patients have responded to chemotherapy. This information can modulate how much of a margin the surgeon feels is necessary in different areas.

At present, there are no tests that will predict with high correlation the percentage of tumor necrosis. Careful assessment with all imaging modalities is important to determine how effective the preoperative chemotherapy has been. Of note, the Response Evaluation Criteria in Solid Tumors (RECIST) rules are not applicable to osteosarcoma and should not be used. Reduction in tumor size, which can be appreciated on X-rays, CT scans, and MRI scans, is definitely a favorable sign, but it occurs variably because the tumor mass may ossify without shrinkage. In addition to tumor size, the vascularity of the tumor is also an indicator of response. Serial arteriograms are important to monitor in this regard. Disappearance of all hypervascular areas is considered a good prognostic sign.

Ossification with sharp delineation of the borders of the tumor is a positive finding. This development usually can be viewed on plain X-rays. CT scans can be helpful in equivocal cases, particularly if the tumor is adjacent to critical neurovascular and soft tissue structures. A smooth, contiguous zone of calcification at the periphery of the tumor is indicative of a good response to chemotherapy. Tissue outside this zone of calcification is not likely to be involved with tumor and can be safely preserved. This assessment is often most critical in determining whether it is safe to preserve nerves and blood vessels in the popliteal fossa for distal femoral and proximal tibial lesions. In areas in which the tumor does not appear to have calcified, it may be necessary to dissect more widely around the tumor and obtain wider margins.

In most cases of conventional osteosarcoma, limb-sparing surgery can be performed. If preoperative MRI and CT scans do not show neurovascular or massive soft tissue involvement, the tumor can be safely resected and the limb reconstructed.

At the time of resection, to ensure the bone margins are negative, the marrow margin is evaluated by frozen section and the tumor is grossly sectioned by the pathologist.

At the common distal femoral and proximal tibial locations, an intra-articular resection can usually be performed. However, first the preoperative MRI scan must be closely studied to ensure the tumor does not extend into the knee joint along the cruciate or collateral ligaments. At MD Anderson, we prefer to reconstruct the distal femur with an endoprosthesis and the proximal tibia with an allograft-prosthesis composite, as discussed in Chap. 9, "Skeletal Reconstruction After Bone Sarcoma Resection." In the proximal humerus, there is an increased possibility of extension into the glenohumeral joint, in which case an extra-articular resection outside the joint capsule must be performed. Also, the deltoid can be directly invaded by the tumor, necessitating resection of that muscle. However, a review of our surgical experience has shown that in most cases, an intra-articular, deltoid-sparing surgery can be performed. If the rotator cuff can be preserved, an allograft-prosthesis composite can provide excellent function. If the cuff cannot be preserved, but the deltoid and axillary nerve remain intact, then a reverse-shoulder prosthesis provides good function.

In a few cases, extensive involvement of the adjacent neurovascular structures or soft tissues precludes obtaining negative margins and mandates an amputation. For osteosarcomas of the distal femur and proximal tibia, an above-knee amputation is performed. An amputation, though traditionally thought to be more difficult for the patient to accept psychologically, does enable quicker mobilization and eliminates the potential prosthesis- and allograft-related complications seen with limb-sparing surgery. The functional level obtained with modern prostheses can be quite high.

Follow-Up

The prognosis for patients with nonmetastatic conventional osteosarcoma is reasonably good. The overall survival rate at 5 years is roughly 65–75% (Fig. 5.3; Meyers et al. 1992; Bacci et al. 1998; Meyers et al. 1998; Le Deley et al. 2007; Meyers et al. 2008; Bielack et al. 2009). As described above, the most important factor that affects survival rate is the response to chemotherapy. Other prognostic variables that affect survival duration include the size of the tumor, the location of the tumor, the age of the patient, and inherited genetic mutations.

Long-term follow-up on a strict schedule is vital to the success of treatment. The general timing for follow-up of high-grade sarcomas is described in Chap. 14, "Follow-up Evaluation and Surveillance After Treatment of Bone Sarcomas"; modified National Comprehensive Cancer Network (NCCN) guidelines are employed. Patients are seen every 3 months during the first 2 years and then gradually less often thereafter. Between years 5 and 10, patients are seen on an annual basis. Our experience suggests that after 10 years the risk of recurrence or secondary malignancy is extremely low, but follow-up may still be worthwhile for other reasons, including evaluation of orthopedic implants, cardiac function, and hearing.

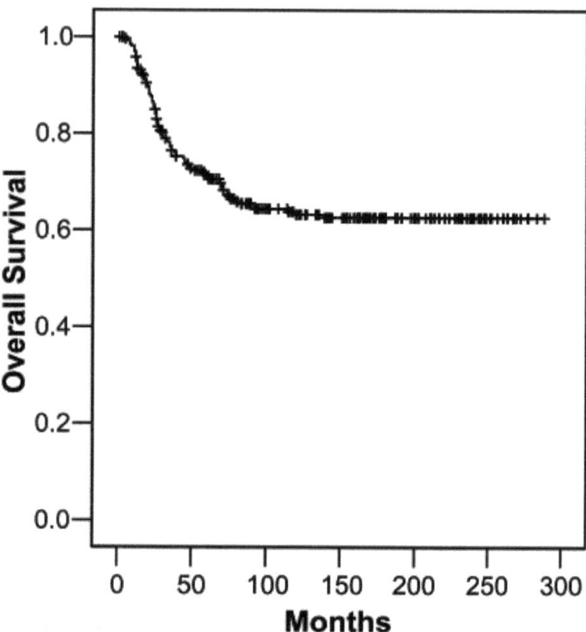

Fig. 5.3 The duration of overall survival for 314 patients with conventional high-grade osteosarcoma who presented with nonmetastatic disease between 1980 and 2005 at MD Anderson.

A few points relevant to osteosarcoma in particular are worth emphasizing here. The reason that patients are evaluated for a minimum of 10 years is that the use of effective chemotherapy has changed the natural history of the disease. Recurrences, which used to occur well within 5 years, are delayed by chemotherapy. Furthermore, treatment-related complications may arise after 5 years. Specific chemotherapy-related complications are important to address. Doxorubicin-induced cardiomyopathy can arise as a function of the cumulative dose and duration of infusion of the drug. Affected patients should undergo echocardiograms and stress tests as clinically indicated. Nephrotoxicity can result from treatment with ifosfamide and cisplatin. The renal effects of ifosfamide may not become evident until well after cessation of treatment, and they are sometimes potentiated by nonsteroidal anti-inflammatory drugs and other nephrotoxic medications. Ototoxicity and sensory neuropathy are prominent side effects of cisplatin. They are consistently present, though to variable degrees, in patients who receive a cumulative dose greater than 300 mg/m². High-dose ifosfamide can exacerbate these effects. As clinically indicated, patients should undergo otologic examinations to assess hearing impairment and the need for hearing-assistive devices.

Surgical complications usually vary according to the type of reconstruction employed. After surgery, all patients with some form of endoprosthesis will need lifelong monitoring for late complications, such as aseptic loosening and hardware failure. Patients with allografts, particularly osteoarticular allografts, may eventually need joint replacement for subsequent arthritis. After amputations, patients also need regular follow-up with a prosthetist for maintenance of their prostheses.

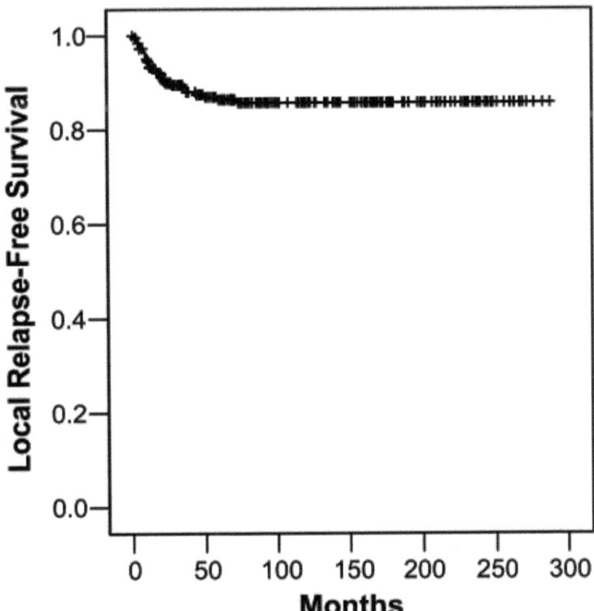

Fig. 5.4 The duration of local relapse-free survival for the same group of 314 patients with conventional high-grade osteosarcoma.

Relapse and Spread of Disease

Local Recurrence

Local recurrence is a significant problem and occurs in approximately 10% of patients (Fig. 5.4; Grimer et al. 2005a; b). To maximize the likelihood of long-term survival, locally recurrent tumors need to be completely resected. If the tumor's size and location are favorable to allowing a wide local excision with negative margins, a limb-sparing surgery should be performed. However, this scenario tends to be more the exception than the rule. Recurrent disease tends to be large and diffuse. The soft tissue involvement can be extensive and difficult to delineate on MRI or other scans. In recurrences in the distal femur and proximal tibia, the popliteal neurovascular structures are often involved. Similarly, proximal humerus recurrences can involve the brachial plexus and artery. Chemotherapeutic options may be limited, thereby decreasing the potential beneficial effect of chemotherapy on the ability to achieve local disease control. Thus, in most cases, local recurrences cannot be treated adequately by a wide excision and warrant an amputation. In two recent series, more than 50% of local recurrences that were managed surgically required an amputation (Grimer et al. 2005a; b; Nathan et al. 2006).

A local recurrence often occurs together with distant metastasis. In such cases, the extent of disease seems to reflect an inherent aggressiveness of the tumor, and the effect of chemotherapy is often noted to be poor. In these cases, the treatment of the locally recurrent tumor may need to be more palliative than curative. Although radiation may be tried, historically it has not been found to be especially effective in controlling disease. Radioactive bone-seeking agents such as samarium might also be considered, but this modality's bone marrow toxicity may limit its usefulness. Although amputation is not necessarily the ideal procedure for a patient with incurable disease, it may offer better control of disease and relief of pain than can be obtained with other measures.

Metastasis

Patients who present with overtly metastatic disease have a significantly worse prognosis, with 5-year survival rates of 30–50% (Bielack et al. 2009; Chou et al. 2009). The definition of metastasis at presentation, however, may need to be reexamined in the future because it is known that most patients have microscopic metastatic disease at the time of presentation. The improvements over the years in CT scanning of the lungs have yielded increasingly higher image resolutions, with the result that tiny pulmonary nodules previously invisible on plain chest X-rays are now noticeable on CT scans. It has yet to be determined how these findings will affect staging and treatment.

There are important therapeutic implications for patients who present with metastases initially in comparison with patients who have metastatic relapses of disease. Patients who present with metastases are chemotherapy naïve and therefore have all treatment options available. The initial preoperative treatment approach for these patients is the same as that for patients with nonmetastatic disease. Surgical resection of the primary tumor and the pulmonary (or other) metastases may be performed if all of the gross disease is considered resectable. Aggressive postoperative chemotherapy is employed until maximal tolerance is reached.

Patients who present with multiple osseous metastases or such extensive pulmonary disease that surgical eradication is not feasible are likely to be incurable. For such patients, enrollment in experimental protocols may be considered. In most cases, however, treatment is directed at palliation and improving quality of life.

Patients who have relapses with metachronous metastases after having been rendered disease-free for a period of time are more difficult to treat than are patients who present with metastasis at initial diagnosis. The disease-free interval and the number of metastases both affect the duration of survival. Approximately 15–20% of patients with metastatic relapses achieve long-term survival beyond 5 years (Harting et al. 2006). Chemotherapeutic options may be limited, particularly for patients who had poor responses previously and received higher cumulative doses of drugs. Nevertheless, retreatment with the standard agents doxorubicin, cisplatin, ifosfamide, and methotrexate can be considered. The combination of gemcitabine and docetaxel can also be given to patients who cannot tolerate further chemotherapy with prior agents. Alternatives include participation in experimental trials of new agents.

Patients who have relapses in the form of a single pulmonary nodule have a relatively favorable prognosis and are sometimes curable by thoracotomy alone. In such patients, it may be worth performing surgery first and giving additional chemotherapy in an adjuvant setting. In most instances, however, there are multiple metastases, and it is more logical to treat with systemic agents before considering surgical resection. In nearly all cases, cure is not possible without surgical excision of the recurrent disease.

Rare Variants of High-Grade Osteosarcoma

Rare histologic variants of high-grade osteosarcoma are *telangiectatic, small cell (round cell), epithelioid,* and *giant cell–rich osteosarcoma.* Like conventional osteosarcoma, these tumors arise from the interior of the bone in the intramedullary cavity, as opposed to the surface of the bone, which characterizes other subtypes such as parosteal osteosarcoma (see below).

Radiographically, these variants produce lytic lesions in bone without the abundant fluffy ossification that is commonly associated with conventional osteosarcoma. As a result, many cases are misdiagnosed as other tumors, such as benign giant cell tumor of bone. The reason for the lack of ossification may be that the tumors tend to produce only a scant amount of osteoid, thus leading to faint calcification on X-rays. Histologically, the tumors are distinguished by features suggested by their names. Telangiectatic osteosarcoma is notable for large vascular-like spaces; small cell osteosarcoma is composed of sheets of small, round, blue cells; epithelioid osteosarcoma is characterized by epithelioid cells; and giant cell–rich osteosarcoma is marked by multinucleated giant cells.

Telangiectatic osteosarcoma, the more common of the rare variants, responds well to the standard chemotherapeutic agents used for conventional osteosarcoma. The other variants do not respond reliably well. Small cell osteosarcoma in particular tends not to respond to standard osteosarcoma protocols, so a different therapeutic approach to this variant may be warranted. Agents that are effective against Ewing sarcoma, rhabdomyosarcoma, and other primitive sarcomas may be worth considering for the small cell variant.

Osteosarcoma of the Craniofacial Bones

Osteosarcoma of the craniofacial bones resembles conventional osteosarcoma histologically but not in its clinical behavior. The reason for this puzzling difference in biological behavior is unknown, but it is believed to relate in part to the fact that the craniofacial bones are formed by membranous ossification, whereas the long bones are formed by enchondral ossification. Of the different craniofacial bones, the mandible is affected most often, followed closely by the maxilla. Compared with conventional osteosarcoma, craniofacial osteosarcomas occur in an older population, with a peak in the third to fourth decade. The craniofacial tumors are more indolent and much less likely to metastasize (Clark et al. 1983). The primary treatment is wide surgical excision, and the strongest predictor for survival is the adequacy of the surgical margins. Craniofacial osteosarcomas tend not to respond to chemotherapy as well as conventional osteosarcomas of the limbs do, but there is a growing recognition that chemotherapy might improve survival for some patients (Smeele et al. 1997). At MD Anderson, if margin-negative surgical resection is not technically feasible, we employ systemic chemotherapy similar to that used for conventional osteosarcoma.

Well-Differentiated Intramedullary and Parosteal Osteosarcoma

There are two types of well-differentiated osteosarcoma (sometimes referred to as low-grade osteosarcoma). *Well-differentiated intramedullary osteosarcoma*, as the name suggests, occurs within the cortical confines of bone. In contrast, *parosteal osteosarcoma* develops on the surface of bone, often with just a small area of contact between the cortical bone and the extraosseous mass; in approximately 25% of cases, there is some penetration of the tumor into the medullary cavity (Okada et al. 1994). Most cases of parosteal osteosarcoma occur in the posterior aspect of the distal femur. While both of these forms of osteosarcoma are rare, parosteal osteosarcoma is seen more frequently than is well-differentiated intramedullary osteosarcoma.

The diagnosis of these tumors may not be straightforward or simple. Both tumor types can present radiographically as densely ossified masses, but areas of fibrous tissue and poor ossification can be present in either lesion (Bertoni et al. 1985). Another difficulty is distinguishing these tumors from other ossified lesions, both radiographically and histologically. The differential diagnosis includes trauma, reactive periosteal bone formation, osteomyelitis, and other tumors, such as osteoid osteoma, which can produce florid cortical bone formation. Parosteal osteosarcoma must be distinguished from heterotopic ossification (also known as myositis ossificans), which arises acutely from direct trauma to muscle.

At MD Anderson, the workup of a suspected case of well-differentiated osteosarcoma is similar to that for conventional osteosarcoma, with one notable exception: an arteriogram is often obtained to assist with the choice of biopsy site. If a region of hypervascularity is encountered, particularly if associated with a less radiodense region, it is given preference as the biopsy site; it may represent an area of dedifferentiation. One of the pitfalls in diagnosing parosteal osteosarcoma is missing such an area of dedifferentiation, which can have grave consequences for the patient because the prognoses and treatments of parosteal osteosarcoma and dedifferentiated parosteal osteosarcoma, which is discussed below, are vastly different.

Well-differentiated osteosarcomas are typically treated with surgery alone. Even though they are low in grade, they still should be completely excised with wide, negative margins. Because parosteal osteosarcomas commonly occur on the surfaces of bones without frank intraosseous invasion, they are amenable to treatment with a hemicortical resection and reconstruction with a hemicortical allograft. In this procedure, the posterior femur is exposed through either a posterior incision or dual medial and lateral incisions. The posterior portion of the distal femur is resected through normal tissue. Reconstruction is then performed using a similarly sized allograft. The advantage of a hemicortical allograft over a circumferential allograft is that with the former, healing is much more prompt and reliable. Normal knee function is typically restored.

A hemicortical allograft may not be appropriate if the parosteal osteosarcoma partially extends into the intramedullary space. If doubt exists as to whether a hemicortical resection can be performed with safe margins, it is preferable to err on the side of resecting the entire circumference of the bone rather than to risk subsequent recurrence. Similarly, well-differentiated intramedullary osteosarcoma is usually not amenable to treatment with a hemicortical resection. In these cases, a conventional resection of a segment of bone is required, and reconstruction with an endoprosthesis or allograft is performed.

The prognosis is excellent for well-differentiated osteosarcomas, and the overall survival rate at 5 years is approximately 95% (Okada et al. 1994). Poor outcomes are generally associated with local recurrence of disease, thus underscoring the importance of wide surgical margins around the primary tumor. When tumors recur, they often become high-grade osteosarcomas. This change in status suggests that either transformation of the low-grade tumor has occurred or that a small, dedifferentiated component of the original tumor was not appreciated.

Periosteal Osteosarcoma

Periosteal osteosarcoma is similar to parosteal osteosarcoma in that the tumor arises on the surface of a long bone, in contrast with conventional osteosarcoma, which arises from the intramedullary cavity of the bone. Despite the similarity in names, periosteal osteosarcoma is distinguished from parosteal osteosarcoma by several features. Periosteal osteosarcoma occurs primarily on the diaphysis, as opposed to the metaphysis, of long bones. Periosteal osteosarcoma tends to be chondroblastic histologically and has less pronounced osteoblastic bone formation. Finally, and most importantly, periosteal osteosarcoma is histologically an intermediate-grade tumor and exhibits a greater degree of atypia and pleomorphism than is seen in parosteal osteosarcoma.

Although it is not disputed that a wide surgical resection is essential to the treatment of periosteal osteosarcoma, the role of chemotherapy is somewhat controversial. The published data are conflicting; some studies purport a benefit, whereas others do not. Some of the discrepancy may arise from diagnostic criteria for periosteal osteosarcoma, which may differ from series to series. It can be challenging to distinguish periosteal osteosarcoma from conventional chondroblastic osteosarcoma of the diaphysis and from periosteal chondrosarcoma.

In the experience of the European Musculoskeletal Oncology Society, the overall prognosis for patients with periosteal osteosarcoma was good. Most patients received doxorubicin-based chemotherapy, and a 5-year overall survival rate of 89% was reported (Grimer et al. 2005a; b). The data for the control arms of this and other retrospective studies, however, are somewhat compromised by potential selection bias. The data at MD Anderson also favor the use of chemotherapy for periosteal osteosarcoma. The same agents used for conventional osteosarcoma (doxorubicin and cisplatin) are employed preoperatively. If a response to the chemotherapy is noted, patients may continue with postoperative chemotherapy. However, if the percentage of necrosis after preoperative chemotherapy is poor (well below 90%), it may not be beneficial to continue with postoperative chemotherapy.

Dedifferentiated Parosteal Osteosarcoma

The diagnosis of dedifferentiated parosteal osteosarcoma requires the presence of a high-grade sarcoma arising from a portion of a low-grade parosteal osteosarcoma. The implication is that the tumor arose as a well-differentiated parosteal osteosarcoma, but a portion of the tumor transformed into a dedifferentiated, high-grade sarcoma. The high-grade portion may be appreciated radiographically as a more lytic, less ossified tumor with permeative, poorly defined borders. On an arteriogram, this portion of the tumor corresponds to the hypervascular region.

Although the dedifferentiated portion of the tumor may represent only a small part of the tumor, it dictates the biological behavior of the tumor. When a metastasis occurs in the lung, it usually recapitulates the morphologic character of the high-grade portion of the tumor. Thus, even if there is only a very small dedifferentiated component, strong consideration must be given to systemic chemotherapy. This approach is controversial, and patients have apparently been cured with wide excision only.

The chemotherapeutic strategy for dedifferentiated parosteal osteosarcoma is similar to that for conventional osteosarcoma, and its response rate is nearly as good. When recognized early, dedifferentiated parosteal osteosarcoma tends to have a favorable outcome. Although the numbers of patients in reported series have been small, published experience suggests that the prognosis is similar to that of conventional osteosarcoma. The long-term overall survival rate in different series has been approximately 50%. The rarity of the disease precludes definitive statements regarding the efficacy of chemotherapy.

Secondary Osteosarcoma

Secondary osteosarcoma arises in the setting of a preexisting lesion (most commonly Paget disease), radiation exposure to bone, fibrous dysplasia, or a bone infarct. Secondary osteosarcomas occur in an older age group, with a peak around the sixth decade. The prognosis is distinctly worse than that of conventional osteosarcoma; the 5-year overall survival rate is 10–20% (Frassica et al. 1991; Shaylor et al. 1999; Longhi et al. 2008). Patients generally respond poorly to chemotherapy. Furthermore, this older patient group does not tolerate chemotherapy as well as younger patients do, and dose reductions may be needed. In a relatively healthy individual with few comorbidities, treatment with standard preoperative chemotherapy, limb-salvage surgery, and postoperative chemotherapy can be tried.

Key Practice Points

- Osteosarcoma encompasses many variants, including low-, intermediate-, and high-grade tumors.
- Conventional osteosarcoma refers to a primary, high-grade sarcoma arising within bone, typically in a patient younger than 30 years.
- The workup of osteosarcoma includes a history and physical examination, laboratory studies, an X-ray of the entire affected bone, an MRI scan of the entire affected bone, a chest X-ray, a chest CT scan, a whole-body technetium bone scan, and a needle biopsy.
- The treatment of conventional osteosarcoma forms the basis for treatment of a number of other high-grade sarcomas of bone, including MFH of bone, dedifferentiated parosteal osteosarcoma, and dedifferentiated chondrosarcoma.
- The treatment of nonmetastatic conventional osteosarcoma includes preoperative induction chemotherapy, wide surgical resection of the primary tumor, quantitative histopathologic assessment of the chemotherapy response, and postoperative chemotherapy.
- The frontline active agents in standard treatment regimens are doxorubicin, cisplatin, ifosfamide, and methotrexate. Second-line agents with activity include gemcitabine and docetaxel.
- Preoperative chemotherapy for conventional osteosarcoma consists of four cycles of intravenous doxorubicin (90 mg/m^2), given as a continuous 72–96 h infusion (to decrease cardiotoxicity), and intra-arterial cisplatin (120 mg/m^2).
- Postoperative chemotherapy for conventional osteosarcoma is based upon the percentage of tumor necrosis in the resected tumor. Patients who do not have an excellent response (at least 95% necrosis) to preoperative chemotherapy are given high-dose ifosfamide (14 g/m^2 for up to six cycles) and high-dose methotrexate (10–12 g/m^2 for six cycles). Patients who have a favorable response are given a shorter course of less intensive chemotherapy, usually consisting of three cycles of doxorubicin (75 mg/m^2) and ifosfamide (10 mg/m^2).
- Resection of pulmonary metastases, whenever feasible, is performed to render the patient free of gross disease.
- Treatment of well-differentiated parosteal osteosarcoma consists of wide surgical excision only, which is associated with greater than 90% survival and excellent prognosis, whereas treatment of dedifferentiated parosteal osteosarcoma includes preoperative and postoperative chemotherapy.
- The prognosis for secondary osteosarcoma is significantly worse than that for conventional osteosarcoma, and these patients do not often have favorable responses to chemotherapy.

Suggested Readings

Bacci G, Picci P, Avella M, et al. Effect of intra-arterial versus intravenous cisplatin in addition to systemic adriamycin and high-dose methotrexate on histologic tumor response of osteosarcoma of the extremities. J Chemother. 1992;4:189–95.

Bacci G, Ferrari S, Mercuri M, et al. Neoadjuvant chemotherapy for extremity osteosarcoma–preliminary results of the Rizzoli's 4th study. Acta Oncol. 1998;37:41–8.

Benjamin RS, Chawla SP, Carrasco CH, et al. Preoperative chemotherapy for osteosarcoma with intravenous adriamycin and intra-arterial cis-platinum. Ann Oncol. 1992;3(Suppl 2):S3–6.

Benjamin RS, Patel SR, Armen T, et al. The value of ifosfamide in postoperative neoadjuvant chemotherapy of osteosarcoma [meeting abstract]. Proc Annu Meet Am Soc Clin Oncol. 1995; 14:A1690.

Bertoni F, Present D, Hudson T, Enneking WF. The meaning of radiolucencies in parosteal osteosarcoma. J Bone Joint Surg Am. 1985;67:901–10.

Bielack S, Jurgens H, Jundt G, et al. Osteosarcoma: the COSS experience. Cancer Treat Res 2009;152:289–308.

Chou AJ, Kleinerman ES, Krailo MD, et al. Addition of muramyl tripeptide to chemotherapy for patients with newly diagnosed metastatic osteosarcoma: a report from the Children's Oncology Group. Cancer. 2009;115:5339–48.

Clark JL, Unni KK, Dahlin DC, Devine KD. Osteosarcoma of the jaw. Cancer. 1983;51:2311–6.

Edge SB, Byrd DR, Compton CC, Fritz AG, Greene FL, Trotti A III (eds). AJCC cancer staging manual, 7th edn. Springer, New York: 2010.

Edmonson JH, Green SJ, Ivins JC, et al. A controlled pilot study of high-dose methotrexate as postsurgical adjuvant treatment for primary osteosarcoma. J Clin Oncol. 1984;2:152–6.

Eilber F, Giuliano A, Eckardt J, et al. Adjuvant chemotherapy for osteosarcoma: a randomized prospective trial. J Clin Oncol. 1987;5:21–6.

Enneking WF, Spanier SS, Goodman MA. A system for the surgical staging of musculoskeletal sarcoma. Clin Orthop Relat Res. 1980;153:106–20.

Fleming ID, Cooper JS, Henson DE, et al (eds). AJCC cancer staging manual, 5th edn. Lippincott-Raven, Philadelphia: 1997.

Frassica FJ, Sim FH, Frassica DA, Wold LE. Survival and management considerations in postirradiation osteosarcoma and Paget's osteosarcoma. Clin Orthop Relat Res. 1991;270:120–7.

Gorlick R, Anderson P, Andrulis I, et al. Biology of childhood osteogenic sarcoma and potential targets for therapeutic development: meeting summary. Clin Cancer Res. 2003;9:5442–53.

Grimer RJ, Bielack S, Flege S, et al. Periosteal osteosarcoma—a European review of outcome. Eur J Cancer. 2005a;41:2806–11.

Grimer RJ, Sommerville S, Warnock D, et al. Management and outcome after local recurrence of osteosarcoma. Eur J Cancer. 2005b;41:578–83.

Harting MT, Blakely ML, Jaffe N, et al. Long-term survival after aggressive resection of pulmonary metastases among children and adolescents with osteosarcoma. J Pediatr Surg. 2005b;41: 194–9.

Jaffe N, Knapp J, Chuang VP, et al. Osteosarcoma: intra-arterial treatment of the primary tumor with cis-diamminedichloroplatinum II (CDP). Angiographic, pathologic, and pharmacologic studies. Cancer. 1983;51:402–7.

Jaffe N, Raymond AK, Ayala A, et al. Effect of cumulative courses of intraarterial cis-diamminedichloroplatinum-II on the primary tumor in osteosarcoma. Cancer. 1989;63:63–7.

Jaffe N, Patel SR, Benjamin RS. Chemotherapy in osteosarcoma. Basis for application and antagonism to implementation; early controversies surrounding its implementation. Hematol Oncol Clin North Am. 1995;9:825–40.

Jaffe N, Carrasco H, Raymond K, Ayala A, Eftekhari F. Can cure in patients with osteosarcoma be achieved exclusively with chemotherapy and abrogation of surgery? Cancer. 2002;95: 2202–10.

Kleinerman ES, Jia SF, Griffin J, et al. Phase II study of liposomal muramyl tripeptide in osteosarcoma: the cytokine cascade and monocyte activation following administration. J Clin Oncol. 1992;10:1310–6.

Le Deley MC, Guinebretiere JM, Gentet JC, et al. SFOP OS94: a randomised trial comparing preoperative high-dose methotrexate plus doxorubicin to high-dose methotrexate plus etoposide and ifosfamide in osteosarcoma patients. Eur J Cancer. 2007;43:752–61.

Link MP, Goorin AM, Miser AW, et al. The effect of adjuvant chemotherapy on relapse-free survival in patients with osteosarcoma of the extremity. N Engl J Med. 1986;314:1600–6.

Longhi A, Errani C, Gonzales-Arabio D, et al. Osteosarcoma in patients older than 65 years. J Clin Oncol. 2008;26:5368–73.

Meyers PA, Heller G, Healey J, et al. Chemotherapy for nonmetastatic osteogenic sarcoma: the Memorial Sloan-Kettering experience. J Clin Oncol. 1992;10:5–15.

Meyers PA, Gorlick R, Heller G, et al. Intensification of preoperative chemotherapy for osteogenic sarcoma: results of the Memorial Sloan-Kettering (T12) protocol. J Clin Oncol. 1998;16:2452–8.

Meyers PA, Schwartz CL, Krailo MD, et al. Osteosarcoma: the addition of muramyl tripeptide to chemotherapy improves overall survival—a report from the Children's Oncology Group. J Clin Oncol. 2008;26:633–8.

Nathan SS, Gorlick R, Bukata S, et al. Treatment algorithm for locally recurrent osteosarcoma based on local disease-free interval and the presence of lung metastasis. Cancer. 2006;107:1607–16.

Okada K, Frassica FJ, Sim FH, et al. Parosteal osteosarcoma. A clinicopathological study. J Bone Joint Surg Am. 1994;76:366–78.

Patel SR. Radiation-induced sarcoma. Curr Treat Options Oncol. 2000;1:258–61.

Patel SR, Papadopolous N, Raymond AK, et al. A phase II study of cisplatin, doxorubicin, and ifosfamide with peripheral blood stem cell support in patients with skeletal osteosarcoma and variant bone tumors with a poor prognosis. Cancer. 2004;101:156–63.

Schajowicz F. Histological typing of bone tumors. World Health Organization international histological classification of tumors. Springer, Berlin: 1993.

Shaylor PJ, Peake D, Grimer RJ, et al. Paget's osteosarcoma: no cure in sight. Sarcoma. 1999;3:191–2.

Smeele LE, Kostense PJ, van der Waal I, Snow GB. Effect of chemotherapy on survival of craniofacial osteosarcoma: a systematic review of 201 patients. J Clin Oncol. 1997;15:363–7.

Chapter 6
Ewing Sarcoma

Patrick P. Lin, Cynthia E. Herzog, Ashleigh Guadagnolo,
and Shreyaskumar Patel

Contents

P.P. Lin (✉)
Department of Orthopaedic Oncology, Unit 1448, Division of Surgery,
The University of Texas MD Anderson Cancer Center, P.O. Box 301402,
Houston, TX 77230, USA
e-mail: plin@mdanderson.org

C.E. Herzog
Department of Pediatrics, Unit 87, Division of Pediatrics, The University of Texas MD
Anderson Cancer Center, 1515 Holcombe Boulevard, Houston, TX 77030, USA
e-mail: cherzog@mdanderson.org

A. Guadagnolo
Department of Radiation Oncology, Unit 97, Division of Radiation Oncology,
The University of Texas MD Anderson Cancer Center, 1515 Holcombe Boulevard,
Houston, TX 77030, USA
e-mail: aguadagn@mdanderson.org

S. Patel
Department of Sarcoma Medical Oncology, Unit 450, Division of Cancer Medicine,
The University of Texas MD Anderson Cancer Center, 1400 Holcombe Boulevard,
Houston, TX 77030, USA
e-mail: spatel@mdanderson.org

P.P. Lin and S. Patel (eds.), *Bone Sarcoma*, MD Anderson Cancer Care Series,
DOI 10.1007/978-1-4614-5194-5_6,
© The University of Texas M. D. Anderson Cancer Center 2013

Chapter Overview Ewing sarcoma is a disease characterized by small, undifferentiated cells. Although their exact histogenesis is not known, it is believed that they may derive from mesenchymal stem cells in bone marrow. The age distribution at diagnosis shows a sharp peak during the second decade, with rare cases in the elderly. Chemotherapy is an essential part of therapy. Vincristine, doxorubicin, cyclophosphamide, dactinomycin, ifosfamide, and etoposide are considered active agents. A positive response to preoperative therapy can be manifested by marked shrinkage of the extraosseous tumor or ossification of the tumor. Local therapy for the primary tumor is usually achieved by wide surgical excision. Radiation is employed without surgery for tumors in certain difficult locations, such as the spine and cranium. Surgery and radiation are occasionally used together, but the risk of complications with the combined treatment is increased. For patients who present with localized disease, the 5-year overall survival rate is approximately 60–70%. The prognosis is markedly worse for patients with metastatic disease.

Introduction

Ewing sarcoma is a distinctive disease that is unlike other sarcomas. Whereas osteosarcomas and chondrosarcomas recapitulate the histologic characteristics of bone and cartilage, Ewing sarcoma appears to be composed of primitive, undifferentiated, small, round cells that bear no resemblance to any recognizable mesodermal tissue (Fig. 6.1). In the past, it was believed that the cell of origin was a primitive neuroectodermal cell, but more recent data suggest that mesenchymal stem cells could acquire the phenotypic features of Ewing sarcoma when genetically altered in a specific fashion. This theory provides a plausible explanation of why the disease arises predominantly in bones and justifies the traditional designation of this malignancy as a sarcoma.

Ewing sarcoma is closely related to several other tumors, including primitive neuroectodermal tumor of soft tissues, peripheral neuroepithelioma, and Askin tumor. The key molecular alteration of these diseases, t(11;22)(q24;q12), is a reciprocal translocation between chromosomes 11 and 22. This translocation results in a fusion gene, *EWSR1-FLI1*, which functions as an aberrant transcription factor. *EWSR1-FLI1* is present in about 90–95% of Ewing sarcoma cases (Mackintosh et al. 2010). In the other cases, a number of variant translocations have been identified, most notably t(21;22), which results in the *EWSR1-ERG* fusion gene. *EWSR1-FLI1* and *EWSR1-ERG* are virtually identical in their DNA sequences because the C-terminal ends of *FLI1* and *ERG* have a high degree of homology.

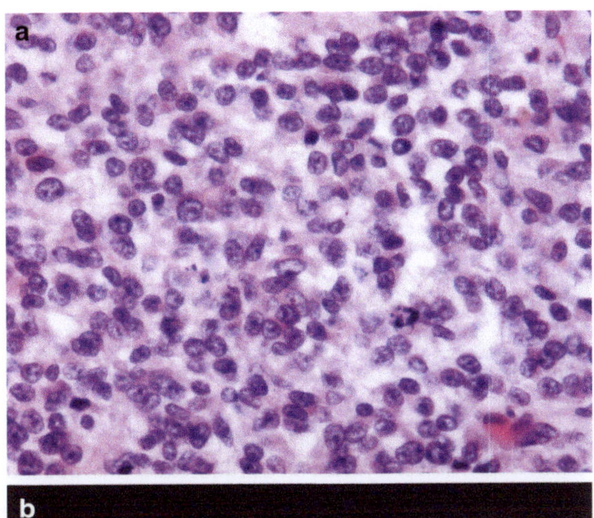

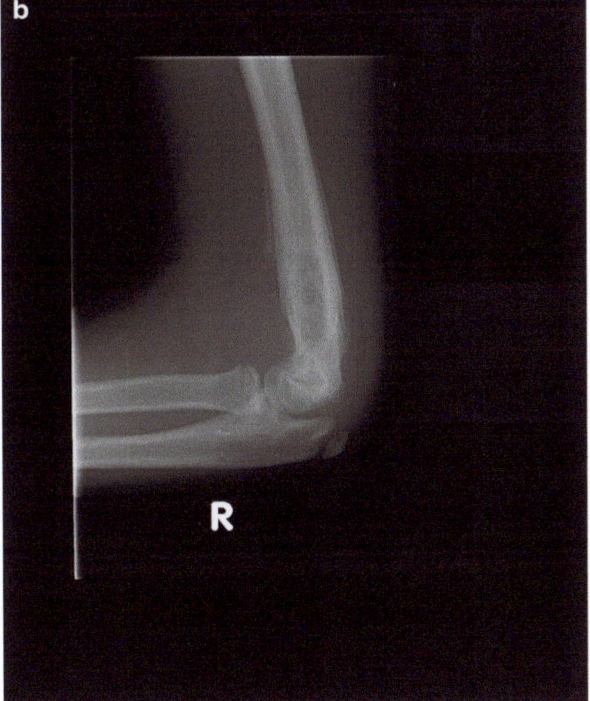

Fig. 6.1 Ewing sarcoma. (**a**) The histologic appearance of Ewing sarcoma is one of small, undifferentiated cells with large nuclei and scant cytoplasm. (**b**) Radiographically, the tumors show periosteal reaction, often in the form of an "onion skin" pattern in the long bones.

Clinical Features

Ewing sarcoma is primarily a disease of young people. Its incidence peaks in the second decade, and the disease is rare after the third decade. There is a predominance in males and whites. The tumor can occur virtually anywhere in the skeleton.

While it is well known to occur in long bones, it is also common in flat bones, such as the pelvis and scapula. A common mode of presentation is a large soft tissue mass that arises out of the pelvis or scapula in a young person. Pain and swelling are common complaints. Fever, anemia, and weight loss that simulate symptoms of infection are also frequent findings, and osteomyelitis is one of the chief diseases that must be distinguished from Ewing sarcoma in the differential diagnosis.

Diagnostic Workup and Staging

The staging of Ewing sarcoma is similar to that for other sarcomas. As for osteosarcoma (Chap. 5), the staging systems from both the Musculoskeletal Tumor Society (MSTS) and the American Joint Committee on Cancer (AJCC) may be used. The MSTS system is simpler and has been traditionally used. The newer AJCC system has not gained widespread acceptance, but it has one advantage: it takes into account tumor size, a well-recognized prognostic factor in this disease (Cotterill et al. 2000).

Neither staging system is entirely satisfactory because neither is specifically designed for Ewing sarcoma. All Ewing sarcomas are undifferentiated (grade G4), and few patients have lymph node metastasis. Furthermore, two important prognostic factors for Ewing sarcoma, axial location of tumor and bone marrow involvement, are not included in the staging systems. The most important distinction in staging is simply whether patients have metastatic disease at the time of presentation. Like osteosarcoma, Ewing sarcoma is characterized by the presence of microscopic metastatic disease in most patients at diagnosis. For the purposes of staging, metastasis refers to gross disease that is visible on imaging studies or present in bone marrow biopsy specimens.

The most common site of metastatic spread is the lung; the next most common is other bones. Thus, chest radiographs, chest computed tomography (CT) scans, and whole-body technetium bone scans are standard tests for staging purposes. Plain radiographs and magnetic resonance imaging (MRI) scans of the affected bone must include the entire length of the bone because skip metastases within the bone can be present.

Ewing sarcoma is different from other bone sarcomas in one important aspect. Whereas in other bone sarcomas bone marrow involvement virtually never occurs, in Ewing sarcoma it is a well-recognized phenomenon. Such involvement generally portends a grave prognosis. Although bone marrow aspiration has been advocated by some authors as part of the staging workup, the rate of positive findings of disease in the aspirate is low, and the utility of the test is not entirely clear. Whether noninvasive tests can detect widespread bone involvement remains to be determined. The role of metabolic scans, such as positron emission tomography scans, is not yet clearly defined, but they may help identify uncommon sites of metastases, including the bone marrow. At present, such scans are considered complementary to other diagnostic tests but do not replace those tests.

Primary Treatment

Systemic Treatment

Ewing sarcoma responds well to chemotherapy; gratifying reductions in tumor size are commonly seen (Fig. 6.2). In some cases, the soft tissue component of the tumor disappears entirely, which portends a good histologic response. In other cases, the tumor mass may ossify completely in the region of "onion skin" periosteal reaction, which also should be recognized as a favorable sign even if there is no reduction in tumor size. Failure of the tumor to disappear completely should not be viewed as a failure of induction chemotherapy, and the Response Evaluation Criteria in Solid Tumors (RECIST) are not directly applicable. Patients with good responses often have a combination of tumor shrinkage and periosteal ossification, which prevents disappearance of the extraosseous mass.

The traditional agents used for treatment include vincristine (V), doxorubicin (A), cyclophosphamide (C), and dactinomycin (Ad). In more recent years, ifosfamide

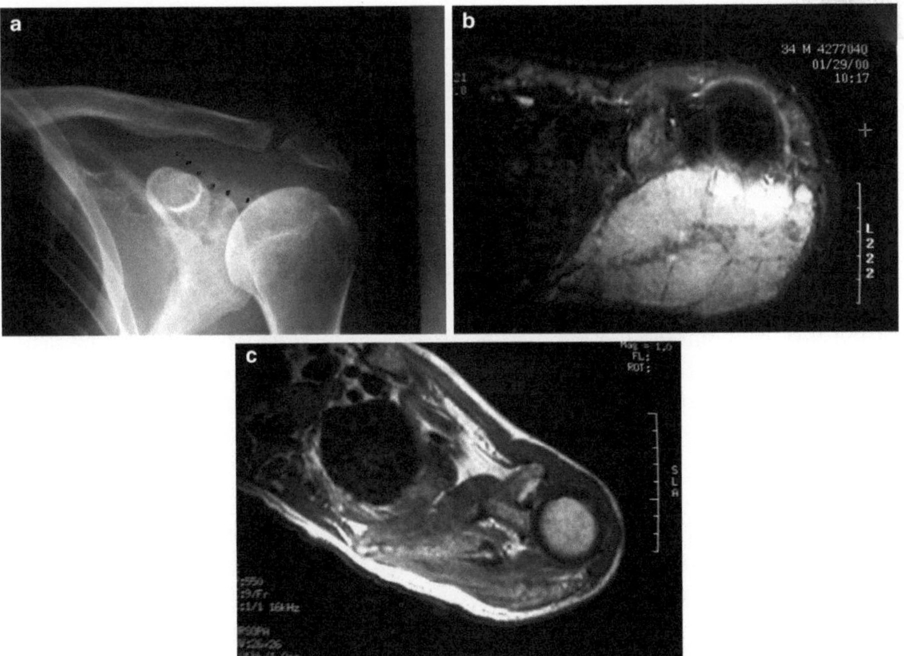

Fig. 6.2 Chemotherapy response in Ewing sarcoma. (**a**) Ewing sarcoma is often seen in the flat bones, including the pelvis and scapula. In this X-ray, a primary tumor of the acromion of the scapula presents as a small lytic lesion. (**b**) An MRI scan at the time of presentation demonstrates a massive soft tissue mass, which is typical for Ewing sarcoma of the flat bones. (**c**) After preoperative chemotherapy, the soft tissue mass has essentially disappeared.

(I) has been recognized as an active agent and incorporated into frontline treatment. Etoposide (E) is frequently combined with ifosfamide with the rationale that the action of ifosfamide as a DNA-alkylating agent could be potentiated by the topoisomerase II–inhibiting effect of etoposide. However, there are scant data substantiating whether etoposide actually increases the efficacy of ifosfamide for Ewing sarcoma. Treatment regimens that have been shown to be efficacious include VAC, VACAd, VAI, VAIAd, and VACAd + IE.

Previous Studies

The results of previous studies are important in terms of the rationale for present-day treatment at MD Anderson Cancer Center. A notable early report was from the first Intergroup Ewing Sarcoma Study (IESS-I) (Nesbit et al. 1990). In this study, a striking benefit for the inclusion of doxorubicin was demonstrated. The basic treatment consisted of vincristine, cyclophosphamide, and dactinomycin. Patients who received doxorubicin in addition to the basic treatment (i.e., VACAd) had a 5-year relapse-free survival rate of 60%, compared with a rate of only 24% for those who received the basic treatment without doxorubicin.

The follow-up study IESS-II was also an important contribution (Burgert et al. 1990). In this study, 214 patients were randomized to receive a high-dose, intermittent dosing schedule or a moderate-dose "continuous" schedule. The agents included were vincristine (1.5 mg/m^2), doxorubicin (high dose, 75 mg/m^2; moderate dose, 60 mg/m^2), cyclophosphamide (high dose, 1,400 mg/m^2; moderate dose, 500 mg/m^2), and dactinomycin (0.45 mg/m^2). (It is worth noting that even in the "high-dose" arm, the doses were still somewhat lower than the doses used today, and that the total length of time for the entire course of treatment extended over 76–78 weeks, which is considerably longer than the typical course of treatment now used at MD Anderson.) The IESS-II study was important not just for validating the effectiveness of the VACAd combination but also for demonstrating the value of dose-intensive scheduling. For patients with localized, nonpelvic disease, there was a significant improvement in survival rate with the intermittent, higher dose schedule. The overall survival rate at 5 years was 77% for the high-dose arm, compared with 63% for the moderate-dose arm. For patients with pelvic disease, the benefit of the dose-intensive schedule was even more striking. The overall survival rate at 5 years was 63% for high-dose treatment, compared with 35% for moderate-dose treatment. However, it was noted that three deaths related to cardiac events occurred in the high-dose arm, and, as expected, greater toxicity occurred with more intensive chemotherapy.

After the IESS-II study, a major advance was the demonstration that ifosfamide was an effective agent for Ewing sarcoma. In the Cooperative Ewing Sarcoma Study (CESS-86) from Europe, ifosfamide was used in the treatment of patients at high risk of relapse (Paulussen et al. 2001). This study employed vincristine, doxorubicin, ifosfamide, and dactinomycin (VAIAd) for high-risk patients, who were defined as those with a tumor volume greater than 100 mL or an axial tumor location. The standard-risk patients received vincristine, doxorubicin, cyclophosphamide, and dactinomycin (VACAd). Although the high-risk patients were expected to have a worse prognosis, the 10-year event-free survival rates were nearly identical, 52% and 51% for the high- and standard-risk groups, respectively. The authors concluded that inclusion of ifosfamide was associated with a better survival rate.

In the large Childhood Cancer Group/Pediatric Oncology Group trial in North America, the addition of ifosfamide and etoposide was found to be beneficial for patients with localized disease (Grier et al. 2003). The basic treatment consisted of VACAd: vincristine ($2\ mg/m^2$), doxorubicin ($75\ mg/m^2$), cyclophosphamide ($1.2\ g/m^2$), and dactinomycin ($1.25\ mg/m^2$), which was substituted for doxorubicin when a cumulative doxorubicin dose of $375\ mg/m^2$ was reached. Patients were randomized to receive ifosfamide ($1.8\ g/m^2$ for 5 days) and etoposide ($100\ mg/m^2$) in addition to the standard agents. A total of 17 courses of treatment over 49 weeks were planned, with surgery or radiation therapy at week 12. Patients with nonmetastatic disease who were randomized to the experimental arm with ifosfamide and etoposide (VACAd + IE) had a significantly superior 5-year event-free survival rate (69%) than that of patients who received the standard agents alone (54%). Interestingly, for patients who presented with metastatic disease, there was no beneficial effect of adding ifosfamide and etoposide.

Corroborative findings with regard to the effectiveness of ifosfamide have been reported in several other studies. In a study from the United Kingdom, treatment with vincristine, doxorubicin, and ifosfamide (VAI) over a 52-week period resulted in a 62% relapse-free survival rate at a median of 58 weeks of follow-up (Craft et al. 1998). Patients with metastatic disease at presentation had a significantly worse survival rate of 23%, which is consistent with other reports. Likewise, in the Italian Cooperative Study, treatment with intensified chemotherapy that included VACAd + IE resulted in a 78% event-free survival rate and 84% overall survival rate at 3 years, which was better than the rates for historical controls, such as those of the original IESS trials (Rosito et al. 1999).

The MD Anderson Experience

The chemotherapy protocols used at MD Anderson for Ewing sarcoma are similar to other published regimens in terms of the agents used, but our treatment approach has several unique features. Specifically, different approaches are utilized for adult and pediatric patients. In part, this difference may stem from the ability of pediatric patients to tolerate higher doses of chemotherapy. The outcome of patients treated at MD Anderson with respect to overall survival (Fig. 6.3) is similar to that of other major centers. Patients with metastatic disease fare significantly worse than patients with localized disease.

As described in Chap. 5, the treatment strategy for osteosarcoma involves choosing a postoperative chemotherapeutic regimen based on the percentage of tumor necrosis found in the surgical specimen; if response was poor, the regimen is

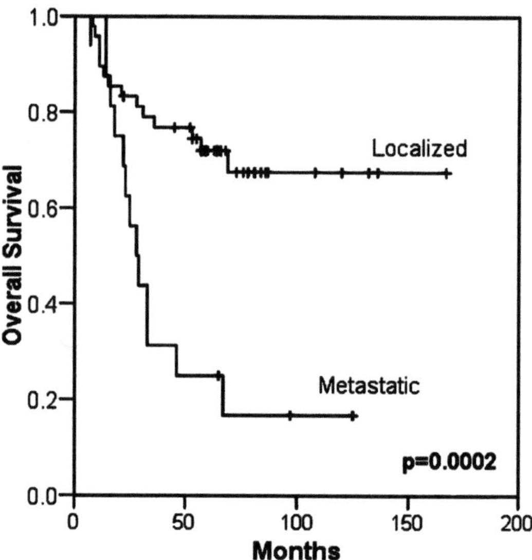

Fig. 6.3 A Kaplan–Meier analysis of overall survival for 48 patients treated at MD Anderson between 1990 and 2000. Patients who presented with nonmetastatic disease had a projected survival rate of 67% at 10 years. Patients who presented with metastasis had a projected survival rate of 17% at 10 years. Reprinted from Lin et al. (2007) with permission.

switched to a different drug combination. In contrast, tailoring of postoperative chemotherapy is not a conventional part of most treatment algorithms for Ewing sarcoma, and there are no published data proving the validity of the concept for Ewing sarcoma. At MD Anderson, some modifications are made to postoperative chemotherapy for Ewing sarcoma, such as increasing the dose of ifosfamide or adding etoposide, on the basis of the percentage of tumor necrosis (see below, "Adult Service"). However, since there are no standard drugs for "crossover" purposes in Ewing sarcoma, this would not be considered "tailoring" in a strict sense.

In certain locations, such as the pelvis, the high complication rate of surgery may have some import for the timing of chemotherapy. If a good clinical and radiographic response to chemotherapy is perceived, most, if not all, chemotherapy may be delivered prior to surgery or local treatment. In such cases, any complications of surgery, such as wound infection, would not cause a significant lapse in chemotherapy or compromise the total cumulative dose of treatment.

Adult Service

In the adult population, the VAI combination is favored at present. Patients receive vincristine (2 mg flat dose), doxorubicin (75 mg/m^2), and ifosfamide (10 mg/m^2) for up to six cycles before surgery, depending upon radiographic response and patient tolerance. Postoperative chemotherapy is continued until maximum tolerance is reached. Patients who respond well to preoperative chemotherapy with near-total necrosis (at least 99%) may continue on the same or a similar regimen for 3–6 more cycles. Patients who have suboptimal necrosis may switch to high-dose ifosfamide (14 mg/m^2) with or without etoposide (100 mg/m^2), based on tolerance. The VAI combination used at MD Anderson is similar to previously reported regimens, but several unique features merit comment. A dose-intensive scheme is employed, with doses that are relatively high compared with those of early studies. This scheme is consistent with the findings of the IESS-II study, in which higher doses and intermittent scheduling had greater effect. Administration of doxorubicin as a continuous infusion over several days significantly reduces its cardiotoxicity, and a higher cumulative dose may thus be tolerated. This method of delivery obviates the need to switch to the weaker agent dactinomycin.

Pediatric Service

In the pediatric population, patients generally are treated with VACAd-type chemotherapy in conventional doses. In addition, an experimental protocol involving an intensified, high-dose regimen (HD-VAC) with or without the immunomodulator ImmTher is currently being tested at MD Anderson. This regimen consists of six cycles of vincristine (2 mg/m^2, with a maximum dose of 2 mg), doxorubicin (90 mg/m^2) with the cardioprotective agent dexrazoxane, and cyclophosphamide (4 g/m^2). The high-dose chemotherapy regimen seems to be better tolerated in pediatric patients than in adults, who seem to have more toxic effects and complications from this protocol.

In addition to HD-VAC, patients are randomized to receive ImmTher, which is a lipophilic disaccharide tripeptide derivative of muramyl dipeptide encapsulated in liposomes. The aim is to stimulate the patient's immune system to help fight the cancer. ImmTher therapy is initiated after completion of chemotherapy and local therapy (surgery and/or radiation therapy). This agent has been shown to activate monocyte-mediated tumor cell killing in vitro and to increase plasma tumor necrosis factor and neopterin levels after intravenous infusion into patients. At the time of this writing, results were not available to determine whether the treatment improves survival.

Local Treatment

Historically, radiation was considered the treatment of choice for the primary tumor, and surgery was reserved for "expendable" bones. In fact, James Ewing himself is credited with advancing the use of radiation for Ewing sarcoma. With the advent of improved techniques for limb preservation, surgery has gradually replaced radiation as the preferred treatment for the primary tumor at many centers, including MD Anderson. Essentially all sites of the appendicular skeleton are considered potentially resectable and reconstructible. In the axial skeleton, resection and reconstruction are more problematic, but even in the spinal, pelvic, sacral, and cranial regions, en bloc resection can be performed and the affected regions repaired in selected favorable cases.

The relative merits of surgery versus radiation have been discussed at length in many articles. In spite of all the attention, it should be recognized that no randomized prospective study has been performed to determine which treatment is superior. Retrospective studies suffer from inherent flaws of potential selection bias. Large, unresectable tumors in the pelvis and sacrum have typically been treated with radiation. Furthermore, differences in chemotherapy regimens compromise the validity of comparisons between institutions and protocols.

The rationale for surgery includes a number of important considerations. Reconstructive methods now offer good or excellent function after surgery for most patients. Removal of the tumor enables the medical oncologist to assess the efficacy of preoperative treatment by quantifying the percentage of necrosis. Excision of the tumor is desirable for the unfavorable cases that are resistant to chemotherapy and radiation therapy, but pretreatment identification of such cases is not yet possible with current imaging modalities. Finally, the risk of late secondary malignancies seems to be higher after combined radiation and chemotherapy for Ewing sarcoma.

The enthusiasm for surgery is tempered somewhat for tumors in central locations, including the pelvis, sacrum, spine, and cranium. In these locations, wide surgical margins may not be feasible without sacrifice of critical structures. For example, resection of high sacral lesions in the S1 and S2 vertebrae may necessitate sacrifice of all the sacral nerve roots, which may result in loss of bowel, bladder, and perineal innervation. Reconstruction in the axial skeleton can be a formidable challenge. Complication rates are high, and the functional results may not be as predictably good as those in the extremities, where modular prostheses and techniques have been refined over the past few decades. In spite of these drawbacks, surgery for tumors in central locations should still be considered on a case-by-case basis. An important reason is the fact that central disease is well established as having a worse prognosis. Aggressive treatment, sometimes with both surgery and radiation, may be indicated to maximize chances for cure (Evans et al. 1991). As surgical techniques improve, resection may become feasible with acceptable morbidity for an increasing number of patients.

Surgery

The planned surgical margins for wide surgical excision are based upon the MRI scan taken after induction chemotherapy. The extraosseous soft tissue tumor mass often has diminished dramatically after chemotherapy, thereby facilitating the surgery. An important aspect of preoperative planning involves assessment of the intramedullary extent of disease. In certain cases, Ewing sarcoma can infiltrate extensively through the bone marrow. The extent of infiltration can be difficult to determine accurately because the widespread use of agents to stimulate marrow production of red blood cells and neutrophils can result in the marrow having abnormal signal characteristics on MRI.

The surgeon must be prepared to resect and reconstruct a lengthy portion of the diaphyseal bone. It is vital during surgery to obtain specimens for frozen-section analysis of the bone marrow to determine whether there is marrow infiltration beyond the site of osteotomy. If infiltration is present, more bone must be removed. The reconstruction may entail rebuilding large segments of bone with custom allograft-prosthetic composites or, in unusual cases, replacing the entire bone with a prosthesis or allograft.

The response to chemotherapy is vitally important to the success of surgery in terms of local control. A recent analysis of patients treated at MD Anderson showed that the response to chemotherapy was the factor most predictive of local recurrence (Lin et al. 2007). Patients who had 99–100% tumor necrosis had better results than did patients with 90–98% tumor necrosis (Fig. 6.4a). Patients who had less than 90% necrosis had significantly worse local recurrence rates.

In the same study, another significant factor that predicted local recurrence was a central site of disease (pelvic girdle, sacrum, shoulder girdle, or chest wall) (Fig. 6.4b). This finding may have reflected thinner surgical margins for these tumors. When outcomes were compared by surgical margin specifically, there was a trend toward better overall results with wider margins (Fig. 6.4c).

In light of these findings, careful consideration must be given to combined surgical and radiation treatment for patients with poor tumor necrosis (less than 90%), central site of disease, and positive surgical margins. The additional toxicity and morbidity of combined treatment must be weighed judiciously before this aggressive treatment is recommended. Fortunately, relatively few patients have these unfavorable characteristics. Further studies will clarify the benefits of combined surgical and adjuvant radiation treatment, enabling refinement of the indications for this multimodality approach.

Radiation Therapy

The decision to use radiation therapy for local control in Ewing sarcoma is a multidisciplinary one. Although surgery is the treatment of choice for addressing the primary tumor after systemic therapy is completed, radiation therapy can be effective in achieving local control in situations in which a surgical procedure would be too morbid or the patient refuses to undergo surgery. Also, adjuvant radiation therapy is recommended when surgical margins are positive for tumor and further surgery to obtain adequate margins is not feasible.

For patients with localized disease who are unable to undergo surgery, involved-field irradiation has been shown to yield results equivalent to those of standard whole-bone irradiation (Donaldson et al. 1998). Therefore, it is not necessary to include the entire bone in the irradiation field unless tumor coverage requires it. However, careful attention must be given to treating an adequate volume. The imaging studies used for planning the treatment volume should include the pretreatment MRI scan so that the original extent of the tumor can be assessed. Coronal and/or

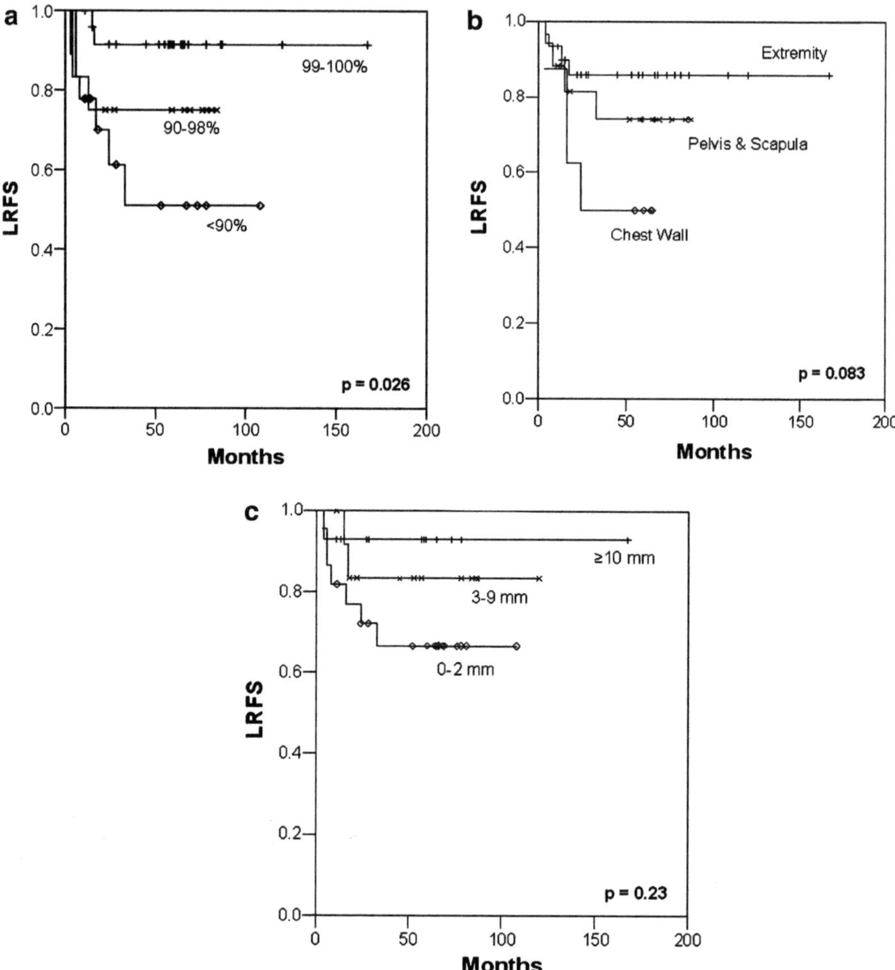

Fig. 6.4 Analyses of factors that have been found to affect the risk of local recurrence for patients treated with surgery at MD Anderson. Sixty-four patients who were surgically treated for Ewing sarcoma between 1990 and 2001 were studied for factors affecting local recurrence. (**a**) The local recurrence–free survival (LRFS) rate depended on the response to chemotherapy. Patients who had near-total necrosis of the tumor, as determined by histopathologic mapping, had the best LRFS (92% at 5 years). (**b**) The site of disease affected the LRFS rate, which was worse in patients with disease in central sites than in patients with disease in the extremities. (**c**) A mild trend toward better LRFS rate was seen with wider surgical margins, but the effect did not reach statistical significance for the number of patients studied. Reprinted from Lin et al. (2007) with permission.

sagittal sequences that survey the entire bone should be part of the analysis to determine the extent of tumor in the marrow space.

Radiation treatment planning requires special attention to immobilization and positioning. A custom cast is preferable to ensure reproducibility of positioning and setup. Dosimetry can vary greatly throughout an extremity because of changes in limb thickness. Therefore, CT scans with multiple slices throughout the limb should be obtained for isodose calculations. For radiation treatment of the extremities, 6-MV photon beams are used, whereas for deep central lesions, 18-MV photons are employed. Appropriate beam modifiers such as wedges or field-in-field techniques should be used to minimize dose inhomogeneities. Intensity-modulated radiation therapy can be used for large lesions in challenging locations or for lesions situated next to dose-limiting structures.

The radiation dose for microscopic disease should be 50 Gy given to the prechemotherapy volume with a 2-cm lateral and/or deep margin and, in an extremity, 5-cm proximal and distal margins. This volume can be modified if there was extension of tumor into a body cavity such as the thorax, abdomen, or pelvis without involvement of adjacent organs. Any infiltrative prechemotherapy abnormality should be covered in the treatment volume. However, if the protruding tumor had displaced normal tissues that were uninvolved by tumor and the chemotherapy has since eliminated the protruding portion of the tumor, the normal tissues do not have to be included in the treatment volume.

Gross disease should be treated with a dose of 55–60 Gy. This dose can be accomplished using a shrinking-field technique: administering 50 Gy to the prechemotherapy volume with the margins described above, followed by a boost to the postchemotherapy volume with a 2-cm margin to bring the dose to 55–60 Gy. During irradiation of lesions involving vertebral bodies, care should be taken to ensure that the dose to the spinal cord does not exceed 45–50 Gy, and individual fractions should be limited to 1.8 Gy.

Additional radiation treatment planning considerations are similar to those employed when treating other extremity sarcomas. When the irradiation fields are designed, a strip of greater than 1 cm of the limb circumference should be spared to allow for preserved lymphatic drainage. If it does not compromise tumor coverage, a strip of bone should also be spared. Unless the joint is violated or the tumor geometry precludes it, half of the joint should be spared. When sparing half the joint is not feasible, efforts should be made to keep the whole-joint radiation dose to less than 40–45 Gy. When radiation therapy is delivered after surgery, the surgical bed and incision should be included in the irradiation field. An exception would be made if the surgical procedure required a remote incision to access the abdominal or thoracic cavity to approach a deep-seated tumor. At MD Anderson, we do not routinely place tissue-equivalent bolus material over the surgical scar unless there is evidence in the individual case for that area being at particularly high risk of recurrence.

Relapse and Spread of Disease

Local Recurrence

The development of local recurrence is a poor prognostic sign. Although local recurrence can occur without distant metastasis, it more often occurs concurrently with or after metastasis. In general, if patients are candidates for systemic chemotherapy, it should be given first, before treatment of the local recurrence.

As with primary tumors, local recurrences can be treated with surgery or radiation. The choice of one or the other depends in part on the clinical situation. If a patient is being treated with curative intent, and the response to the salvage chemotherapy is good, consideration should be given to aggressive surgery. In many cases, such an approach may mean radical amputation. Unfortunately, the number of patients with recurrent disease who have a reasonable chance of complete disease eradication is small. In most instances, the treatment becomes more palliative than curative. In such instances, a more conservative operation combined with radiation may be adequate to control the local disease and pain for the duration of the patient's life.

Metastasis

Metastatic disease may be present at the time of presentation, or it may develop after initial treatment. In either case, the prognosis is not favorable, and the chances for cure are markedly diminished. Patients with metastasis only in the lung may have better survival rates than those of patients with metastatic disease in the bone or bone marrow. Approximately 20–30% of patients who present with pulmonary disease might achieve survival beyond 5 years (Paulussen et al. 1998), whereas very few patients with bone or bone marrow metastases are expected to survive that long.

At the time of presentation, CT findings with regard to pulmonary metastatic disease may be equivocal, especially with the increased sensitivity of modern, high-resolution scanners. It is quite common now for small, 1–2-mm indeterminate nodules to be visualized on staging studies. The mere presence of such nodules does not qualify the patient as having metastases. If the nodules disappear with induction chemotherapy, it may be justifiable to consider the patient to have had metastatic disease. Conversely, if the nodules persist and do not change after cessation of all chemotherapy, it is likely that they represent granulomas or other benign entities.

The treatment of patients with metastatic disease at presentation may differ from that of patients who have relapses of disease. Patients who present with metastatic disease have more chemotherapeutic options because they have not accumulated any treatment-related toxic effects. In general, such patients would start with the same chemotherapeutic regimen as is given to patients who present with localized disease. The need for postoperative chemotherapy would be guided by the chemotherapeutic response evident in the tumor specimen and the amount of residual tumor at the metastatic sites. Patients who have a positive response to chemotherapy may be candidates for thoracotomy and resection of residual disease.

Patients who have disease relapses may have fewer treatment options than those of patients with untreated disease. If they have been treated with either VAI or

HD-VAC, they may have reached the near-maximum cumulative dose of doxorubicin that can be tolerated. In this situation, high-dose ifosfamide, with or without etoposide, may be tried. Salvage treatment may also include irinotecan, gemcitabine/docetaxel, and other protocol-based therapeutic options. Recently, in pediatric patients, a combination of vincristine, temozolomide, and irinotecan has been employed with good preliminary results. A phase I trial of temozolomide and aerosol rubitecan is presently being evaluated in patients with recurrent pulmonary metastatic disease.

More recently, there has been much interest in the use of anti–insulin-like growth factor-1 receptor (IGF-1R) antibodies to treat relapsed Ewing sarcoma. The initial experience has been encouraging, and some dramatic responses have been achieved using humanized monoclonal antibodies (Olmos et al. 2010). However, the response may not be durable, and relapses may occur with either cessation of the drug or prolonged treatment (Subbiah et al. 2011).

It is not our practice at MD Anderson to routinely offer whole-lung irradiation to adult patients with isolated pulmonary metastases. However, radiation therapy is an effective modality for palliation of symptoms of metastatic disease, particularly for bone metastasis. Dose and fractionation considerations for palliation of Ewing sarcoma are similar to those for other tumors. Most commonly, 30 Gy would be given for symptomatic bone metastases.

The results of trials employing myeloablation and stem cell rescue have not been especially encouraging. Although early reports suggested some promise, late relapse and high toxicity have demonstrated the inherent limitations of this approach. Kushner and Meyers (2001) at Memorial Sloan-Kettering Cancer Center reported on a study of the dose-intensive, myeloablative P6 protocol for patients with bone or bone marrow metastasis. The P6 protocol alternated cycles of HD-VAC, consisting of vincristine (2 mg/m^2), doxorubicin (75 mg/m^2), and cyclophosphamide (4.2 g/m^2), with cycles of ifosfamide (9 g/m^2) and etoposide (500 mg/m^2). Some patients received radiation for control of local disease. After induction therapy, consolidation with myeloablative therapy (either total-body irradiation plus melphalan or thiotepa plus carboplatin) was performed. Of the 21 patients enrolled in the study, there was only one long-term survivor, who remained in complete remission beyond 7 years. The authors concluded that dose-intensive use of current chemotherapeutic agents had reached their limits of efficacy and toxicity and that further advances in treatment would have to await the development of entirely novel therapies.

Follow-Up

After treatment, strict monitoring of patients for relapse of disease and complications of treatment is performed at regular intervals. The National Comprehensive Cancer Network (NCCN) guidelines offer a good general framework for follow-up visits (see Chap. 14, "Follow-up Evaluation and Surveillance after Treatment of Bone Sarcomas"). For the first 2 years, patients are seen at 3-month intervals for disease surveillance. For the next 3 years, the interval between follow-up visits is gradually increased to every 4–6 months. After the fifth year, patients are seen yearly. Late relapses between 5 and 10 years have been observed for Ewing sarcoma.

The patient's medical history, physical examination, chest X-ray, and X-rays of the affected extremity are all vital components of the follow-up evaluation. The examination of the primary site includes both careful palpation of the soft tissues for masses that would signal recurrence and assessment of the function of the limb. The use of metallic hardware in many patients compromises the ability to visualize recurrent disease on MRI and CT scans. In general, these scans and ultrasound examination are not routinely used to evaluate the soft tissues. Most local recurrences are either palpable during physical examination or visible on plain radiographs.

CT scans of the chest are not routinely obtained unless there were specific indeterminate small nodules seen preoperatively, which demand follow-up. If such nodules remain stable for 1 year after cessation of treatment, it is unlikely that they are related to the disease.

In addition to being monitored for recurrence of disease, patients must be assessed for function and complications of treatment (see Chap. 12, "Perioperative Management of Patients with Bone Sarcomas"). Younger patients may need to have radiographic measurements of limb lengths. Range of motion, gait, muscle strength, pain, and limitations of activities should be noted. Radiographs should be analyzed for signs of hardware failure or loosening, bone healing, and infection. All patients who are treated with doxorubicin need regular assessments of cardiac function and possible cardiomyopathy.

Long-term surveillance is necessary in patients treated with radiation therapy for Ewing sarcoma because the combination of alkylating agents with radiation therapy has been associated with an increased cumulative lifetime risk of a secondary malignancy in survivors of Ewing sarcoma. It should be noted that secondary malignancies can also occur if radiation was not used. Sarcomas, leukemias, and other hematologic malignancies account for the majority of the new diseases.

Patients who are treated surgically for the primary disease require long-term follow-up beyond 10 years for somewhat different reasons. For these patients, late complications pertaining to the reconstruction are a greater concern than is development of a new neoplasm. Most patients nowadays have reconstruction with metallic endoprostheses, bone allografts, or composites of both. Each of these types is prone to late failures by different mechanisms (see Chap. 9, "Skeletal Reconstruction after Bone Sarcoma Resection") and therefore requires regular long-term monitoring.

Key Practice Points

- Although many different chemotherapy regimens have been described, the preferred protocol at MD Anderson involves dose-intensive treatment consisting of vincristine, doxorubicin, and ifosfamide (VAI) or vincristine, doxorubicin, and cyclophosphamide (VAC).
- The VAI regimen, which is given over a longer course of treatment, is tolerated better and preferred in adult patients.
- High-dose ifosfamide, either alone or in combination with etoposide and other agents, can be employed for patients who have poor response to chemotherapy or relapsed disease.
- Surgical resection is preferred for local control in most cases that present in the extremities without metastasis.
- The percentage of tumor necrosis is an important prognostic guide, but it is not certain whether it can be utilized effectively to guide postoperative treatment.
- Radiation treatment is a valuable modality in difficult cases, particularly those involving central location of disease, metastatic disease, and unresectable primary tumors.
- The rate of local recurrence is highest in patients with central tumor location, poor tumor necrosis after preoperative chemotherapy, and positive surgical margins.
- Despite the added morbidity of combined surgery and adjuvant radiation, this approach should be strongly considered in patients deemed to be at high risk of local recurrence.

Suggested Readings

Burgert Jr EO, Nesbit ME, Garnsey LA, et al. Multimodal therapy for the management of nonpelvic, localized Ewing's sarcoma of bone: intergroup study IESS-II. J Clin Oncol. 1990;8:1514–24.

Cotterill SJ, Ahrens S, Paulussen M, et al. Prognostic factors in Ewing's tumor of bone: analysis of 975 patients from the European Intergroup Cooperative Ewing's Sarcoma Study Group. J Clin Oncol. 2000;18:3108–14.

Craft A, Cotterill S, Malcolm A, et al. Ifosfamide-containing chemotherapy in Ewing's sarcoma: the Second United Kingdom Children's Cancer Study Group and the Medical Research Council Ewing's Tumor Study. J Clin Oncol. 1998;16:3628–33.

Donaldson SS, Torrey M, Link MP, et al. A multidisciplinary study investigating radiotherapy in Ewing's sarcoma: end results of POG #8346. Pediatric Oncology Group. Int J Radiat Oncol Biol Phys. 1998;42:125–35.

Evans RG, Nesbit ME, Gehan EA, et al. Multimodal therapy for the management of localized Ewing's sarcoma of pelvic and sacral bones: a report from the second intergroup study. J Clin Oncol. 1991;9:1173–80.

Grier HE, Krailo MD, Tarbell NJ, et al. Addition of ifosfamide and etoposide to standard chemotherapy for Ewing's sarcoma and primitive neuroectodermal tumor of bone. N Engl J Med. 2003;348:694–701.

Kushner BH, Meyers PA. How effective is dose-intensive/myeloablative therapy against Ewing's sarcoma/primitive neuroectodermal tumor metastatic to bone or bone marrow? The Memorial Sloan-Kettering experience and a literature review. J Clin Oncol. 2001;19:870–80.

Lin PP, Jaffe N, Herzog CE, et al. Chemotherapy response is an important predictor of local recurrence in Ewing sarcoma. Cancer. 2007;109:603–11.

Mackintosh C, Madoz-Gurpide J, Ordonez JL, et al. The molecular pathogenesis of Ewing's sarcoma. Cancer Biol Ther. 2010;9:655–67.

Nesbit Jr ME, Gehan EA, Burgert Jr EO, et al. Multimodal therapy for the management of primary, nonmetastatic Ewing's sarcoma of bone: a long-term follow-up of the First Intergroup study. J Clin Oncol. 1990;8:1664–74.

Olmos D, Postel-Vinay S, Molife LR, et al. Safety, pharmacokinetics, and preliminary activity of the anti-IGF-1R antibody figitumumab (CP-751,871) in patients with sarcoma and Ewing's sarcoma: a phase 1 expansion cohort study. Lancet Oncol. 2010;11:129–35.

Paulussen M, Ahrens S, Craft AW, et al. Ewing's tumors with primary lung metastases: survival analysis of 114 (European Intergroup) Cooperative Ewing's Sarcoma Studies patients. J Clin Oncol. 1998;16:3044–52.

Paulussen M, Ahrens S, Dunst J, et al. Localized Ewing tumor of bone: final results of the Cooperative Ewing's Sarcoma Study CESS 86. J Clin Oncol. 2001;19:1818–29.

Rosito P, Mancini AF, Rondelli R, et al. Italian cooperative study for the treatment of children and young adults with localized Ewing sarcoma of bone: a preliminary report of 6 years of experience. Cancer. 1999;86:421–8 [Note: dosage error in text. Erratum appears in *Cancer* 2005;104:667.].

Subbiah V, Naing A, Brown RE, et al. Targeted morphoproteomic profiling of Ewing's sarcoma treated with insulin-like growth factor 1 receptor (IGF1R) inhibitors: response/resistance signatures. PLoS One. 2011;6:e18424.

Chapter 7
Chondrosarcoma

Alan W. Yasko, Vinod Ravi, and Ashleigh Guadagnolo

Contents

Dr. Yasko died during production of this volume. Further revisions to the chapter were made by Vinod Ravi, Ashleigh Guadagnolo, and Patrick P. Lin.

A.W. Yasko
Department of Orthopaedic Surgery, Northwestern University,
Feinberg School of Medicine, Chicago, IL, USA

V. Ravi (⊠)
Department of Sarcoma Medical Oncology, Unit 450, Division of Cancer Medicine,
The University of Texas MD Anderson Cancer Center, 1400 Holcombe Boulevard,
Houston, TX 77030, USA
e-mail: vravi@mdanderson.org

A. Guadagnolo
Department of Radiation Oncology, Unit 97, Division of Radiation Oncology,
The University of Texas MD Anderson Cancer Center, 1515 Holcombe Boulevard,
Houston, TX 77030, USA
e-mail: aguadagn@mdanderson.org

P.P. Lin and S. Patel (eds.), *Bone Sarcoma*, MD Anderson Cancer Care Series,
DOI 10.1007/978-1-4614-5194-5_7,
© The University of Texas M. D. Anderson Cancer Center 2013

Chapter Overview Chondrosarcomas constitute a heterogeneous group of rare malignancies that produce a cartilaginous matrix. These tumors exhibit a wide spectrum of clinical behavior. The overwhelming majority are relatively chemo- and radioresistant; therefore, surgery is presently the mainstay of treatment. Intratumoral heterogeneity can confound the determination of an accurate diagnosis, which can result in inappropriate surgery. In the absence of novel effective adjuvant therapies, treatment generally has remained unchanged, and clinical outcomes have been relatively stable for decades. Current issues that remain unresolved include the value of pretreatment biopsy, the role of intralesional curettage of histologically low-grade tumors, the role of adjuvant radiation therapy, and the identification of effective systemic therapies.

Introduction

Chondrosarcoma of bone is the second most common primary malignancy of bone after osteosarcoma (excluding myeloma), accounting for approximately 25% of all primary osseous malignancies (Unni and Inwards 2010a). Among chondrosarcomas, approximately 80% are of the conventional subtype, in which tumor cells produce hyaline cartilage (Unni and Inwards 2010a). The remainder of chondrosarcomas consist of rare variants, including dedifferentiated, mesenchymal, clear cell, and periosteal chondrosarcomas.

The age distribution of chondrosarcoma is broad, and the highest incidence is in the fifth and sixth decades. Chondrosarcomas occur slightly more often in males than in females. Presenting signs and symptoms typically include dull, persistent pain; a palpable mass; and occasionally a pathologic fracture.

The majority of primary chondrosarcomas arise de novo within the medullary canals of long bones, but the pelvis, scapula, and other flat bones are also common sites of disease. Secondary chondrosarcomas arise from preexisting benign cartilaginous neoplasms (most commonly osteochondromas) in the flat bones. Histologically, conventional chondrosarcomas can present as low-, intermediate-, or high-grade lesions but not uncommonly have a heterogeneous histologic makeup. (For a full description of the histopathologic and radiologic characteristics of chondrosarcoma, see Bertoni et al. 2002; Huvos 1991; Unni and Inwards 2010a.)

Very little progress has been made in the treatment of chondrosarcoma. Treatment for most cases continues to be surgical excision. The lack of advances in nonsurgical therapies has been the factor most limiting improvement in disease-specific survival rates. The most powerful predictor of outcome for patients with localized disease remains histologic grade (Fig. 7.1). Recent investigations have focused on defining and applying rigor to the analysis of the appropriate level of surgical aggressiveness for low-grade chondrosarcomas to minimize local recurrence and patient morbidity. However, for patients with high-grade chondrosarcomas, no substantive progress has been made on the development of therapies to improve outcomes.

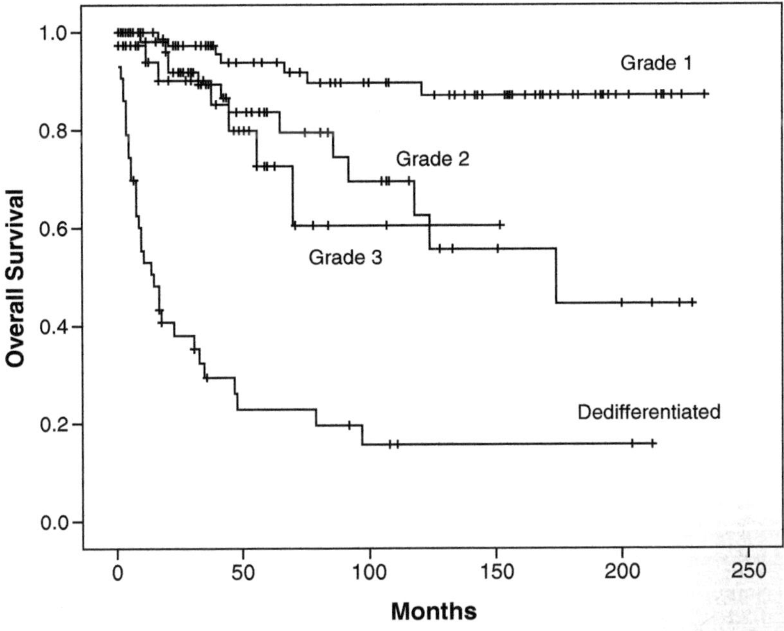

Fig. 7.1 Overall survival of 253 patients with primary nonmetastatic chondrosarcoma treated at MD Anderson from 1986 to 2008. Patients with grade 1 tumors had an excellent long-term survival rate, whereas patients with grades 2 and 3 tumors had significantly worse survival rates. Patients with dedifferentiated chondrosarcoma had the worst prognosis, with a long-term survival rate of 18% (unpublished data) (image courtesy of Patrick P. Lin).

Diagnostic Workup

The value of biopsy for rare musculoskeletal tumors is indisputable. Few clinicians, including radiologists and pathologists, have sufficient experience with any one tumor type to feel comfortable making a diagnosis without tissue confirmation. The accurate diagnosis of a chondrosarcoma is critical to formulating appropriate treatment recommendations. However, the intratumoral heterogeneity of large primary and secondary chondrosarcomas can confound diagnosticians because nonselective biopsy samples may not reflect accurately the biological behavior of the tumor. As with other musculoskeletal tumors, but more so with chondrosarcoma, the biopsy diagnosis must be correlated with radiographic imaging studies before a final treatment recommendation can be made.

The intralesional heterogeneity has raised concerns about the value of biopsy for large chondrosarcomas. As described in Chap. 3, image-guided percutaneous needle biopsy techniques are applied routinely at MD Anderson in the evaluation of the overwhelming majority of musculoskeletal neoplasms. In using these techniques, selective sampling is critical for an adequate diagnosis. Nonselective tumor sampling performed using percutaneous needle techniques or surgery can result in an incorrect grade and diagnosis that do not reflect the tumor's true biologic level of aggressiveness. This inaccuracy can result in under- or overtreatment of the tumor. Although selective biopsies may yield more accurate histologic characterization and surgical biopsies may yield greater amounts of tissue for rendering a diagnosis, the possibility of misdiagnosis remains a concern unless a high-grade histologic component is diagnosed. A diagnosis of a low-grade tumor carries the risk of underdiagnosis of a heterogeneous tumor that also has high-grade components. Furthermore, distinguishing an apparent low-grade chondrosarcoma from benign enchondroma can be challenging despite adequate tumor sampling. Interobserver variability in identifying these tumors remains problematic even among experienced bone pathologists.

The correlation between the biopsy diagnosis and the final diagnosis after definitive surgery was recently analyzed at MD Anderson to determine how much reliable information can be obtained from the biopsy of cartilaginous lesions in the long bones, scapula, and pelvis (unpublished data). For determining whether cartilage was present, there was a 90–100% correlation between pre- and postoperative histologic diagnoses. A distinction between high- and low-grade tumor designations correlated much less, yielding concordance in only 35–70% of cases. The histologic grade (when the biopsy specimen was compared to the final resection specimen) was determined successfully in only 30–40% of biopsy samples. The greatest drop-off in agreement from the diagnosis of cartilage to the diagnosis of the exact grade of chondrosarcoma was in tumors of the pelvis. No difference was noted between outcomes based on biopsy techniques used and whether the biopsy was performed at our institution or another. Overall diagnostic errors (when the biopsy specimen was compared to the final resection specimen) occurred in 66% of cases, two-thirds of which were underdiagnosed. The uncertainty attendant with the histologic diagnosis based on small tumor samples is underscored by the common inclusion in final pathology reports of a notation that suggests correlation of the histologic findings with radiographic features of the lesion.

Given these data, it can be stated that the biopsy is important for establishing the presence of a cartilaginous tumor but not necessarily for pinpointing the specific nature of such a tumor. Therefore, at MD Anderson and other sarcoma referral centers, a biopsy in some cases is not considered as critical a component of the pretreatment evaluation if the diagnosis of a cartilaginous tumor (chondrosarcoma) can be made confidently by using radiologic studies. In cases in which the diagnosis of a cartilaginous tumor by using one or more imaging modalities is in doubt, the presence of cartilage should be established by biopsy.

Radiologic Studies

The data on histologic discordance described above suggest that reliance on the radiographic appearance of the lesion may be paramount to the decision-making process about the nature and extent of surgery. The accurate interpretation of

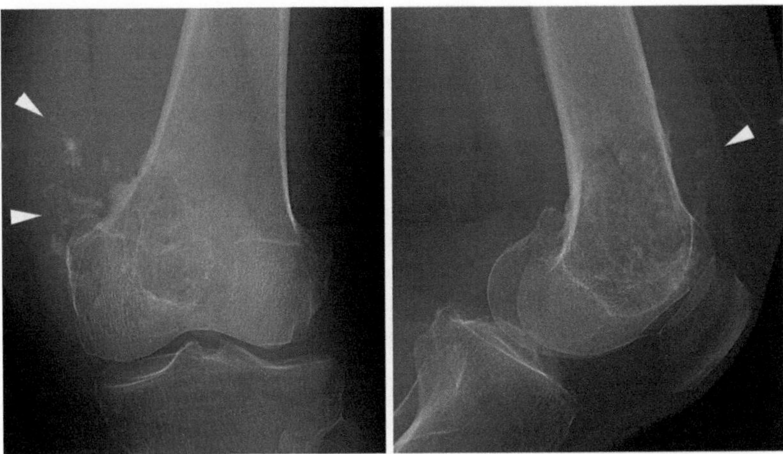

Fig. 7.2 X-rays (anteroposterior and lateral) showing calcifications within a grade 3 chondrosarcoma in the distal femur. Such calcifications are a common feature of cartilaginous tumors, both benign and malignant. The aggressive nature of this tumor is demonstrated by the growth of the tumor out of the bone and its invasion into the surrounding soft tissues. Small "popcorn" or "ring" calcifications (*arrowheads*) are visible in the tumor (image courtesy of Patrick P. Lin).

radiographic features to provide critical treatment-determining information in the absence of confirming histologic findings is one unique feature of the management of chondrosarcoma that has evolved at MD Anderson through the analysis of histologic, radiographic, and clinical data for hundreds of patients treated over a period of 30 years.

Biplanar radiographs remain a critical first step in the evaluation of a suspected chondrosarcoma. The feature that calls attention to the presence of a cartilaginous neoplasm is intralesional matrix calcification that appears consistently and characteristically on all imaging modalities, including plain radiographs (Fig. 7.2), computed tomography (CT) scans, and magnetic resonance imaging (MRI) scans. The pattern of calcification is described variably as dense, stippled, or punctate. The calcifications show a lobular distribution and as a result can resemble popcorn or rings.

Despite the various imaging modalities available for diagnosis, the distinction between benign and low-grade malignant cartilage can be difficult. The clinical context in which the radiographs are obtained must be considered. Low-grade chondrosarcoma of the long bones commonly has uniform tumor matrix calcification; focal, shallow endosteal scalloping; and bone lysis. In the presence of localized pain, it can be assumed to be a lesion of low aggressiveness. Cortical thickening, expansion of the involved region of the long bone, and soft tissue extension are uncommon in low-grade cases. Enchondromas are more commonly asymptomatic with minimal or no activity at the leading margin of the tumor.

In the long bones, some lesions may have radiographic findings consistent with activity (endosteal scalloping or lytic areas) without adaptive or aggressive changes (cortical thickening, cortical thinning, or focal bone destruction with soft tissue extension). Such active but nonaggressive lesions have been categorized by clinicians, pathologists, and radiologists as being of borderline malignancy, variably assigned such nomenclature as *grade ½ chondrosarcoma, cartilaginous neoplasm of uncertain malignant potential, atypical enchondroma, grade 1 cartilage lesion, grade 0 chondrosarcoma,* and *chondrosarcoma* in situ. The indeterminate nature of these terms clearly defines the need for more precise diagnostic modalities for low-grade tumors. For the present, however, a surrogate for a definitive pathologic diagnosis is the presence or absence of radiographic signs of aggressiveness.

For those unusual chondrosarcomas that are void of matrix calcification, cross-sectional imaging with CT and/or MRI may be helpful. CT is preferable to MRI for the diagnosis of chondrosarcoma, especially in the pelvis, scapula, and spine, where it is difficult to discern the pattern of bone destruction and the presence of matrix mineralization. In the long bones, the distribution of the calcified cartilage, activity at the endosteal surface of the bone (scalloping), and presence of focal cortical thinning, expansion, or breach are also better delineated by CT. MRI is useful in delineating the pattern of bone involvement (usually lobular) of intramedullary tumors and the extent of soft tissue involvement for tumors that have invaded through the cortex.

Intermediate- and high-grade chondrosarcomas exhibit adaptive changes characterized by localized cortical expansion and thickening or aggressive features such as deep endosteal scalloping, cortical disruption, pathologic fracture, periosteal reaction, and soft tissue extension with faint amorphous calcifications and variable areas of noncalcified tumor matrix. Dedifferentiated chondrosarcoma commonly has non-aggressive calcified tumor matrix juxtaposed with lytic, destructive changes consistent with a high-grade tumor. For this bimorphic tumor, MRI can be helpful for identifying the high-grade component that should be the target of selective biopsy. In some dedifferentiated tumors, the low-grade component can be obliterated by the high-grade component.

The question as to whether the radiographic distinction of aggressiveness is sufficiently evident to an experienced observer to conclude that an intermediate- or high-grade tumor is present was analyzed in a study of 100 cartilaginous tumors in which the observers (8 MD Anderson musculoskeletal radiologists and orthopedic oncologists) were asked to determine the histologic grade and recommend treatment based solely on plain radiographs. There was substantial agreement among both the radiologists and the surgeons. Hypothetical overtreatment of low-grade tumors was deemed to have occurred in 15% of patients based on the results of this analysis, but no undertreatment of high-grade tumors would have occurred (unpublished data). The strength of the agreement increased with the surgeons' and radiologists' years of clinical experience with musculoskeletal tumors. Based on these data, we routinely incorporate findings from the radiographic evaluation of the tumor into the surgical decision-making process.

Primary Treatment

Surgery

Given the absence of reliably effective adjuvant therapies for chondrosarcoma, surgery presently provides the only chance for long-term disease-free survival for patients with chondrosarcoma. For any given tumor, the surgical management may include intralesional excision by curettage with or without a surgical adjuvant, or wide resection. Ultimately, the surgeon must consider the radiographic features of the tumor together with the histologic findings, if a biopsy was performed, to formulate the appropriate surgical plan. Wide en bloc excision to achieve tumor-free surgical margins is recommended for histologically intermediate- and high-grade chondrosarcoma, as well as for the rare variants of dedifferentiated, clear cell, and mesenchymal chondrosarcoma. In the absence of an established histologic diagnosis, radiographically aggressive cartilaginous-appearing tumors should be widely excised.

Although complete excision is recommended for all grades and subtypes of chondrosarcoma, the optimal method of achieving this goal for some low-grade tumors is debatable. Not all of these tumors behave similarly, and wide excision may be appropriate for some patients with low-grade tumors but may be excessive for others (Bauer et al. 1995). In the long bones, active but nonaggressive tumors (those considered to be of borderline malignancy) can be treated with intralesional excision by curettage and high-speed burring of the walls of the cavity. Surgical adjuvants such as intracavitary administration of phenol, liquid nitrogen, and thermal cautery can be used to extend the margins of excision. In contrast, for long-bone chondrosarcomas with adaptive or aggressive changes, wide resection is recommended irrespective of the histologic grade.

Pelvic and scapular chondrosarcomas also are addressed through wide resection, which is dictated by their consistently large extraosseous components rather than by histologic grade. Local control in our analyses was achieved consistently only with an aggressive resection (Pant et al. 2005; Sheth et al. 1996). There is no role for intralesional excision in such cases because tumor spillage in the soft tissues would be inevitable with piecemeal excision, and the likelihood of local recurrence would be unacceptably high. In our experience, given the central locations of these tumors and their generally large size, local recurrence is more common for these tumors than for intramedullary chondrosarcomas of similar histologic grade in the long bones of the limbs, even after complete surgical extirpation.

Radiation Therapy

As described above, the first-line modality for definitive management of chondrosarcoma is wide excision. Radiation therapy may be considered in some cases of chondrosarcomas of the skull base and sacral regions that are deemed to be unresectable. However, radiation therapy in the absence of surgery offers inferior prospects for local control. These tumors can present similarly to chordomas, and misdiagnosis of the two is possible. Biopsy of the tumor and review of the specimen by an experienced pathologist are critical because the prognosis of chondrosarcoma tends to be better than chordoma in these locations, and it may also be controlled with a lower radiation dose. Outcomes after radiation therapy for chondrosarcoma in the base of the skull and sacrum are often reported along with outcomes of treatment for chordoma, given their similar presentations. Treatment planning and techniques for the two types of tumors are similar (see the chordoma section in Chap. 8, "Rare Tumors"). However, multiple investigators have found that a lower radiation dose, in the range of 70 cobalt gray equivalents (CGE) for gross disease, is needed to control chondrosarcoma.

Radiation therapy may also have application as an adjuvant therapy after en bloc resection when there are positive surgical margins and for symptom palliation when procedure morbidity or tumor unresectability precludes further surgery. However, because chondrosarcomas tend to be radioresistant, radiation has not been applied on a consistent basis as an adjuvant after surgery for primary tumors. Indeed, external-beam radiation for such tumors, even if negative surgical margins are not achieved, is not a routine component of the treatment paradigm applied at MD Anderson. The low mitotic index and relatively anaerobic matrix environment for these tumors are thought to contribute to the radiation insensitivity. If radiation is used, a dose greater than 60 Gy has been recommended but has limited utility for tumors resected in the vicinity of critical normal structures whose radiation tolerance would be exceeded by that dose. The role of intensity-modulated radiation therapy (IMRT) or proton therapy to address these tumors remains undefined but continues to be studied in selected centers.

Chemotherapy

The role of chemotherapy in the multidisciplinary management of chondrosarcoma remains under investigation. While chemotherapy has been largely ineffective in the management of conventional chondrosarcoma, it may have a role in the management of mesenchymal and dedifferentiated chondrosarcomas. Multiagent chemotherapy has been administered to target the high-grade components of these unique subtypes, whose histologic features bear similarities to osteosarcoma, Ewing sarcoma, and other high-grade spindle cell malignancies. Chemotherapy experience for specific chondrosarcoma subtypes is described below.

Conventional Chondrosarcoma

Conventional chondrosarcoma, regardless of grade, is primarily treated with surgery and radiation, as effective systemic therapeutic options are unavailable. In retrospective studies, systemic therapy has been shown to be ineffective, with no changes in the outcomes when compared with no systemic therapy (Lee et al. 1999). Systemic chemotherapy should only be used in the management of conventional chondrosarcoma (any grade) in the setting of a clinical trial.

Mesenchymal Chondrosarcoma

Mesenchymal chondrosarcoma has a biphasic histologic appearance, with a combination of highly cellular areas interspersed with islands of relatively bland-appearing chondroid matrix. The cellular areas are composed of small anaplastic cells, reminiscent of those seen in Ewing sarcoma (Unni and Inwards 2010b). Mesenchymal chondrosarcoma is treated with the same strategy used for Ewing sarcoma because of its small, round, blue cell component and its sensitivity to the drugs used for Ewing sarcoma.

A multidisciplinary approach is suggested for mesenchymal chondrosarcoma; it should include multiagent chemotherapy using at least three of the following agents: ifosfamide and/or cyclophosphamide, etoposide, doxorubicin, and vincristine. The evidence to support the use of chemotherapy in mesenchymal chondrosarcoma comes from a 26-patient retrospective study by Cesari et al. from the Rizzoli Institute (2007). This study demonstrated that among patients who had a complete surgical remission, the 10-year disease-free survival rates were 76% for patients who received chemotherapy and 17% for those who did not ($P=0.008$). Margin-negative resection was noted to be a strong predictor of long-term survival, especially when multiagent chemotherapy was given. Among all patients in the study, regardless of surgical remission status, there was a trend toward a higher survival rate in the chemotherapy group. The 10-year disease-free survival rate in patients who received chemotherapy was 31%, compared with 19% in those who did not receive chemotherapy (the difference did not reach statistical significance) (Cesari et al. 2007). Additional evidence to support the use of chemotherapy in the management of mesenchymal chondrosarcoma comes from a pediatric study that looked at the treatment of patients ages 1–25 years who were enrolled in various clinical trials with multiagent chemotherapy. All patients in the study ($n=15$) received chemotherapy, and only one patient had metastatic disease. Their overall 10-year survival rate was 67%. Among eight patients who had a margin-negative resection, seven (87.5%) were reported to be alive at the time of the report (median follow-up, 14.6 years) (Dantonello et al. 2008).

Given the inherent difficulty in conducting a prospective randomized trial in a rare disease, these two studies and the consensus opinion of experts support a role for chemotherapy in patients with mesenchymal chondrosarcoma. Preoperative therapy lasting 12–24 weeks is recommended, with imaging every two cycles. After local control (surgery and/or radiation therapy), further adjuvant chemotherapy is recommended until maximal tolerance is reached. At our institution, a combination of vincristine (2 mg/m^2; maximal dose, 2 mg), ifosfamide (10 g/m^2), and doxorubicin (75 mg/m^2) is used every 21 days with growth-factor support.

Dedifferentiated Chondrosarcoma

Treatment of dedifferentiated chondrosarcoma remains a challenge because of the high propensity of these tumors to metastasize. Although local control can be accomplished in the majority of cases, 90% of patients develop distant disease (Dickey et al. 2004). Current consensus is to treat dedifferentiated chondrosarcoma using a multidisciplinary approach similar to that used for osteosarcoma, which typically includes preoperative chemotherapy employing doxorubicin and cisplatin, followed by wide surgical excision and further chemotherapy. This approach is based on retrospective data as no prospective trials have examined its utility. In 1995, Benjamin et al. presented their experience with continuous infusion of doxorubicin and intra-arterial cisplatin in 15 patients with dedifferentiated chondrosarcoma. They reported a 51% relapse-free survival rate at 30 months of follow-up (Benjamin et al. 1995). Some of the patients were also treated with ifosfamide and/or methotrexate. That study did not have a control group that did not receive chemotherapy, but a previous report from MD Anderson Cancer Center looked at the outcomes of 17 patients with resectable dedifferentiated chondrosarcoma treated with local therapy alone and reported a median time to relapse of 5 months and median survival of 10 months. All patients died within 25 months (Johnson et al. 1986). Using that study as a historical control, the outcomes in patients treated with chemotherapy appear to be better.

In another retrospective study of 22 patients with dedifferentiated chondrosarcoma from the Royal Orthopaedic Hospital in Birmingham, England, the median overall survival was 9 months, and the 5-year survival rate was 18%. In the subset of patients who had chemotherapy, either preoperatively or postoperatively, the median survival was 14 months, and the 5-year survival rate was 36%. Six patients who were treated with excision only (without chemotherapy) died within a year, with a median survival of 8 months. This study, therefore, suggests better outcomes for patients who received chemotherapy. Among the patients who received chemotherapy, the combination of doxorubicin and cisplatin was most commonly used (Mitchell et al. 2000).

Two retrospective studies from the Mayo Clinic have questioned the benefit of chemotherapy for dedifferentiated chondrosarcoma. The first was published in 1986 and reviewed treatment outcomes of 78 patients with the disease. The authors reported no statistically significant difference in the 5-year survival rates of patients who were treated with and without adjuvant therapy (chemotherapy and/or radiation). However, among the subset of patients who received both surgery and chemotherapy ($n=9$), 22% were alive at 5 years, while among the surgery-only subset ($n=41$), only 10% were alive at 5 years (Frassica et al. 1986). In 2004, an extension to the first study was published; it reviewed the treatment outcomes of 42 patients between 1986 and 2000. Patients who received surgery and chemotherapy had a median survival of 8.4 months, compared with 6.4 months for the surgery-only group, but the difference was not statistically significant ($P=0.69$). The disease-free survival time also did not improve with the administration of chemotherapy ($P=0.54$). Patients were treated with chemotherapy consisting of doxorubicin, ifosfamide, cisplatin, methotrexate, or a combination of these drugs (Dickey et al. 2004). Along similar lines, another large retrospective study from the European Musculo-Skeletal Oncology Society (EMSOS) looked at outcomes of 337 patients with dedifferentiated chondrosarcoma and did not find a statistically significant improvement in survival for patients who received chemotherapy. However, among 242 patients who were considered potentially curable (without identifiable metastases at presentation), a trend was noted in favor of chemotherapy; the 5-year survival rate was 33% for patients who received chemotherapy, compared with 25% for those who did not. Similarly, among patients with metastatic disease, the use of chemotherapy and surgery suggested longer survival times when compared with supportive care (7 months vs. 3 months, respectively); the difference was, however, not statistically significant and could have been attributable to the difference in performance status at diagnosis rather than to treatment (Grimer et al. 2007).

Overall, the diagnosis of dedifferentiated chondrosarcoma portends a poor prognosis. The response to cytotoxic chemotherapy and overall survival are worse than those for de novo osteosarcoma. Nevertheless, at MD Anderson, patients with localized disease are treated aggressively with chemotherapy regimens similar to those used for osteosarcoma. Our current standard approach consists of preoperative chemotherapy with doxorubicin and cisplatin, followed by limb-sparing surgery, followed by additional postoperative chemotherapy that may include drugs such as ifosfamide and high-dose methotrexate (see Chap. 5, "Osteosarcoma").

Follow-Up

Patients with low-grade tumors of the long bones are monitored by physical examination, plain radiographs of the affected region, and chest imaging every 6 months for 5 years after completion of treatment and then yearly for a minimum of 10 years. Patients with intermediate- and high-grade tumors are followed up in a similar fashion but more frequently, every 3–6 months for 5 years, then yearly for a minimum of 10 years. Local imaging with MRI with or without CT of the pelvis, scapula, and spine is recommended as an adjunct to plain radiographs to identify small recurrences that can be difficult to define within the disrupted, complex anatomy after resection; these modalities also help to define resectability if a recurrence is found.

Relapse and Spread of Disease

Local Recurrence

The likelihood of local recurrence of chondrosarcoma depends upon a number of factors, including the completeness of the tumor excision and the histologic grade of the primary tumor. Low-grade tumors can recur locally up to 10 years after surgery and rarely recur thereafter. Pelvic and vertebral tumors have higher recurrence rates than do long-bone tumors (Fig. 7.3). Published data of a series of 67 patients with pelvic chondrosarcoma treated at MD Anderson showed a 28% local recurrence rate, with recurrences noted at a median of 23 months (range, 1–111 months) after definitive surgery (Sheth et al. 1996). These data are consistent with other site-specific analyses of pelvic chondrosarcomas.

The treatment recommendation for local recurrence in the extremity, pelvis, or scapula is wide resection, if feasible (Lin et al. 2012). Amputation may be recommended for local tumor control if the recurrent tumor is unresectable or negative surgical margins cannot be achieved with a limb-sparing procedure. Experience

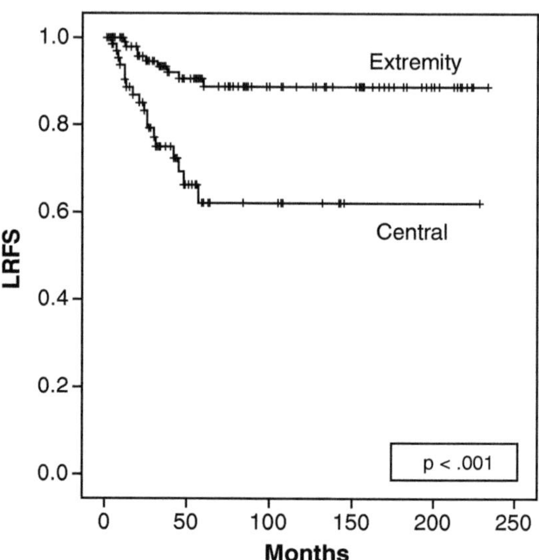

Fig. 7.3 Local recurrence-free survival (LRFS) rates in 182 patients with conventional chondrosarcoma treated at MD Anderson. In this patient group, the LRFS rate was significantly better for patients with extremity tumors than for patients with centrally located tumors (unpublished data) (image courtesy of Patrick P. Lin).

with amputation has been reported most frequently for recurrent pelvic or periscapular chondrosarcoma. In our experience, amputation has been deemed necessary in only rare cases of multifocal recurrent disease for which en bloc excision cannot be executed effectively. Radiation has been recommended for symptom palliation for unresectable locally recurrent disease in the axial skeleton in cases in which surgery would be ineffective at controlling disease. Data are lacking regarding the effectiveness and durability of palliative radiation.

Metastasis

Metastasis at presentation is uncommon in chondrosarcoma. Systemic disease relapse after successful treatment of the primary tumor is more common and poses a unique challenge given the absence of effective systemic therapies. Distant relapse rates of 20–60% have been reported, with higher rates associated with higher histologic grade of the primary tumor (Sheth et al. 1996). The survival rate for conventional chondrosarcoma (all grades combined) has been reported to be approximately 70% in large series (Bjornsson et al. 1998; Fiorenza et al. 2002; Lee et al. 1999; Sheth et al. 1996). Histologic grade-dependent survival varies, with patients diagnosed with dedifferentiated chondrosarcoma experiencing the worst prognosis (5-year survival rate, 10–36%) and patients with clear cell chondrosarcoma and low-grade conventional chondrosarcoma exhibiting the most favorable prognosis (5-year survival rate, >90%). In our institutional experience and reports of other large series of patients, tumor relapse after a continuously disease-free interval of 10 years is rare. Patients with advanced disease should be considered for enrollment in clinical trials of novel systemic therapies.

Key Practice Points

- Chondrosarcoma is biologically and histologically diverse.
- Biopsy-obtained tissue can misrepresent the aggressiveness of large chondrosarcomas.
- Radiographic characteristics are a key determinant of the appropriate surgical approach to chondrosarcoma.
- Conventional chondrosarcoma has no consistently effective adjuvant therapies to surgery.
- Radiation therapy is sometimes used in surgically inaccessible sites, such as the base of the skull.
- Chemotherapy does not have an established role in the treatment of conventional chondrosarcoma but may offer some benefit in mesenchymal and dedifferentiated chondrosarcoma.
- Regular surveillance (at least 10 years after treatment) is recommended to monitor for tumor relapse.

Suggested Readings

Bauer HC, Brosjo O, Kreicbergs A, Lindholm J. Low risk of recurrence of enchondroma and low-grade chondrosarcoma in extremities. 80 patients followed for 2–25 years. Acta Orthop Scand. 1995;66:283–8.

Benjamin RS, Chu P, Patel SR, et al. Dedifferentiated chondrosarcoma: a treatable disease. Proc Am Assoc Cancer Res. 1995;36:243 [abstract].

Bertoni F, Bacchini P, Hogendoorn PC. Chondrosarcoma. In: Fletcher CDM, Unni KK, Mertens F, editors. World Health Organization classification of tumours. Pathology and genetics of tumours of soft tissue and bone. Lyon: IARC Press; 2002. p. 247–51.

Bjornsson J, McLeod RA, Unni KK, Ilstrup DM, Pritchard DJ. Primary chondrosarcoma of long bones and limb girdles. Cancer. 1998;83:2105–19.

Cesari M, Bertoni F, Bacchini P, Mercuri M, Palmerini E, Ferrari S. Mesenchymal chondrosarcoma. An analysis of patients treated at a single institution. Tumori. 2007;93:423–7.

Dantonello TM, Int-Veen C, Leuschner I, et al. Mesenchymal chondrosarcoma of soft tissues and bone in children, adolescents, and young adults: experiences of the CWS and COSS study groups. Cancer. 2008;112:2424–31.

Dickey ID, Rose PS, Fuchs B, et al. Dedifferentiated chondrosarcoma: the role of chemotherapy with updated outcomes. J Bone Joint Surg Am. 2004;86:2412–8.

Eefting D, Schrage YM, Geirnaerdt MJ, et al. Assessment of interobserver variability and histologic parameters to improve reliability in classification and grading of central cartilaginous tumors. Am J Surg Pathol. 2009;33:50–7.

Fiorenza F, Abudu A, Grimer RJ, et al. Risk factors for survival and local control in chondrosarcoma of bone. J Bone Joint Surg Br. 2002;84:93–9.

Frassica FJ, Unni KK, Beabout JW, Sim FH. Dedifferentiated chondrosarcoma. A report of the clinicopathological features and treatment of seventy-eight cases. J Bone Joint Surg Am. 1986;68:1197–205.

Giuffrida AY, Burgueno JE, Koniaris LG, Gutierrez JC, Duncan R, Scully SP. Chondrosarcoma in the United States (1973 to 2003): an analysis of 2890 cases from the SEER database. J Bone Joint Surg Am. 2009;91:1063–72.

Grimer RJ, Gosheger G, Taminiau A, et al. Dedifferentiated chondrosarcoma: prognostic factors and outcome from a European group. Eur J Cancer. 2007;43:2060–5.

Huvos AG. Chondrosarcoma. In: Bone tumors: diagnosis, treatment, and prognosis. 2nd ed. Philadelphia: W.B. Saunders Company; 1991. p. 343–61.

Johnson S, Tetu B, Ayala AG, Chawla SP. Chondrosarcoma with additional mesenchymal component (dedifferentiated chondrosarcoma). I. A clinicopathologic study of 26 cases. Cancer. 1986;58:278–86.

Lee FY, Mankin HJ, Fondren G, et al. Chondrosarcoma of bone: an assessment of outcome. J Bone Joint Surg Am. 1999;81:326–38.

Leerapun T, Hugate RR, Inwards CY, Scully SP, Sim FH. Surgical management of conventional grade I chondrosarcoma of long bones. Clin Orthop Relat Res. 2007;463:166–72.

Lin PP, Alfawareh MD, Takeuchi A, Moon BS, Lewis VO. Sixty percent 10-year survival of patients with chondrosarcoma after local recurrence. Clin Orthop Relat Res. 2012;470:670–6.

Mitchell AD, Ayoub K, Mangham DC, Grimer RJ, Carter SR, Tillman RM. Experience in the treatment of dedifferentiated chondrosarcoma. J Bone Joint Surg Br. 2000;82:55–61.

Normand AN, Cannon CP, Lewis VO, Lin PP, Yasko AW. Curettage of biopsy-diagnosed grade 1 periacetabular chondrosarcoma. Clin Orthop Relat Res. 2007;459:146–9.

Pant R, Yasko AW, Lewis VO, Raymond K, Lin PP. Chondrosarcoma of the scapula: long-term oncologic outcome. Cancer. 2005;104:149–58.

Sheth DS, Yasko AW, Johnson ME, Ayala AG, Murray JA, Romsdahl MM. Chondrosarcoma of the pelvis. Prognostic factors for 67 patients treated with definitive surgery. Cancer. 1996;78:745–50.

Skeletal Lesions Interobserver Correlation among Expert Diagnosticians (SLICED) Study Group. Reliability of histopathologic and radiologic grading of cartilaginous neoplasms in long bones. J Bone Joint Surg Am. 2007;89:2113–23.

Unni KK, Inwards CY. Chondrosarcoma (primary, secondary, dedifferentiated, and clear cell). In: Dahlin's bone tumors: general aspects and data on 10,165 cases. 6th ed. Philadelphia: Lippincott Williams & Wilkins; 2010a. p. 60–91.

Unni KK, Inwards CY. Mesenchymal chondrosarcoma. In: Dahlin's bone tumors: general aspects and data on 10,165 cases. 6th ed. Philadelphia: Lippincott Williams & Wilkins; 2010b. p. 92–7.

van der Geest IC, de Valk MH, de Rooy JW, Pruszczynski M, Veth RP, Schreuder HW. Oncological and functional results of cryosurgical therapy of enchondromas and chondrosarcomas grade 1. J Surg Oncol. 2008;98:421–6.

Chapter 8
Rare Bone Sarcomas

**Valerae O. Lewis, Ashleigh Guadagnolo, Laurence D. Rhines,
and Shreyaskumar Patel**

Contents

V.O. Lewis (✉)
Department of Orthopaedic Oncology, Unit 1448, Division of Surgery, The University of Texas
MD Anderson Cancer Center, P.O. Box 301402, Houston, TX 77230, USA
e-mail: volewis@mdanderson.org

A. Guadagnolo
Department of Radiation Oncology, Unit 97, Division of Radiation Oncology, The University
of Texas MD Anderson Cancer Center, 1515 Holcombe Boulevard, Houston, TX 77030, USA
e-mail: aguadagn@mdanderson.org

L.D. Rhines
Department of Neurosurgery, Unit 442, Division of Surgery, The University of Texas MD
Anderson Cancer Center, 1400 Holcombe Boulevard, Houston, TX 77030, USA
e-mail: lrhines@mdanderson.org

S. Patel
Department of Sarcoma Medical Oncology, Unit 450, Division of Cancer Medicine,
The University of Texas MD Anderson Cancer Center, 1400 Holcombe Boulevard,
Houston, TX 77030, USA
e-mail: spatel@mdanderson.org

P.P. Lin and S. Patel (eds.), *Bone Sarcoma*, MD Anderson Cancer Care Series,
DOI 10.1007/978-1-4614-5194-5_8,
© The University of Texas M. D. Anderson Cancer Center 2013

Chapter Overview Rare tumors of bone include chordoma, adamantinoma, hemangioendothelioma, hemangiopericytoma, low-grade fibrosarcoma of bone, and malignant fibrous histiocytoma (MFH). These are distinctive and interesting diseases with unique features. They bear some relationship to a spectrum of different mesenchymal tissues. Chordomas are probably derived from notochordal cells and thus are found primarily in the sacrum and sphenoocciput. Adamantinomas, on the other hand, are found predominantly in the tibia and show a peculiar tendency toward epithelial differentiation. The other tumors are more widely located within the body; hemangioendothelioma and hemangiopericytoma are tumors related to vascular tissue, whereas low-grade fibrosarcoma and MFH are most likely derived from spindle-shaped, fibroblast-like cells.

Introduction

There are several primary tumors of bone that defy classification in a specific group. However, these tumors—chordoma, adamantinoma, hemangioendothelioma, hemangiopericytoma, and low-grade fibrosarcoma of bone—are often discussed together because they share several characteristics: they are rare, they tend to be low grade with low metastatic potential, and when they are localized, surgery is often considered the best treatment option. When treated appropriately, the overall prognosis for patients with these lesions is good. This chapter discusses the above-mentioned tumors, as well as malignant fibrous histiocytoma (MFH). Although the latter is a high-grade lesion and is treated with a combination of surgery and chemotherapy, it is included in this chapter because of its rarity and the possibility that it constitutes one end of the spectrum of fibrosarcoma of bone.

Chordoma

Clinical Features

Chordomas are rare tumors of bone that arise from malignant transformation of notochordal remnants. They are low- to intermediate-grade malignancies that represent approximately 1–4% of all primary bone tumors (Healey and Lane 1989). Chordomas occur in males more often than in females, occur in whites more often than in African Americans, and are most commonly diagnosed in the fifth to seventh decades of life.

Since chordomas arise from notochord remnants, they are found in the midline of the spine. Chordomas most commonly occur at the ends of the spine—in the sacrococcygeal and sphenooccipital regions. Only about 15% of chordomas occur in the mobile spine (Bergh et al. 2000). Although chordomas represent less than 5% of all primary bone tumors, they are the most common primary malignant bone tumor found in the spine (Boriani et al. 2006; Sundaresan et al. 2009).

Diagnostic Workup and Staging

The most common presenting symptom of chordomas is pain. The pain tends to develop gradually and progressively. Other symptoms depend on the location of the tumor and what it is compressing. Lesions in the sacrum can cause rectal dysfunction, including obstipation or constipation; lesions in the sphenooccipital region can cause symptoms of compression of the cranial nerve; and lesions of the vertebral bodies can cause symptoms of cord or nerve root compression. Both the pain and the symptoms are generally insidious in onset.

Radiographically, chordomas present as midline, poorly marginated, lytic lesions. Three-dimensional imaging (computed tomography [CT] or magnetic resonance imaging [MRI]) often reveals a soft tissue mass, which is calcified in approximately 50% of cases. CT and MRI are helpful in delineating the lesion and defining its extension into the surrounding soft tissues.

When a patient presents to our clinic with a potential primary bone tumor of the spine, a histologic diagnosis is mandatory to determine the next phases of the treatment. CT-guided core biopsy is our method of choice for obtaining the tissue diagnosis because fine-needle aspiration (FNA) specimens lack the cytoarchitectural detail that is critical for diagnostic accuracy. Every effort should be made to plan the trajectory of this biopsy such that the biopsy track can subsequently be resected with the tumor. Transvisceral biopsies, such as a transoral approach for upper cervical tumors or transrectal approach for sacral tumors, should be avoided at all costs. These biopsy routes risk contaminating an additional anatomic compartment that would otherwise not need to be resected.

Histologically, chordomas appear as lobules of myxoid tissue with spindle cell septation. The characteristic cell is the physaliferous cell, which has abundant cytoplasm, multiple intracytoplasmic vacuoles, and a small, round nucleus. This composition gives the cell its clear, "soap bubble" appearance. The cells are surrounded by a mucin-containing myxoid stroma. One-third of sphenooccipital lesions contain chondroid; a variant of chordoma contains bland-appearing hyaline cartilage.

Chordomas should be differentiated from benign notochordal rests, which are intraosseous lesions that have the same anatomic distribution as chordomas. Histologically, these two types of lesions appear similar because they are both made up of sheets of vacuolated cells, but benign notochordal rests lack mitotic activity and surrounding myxoid stroma. The differential diagnosis of chordoma also includes myeloma, melanoma, and chondrosarcoma.

As with other bone tumors, staging modalities consist of radiographs and MRI scans of the involved site (in this case, the spine), a bone scan, and a chest CT scan. Under the Enneking staging system (Enneking 1986; Enneking et al. 1980), chordomas most commonly present as stage IB, low-grade malignant tumors that have invaded another compartment (broken out of the vertebral body).

Treatment

Surgery

As with primary malignant bone tumors outside the spine, the optimal surgical management of chordoma is en bloc resection with as wide a margin of normal tissue as possible. Surgery to remove chordomas is quite challenging and fraught with complications. The risks of infection, wound-healing problems, blood loss, and injury to local structures are high during these complex cases.

Our surgical approach was described in detail in a previous publication (Bohinski and Rhines 2003). Although techniques for resecting spinal tumors en bloc have improved significantly in the last two decades (Boriani et al. 1996; Tomita et al. 1997; Marmor et al. 2001), these operations remain technically demanding and require a high degree of training and experience on the part of the surgical team. The spine surgeon performing en bloc resection of chordomas of the spine must be knowledgeable about the spinal and paraspinal anatomy. The team should also include a surgical oncologist, a vascular surgeon, a plastic surgeon, an orthopedic surgeon, and, when appropriate, a neurologist. The value of a multidisciplinary surgical approach to these tumors cannot be overemphasized (Bohinski and Rhines 2003).

With respect to chordoma, en bloc resection with negative margins, either marginal or wide, offers the patient the best chance at prolonged disease-free survival and the only chance at surgical cure. An increasing number of surgical series have demonstrated better outcomes with en bloc resection than with intralesional techniques (Rich et al. 1985; Tomita et al. 1997; York et al. 1999; Boriani et al. 2000, 2006). As noted previously (Bohinski and Rhines 2003), in some cases, the anatomic arrangement of the tumor may necessitate some intralesional dissection, which will result in partially contaminated surgical margins; in such circumstances, en bloc resection may result in better outcomes than intralesional resection alone (Boriani et al. 1996; Tomita et al. 1997).

In most cases of chordoma, the tumor has not metastasized at the time of diagnosis. Obviously, in the case of metastatic disease, the role of en bloc resection for potential cure or prolongation of disease-free survival becomes less critical. Once it is determined through chest CT and bone scans that a tumor represents a solitary site of disease within the spine, the tumor imaging is rigorously evaluated in order to plan a method of en bloc resection, including the osteotomies and soft tissue dissection that will be required. Part of this rigorous planning is assessing the involvement of paraspinal structures, including the viscera and vascular structures that are adjacent to the spine. Moreover, involvement of the nerve roots must also be assessed. To achieve an en bloc resection with negative margins, it may be necessary to resect portions of the visceral and vascular structures, as well as neurological elements. The patient must be counseled accordingly. As an example, it is not uncommon when operating on chordomas of the sacrum to sacrifice the sacral nerve roots that run through the tumor, in an effort to achieve an en bloc resection.

Although such nerve root loss may cost the patient significant bowel, bladder, and sexual function, it may be necessary in order to offer the potential for cure. These trade-offs must be discussed openly with the patient over several visits, and ultimately the patient must be comfortable with the consequences of the proposed operation. It is our experience that if these sacrifices are not made at the time of the initial surgery, then the tumor is much more likely to recur, and when it does, it is likely to cause the very complications that we tried to avoid.

Chordomas of the Mobile Spine

As noted previously (Bohinski and Rhines 2003), to safely remove a vertebral body in an en bloc fashion, the surgeon must resect the vertebral arch either across one pedicle and the contralateral lamina or across both pedicles to completely free the posterior element complex from the dural tube. The resultant gap in the ring of the spine should allow release of the dural tube during en bloc resection of the diseased vertebra.

We utilize the Weinstein–Boriani–Biagini (WBB) system (Boriani et al. 1997), originally described for staging spinal tumors, during our preoperative planning for en bloc resection of chordoma in the mobile spine. In this system, the spine is divided into 12 radiating zones and 5 concentric layers. By superimposing the tumor geometry upon the WBB diagram, the optimum location for vertebral osteotomies can be selected. Use of this system not only aids surgical planning but also facilitates communication.

En bloc resection is usually performed using a posterior approach followed by an anterior approach (Bohinski and Rhines 2003). Tumors with extensive involvement of the paraspinal structures (either the psoas muscle in lumbar spine cases or the chest wall in thoracic spine cases) may require a simultaneous two-pronged approach to allow direct visualization of the posterior, lateral, and anterior aspects of the spine at the same time. In the thoracic spine, where the nerve roots are expendable, Tomita et al. (1997) have described an approach by which the vertebra can be removed in en bloc fashion entirely from a posterior approach.

Chordomas of the Sacrum

Chordomas of the sacrum are considered separately from chordomas of the mobile spine because of significant differences in anatomy and approach. Understanding the anatomy, particularly the course of the lumbosacral nerve roots and the relationship of the tumor to the iliac vessels, ureters, and rectum, is requisite to performing surgery in this complex and hazardous region. A combination of surgical approaches is often employed to expose the sacrum. These may include posterior, anterior, transperineal, and lateral retroperitoneal planes of dissection. Because of the large size that tumors may attain (Fig. 8.1) and the length of time needed for surgery, the operations are sometimes staged in two or even more different settings.

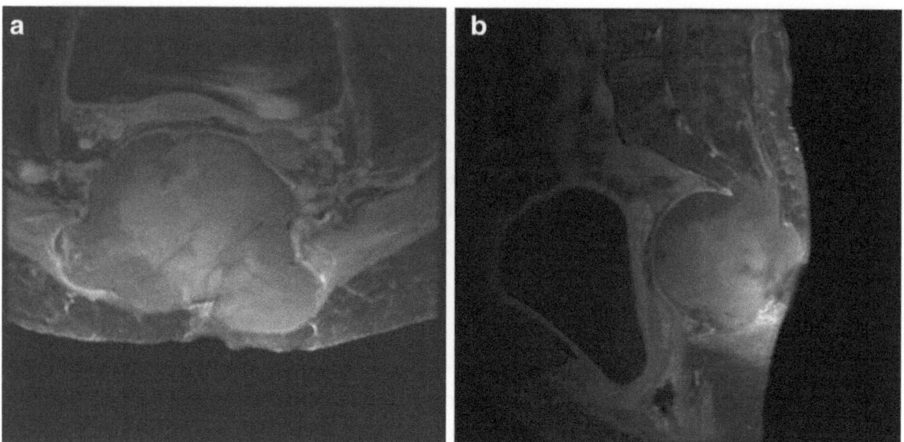

Fig. 8.1 Chordoma. (**a**) T1 axial and (**b**) sagittal images of a large sacral tumor.

In our experience, low (S3 and below) and mid (S2–S3) sacral amputations can be performed entirely from a posterior approach. The dorsal exposure is extended inferiorly beyond the tip of the coccyx, and, via a Kraske approach, the levator ani muscles can be taken down, and a plane can be created between the posterior aspect of the rectum and the ventral aspect of the sacrum and tumor. This strategy allows the anterior aspect of the tumor to be palpated, and the sacral amputation can be guided by this tactile feedback. With the rectum protected and the superior aspect of the tumor identified, the osteotomies and soft tissue dissection necessary for en bloc resection can be performed entirely from a posterior approach.

Spinal stabilization is generally not necessary with mid or low sacral resections. Obviously, sacral amputation performed at the mid S1 level or higher raises concerns regarding the mechanical stability of the lumbosacral junction. In these cases, the resection generally needs to be supplemented with an extensive lumbopelvic spinal stabilization and arthrodesis.

For high and total sacrectomies, we utilize a staged approach beginning with an anterior operation. This transperitoneal approach is necessary to free the more superior aspects of the rectum, mobilize the lumbosacral trunks, and divide the internal iliac vessels so that these structures can be protected in anticipation of the osteotomies created in the second-stage posterior procedure. The other benefit of the anterior approach is to provide a source of soft tissue coverage. Resection of a large portion of the sacrum can leave a sizable soft tissue defect, and we rely on our plastic surgeons to mobilize soft tissues to fill this defect. The smaller defects created during low and mid sacral amputations can typically be filled using local advancement flaps, including advancement of the gluteal muscles or posterior thigh flaps. The larger defects created through high sacral amputation or total sacrectomy require larger soft tissue reconstruction. In these cases, a vertical rectus abdominis myocutaneous (VRAM) flap can be harvested during the anterior

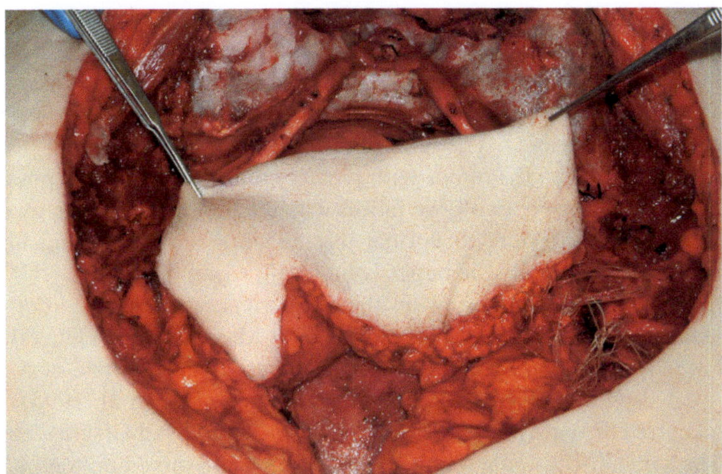

Fig. 8.2 Chordoma resection and reconstruction. This intraoperative photograph shows the resected sacrum edge, the S1 nerve roots lateral to the sacrum, and the tied-off cauda equina. The VRAM flap is in the foreground.

approach, maintained on its pedicle, placed into the pelvis, and then retrieved during the second-stage operation following removal of the sacral tumor. It can then be used to reconstruct the defect (Fig. 8.2).

Radiation Therapy

As described above, the first-line modality for definitive management of chordoma is wide excision. However, complete resection of these tumors can often be difficult given their location (when they occur in the base of the skull) or their size (when they occur in the sacral region). Because of the infiltrative nature of these tumors and their close proximity to critical structures, residual tumor is often unavoidable after surgery. Such residual disease almost invariably leads to recurrence. Tumor spillage during surgery can also increase the risk of local recurrence. In such cases, radiation therapy can be useful in combination with surgery to optimize local control or to increase the time interval to recurrence. Neoadjuvant radiation therapy can be employed in some cases if positive margins are expected after surgery or to reduce the risk of intraoperative tumor spillage. More commonly, radiation therapy follows surgery, either adjuvantly or at first relapse. Decisions regarding the use and timing of radiation therapy require discussion between the radiation oncologist and the treating surgeon.

For radiation treatment planning for tumors in the base of the skull, diagnostic CT and MRI are recommended to evaluate the extent of tumor. Three-dimensional CT–based planning is essential to delivering radiation therapy for these tumors.

Relatively high doses of radiation therapy are needed to control local disease. Conventional photon irradiation techniques often preclude delivery of an adequate dose to the tumor because of resultant unacceptably high doses to adjacent critical normal structures. Multiple centers now offer mixed proton- and photon-beam radiation therapy for chordoma. The addition of protons to the radiation plan allows delivery of high doses to the tumor with greater conformality than is possible with photons because of sharper exit-dose falloff with the proton beam. The mixed-beam approach decreases exposure to normal tissues while still delivering high-linear energy transfer irradiation to the target volume.

Multiple centers have reported on their experience treating chordomas using proton-beam irradiation. Clinical investigators at Massachusetts General Hospital reported a 53% local control rate and a 50% overall survival rate at 5 years for patients treated with mixed proton/photon irradiation (Hug et al. 1995). All local failures occurred in patients who received less than 77 cobalt gray equivalents (CGE). The same institution's report on outcomes using mixed proton/photon irradiation for sacral chordomas recommended 70.2 CGE in cases of microscopically negative margins after surgery, 73.8 CGE for microscopically positive margins, and 77.4 CGE for gross disease (Park et al. 2006). Acute and late toxic effects from these series showed that the high-dose, mixed-beam radiation therapy was well tolerated. Other investigators have confirmed the safety and efficacy of these doses using mixed proton/photon irradiation in both base-of-skull and sacral chordomas (Igaki et al. 2004; Noel et al. 2005; Weber et al. 2005). Consideration should be given to referring patients with chordoma to one of the growing number of cancer centers with proton therapy capabilities, if feasible.

Stereotactic fractionated radiation therapy has also been studied as a potential treatment modality for base-of-skull chordomas (Debus et al. 2000). The reported 5-year local control rate was 50% with a median dose to isocenter of 66.6 Gy. The outcomes in this small series reinforce the importance of a high radiation dose for local control. No study has compared stereotactic photon irradiation to proton-beam therapy for chordoma. In all radiation treatment planning, tolerance doses of critical normal structures should be respected to minimize acute and long-term toxicity.

Adamantinoma

Adamantinomas are rare tumors of bone; they account for less than 1% of primary malignant bone tumors (Unni 1996; Qureshi et al. 2000). This tumor has a male predominance (male-to-female ratio, 3:2) and is most common in the third and fourth decades of life. These tumors most commonly occur in the lower extremity, with more than 90% of cases found in the tibia.

Radiographically, adamantinomas have a characteristic appearance. They tend to be cortical bone–based lesions in the mid-diaphysis of the tibia (Fig. 8.3). They are typically multilocular lytic lesions with well-defined margins that give the lesion a "soap bubble" appearance (Mori et al. 1981; Moon and Mori 1986). They tend to

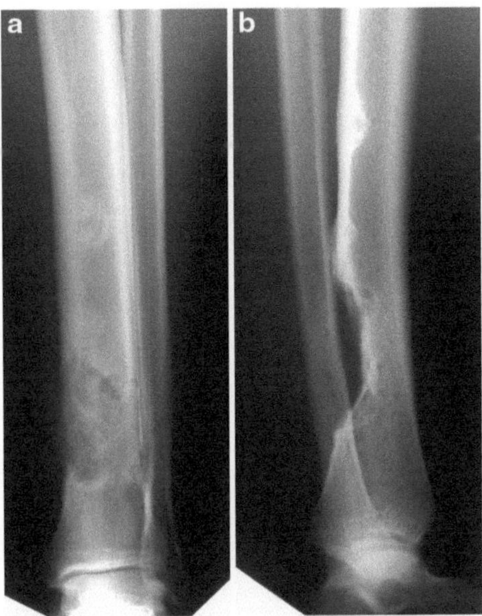

Fig. 8.3 Adamantinoma. (**a**) Anteroposterior and (**b**) lateral radiographs of a tibial adamantinoma. Note the cortically based lesion with a sclerotic border.

expand into the medullary canal with a thinned outer cortex, and periosteal reaction tends to be absent.

Histologically, adamantinomas consist of nests of epithelial or epithelioid cells surrounded by a fibrous stroma (Unni 1996). The tumors contain two cell populations: neoplastic, cytokeratin-positive epithelial cells and bland, spindled cells. Several histologic variants of classic adamantinoma have been described, including tubular, basaloid, squamous, and spindled variants (Dorfman and Czerniak 1997). These variants are based on the appearance, orientation, and architecture of the epithelial cells. Mitotic activity is usually low. The differential diagnosis for adamantinoma includes metastatic carcinoma, vascular neoplasms, fibrous dysplasia, osteofibrous dysplasia, and malignant mixed tumor of the bone. The diagnosis is reached in a multidisciplinary manner using radiologic and clinical assessment in combination with the histologic findings.

On the whole, adamantinomas are slow-growing tumors with a limited propensity for metastasis and local recurrence. If treated appropriately, patients with adamantinomas have an excellent prognosis (Qureshi et al. 2000). The tumors are radioresistant, and chemotherapy has not been shown to be effective for primary localized disease. Surgical resection is the treatment of choice. The operative treatment depends on the extent and location of the lesion; options are amputation and en bloc resection with wide margins (Campanacci et al. 1981; Gebhardt et al. 1987; Qureshi et al. 2000) (Fig. 8.4). The 10-year survival rate has been noted to be

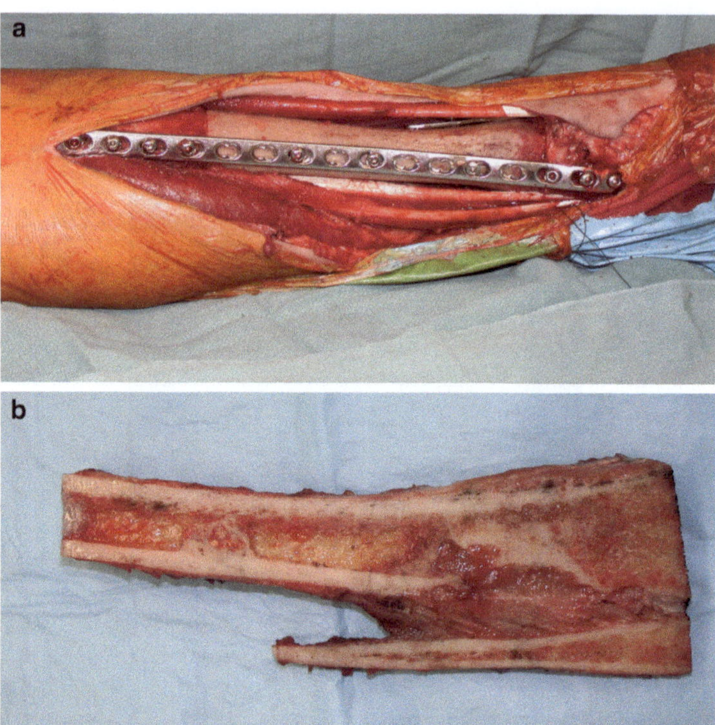

Fig. 8.4 Adamantinoma resection and reconstruction. (**a**) Intraoperative photograph of a reconstruction with an intercalary allograft after resection of an adamantinoma. (**b**) The resected specimen. Note the cortically based lesion.

80–90% (Qureshi et al. 2000). Negative margins are associated with a significantly lower risk of local recurrence. Some studies have found that male sex, pain at presentation, and duration of symptoms of less than 5 years are associated with an increased risk of recurrence or metastatic disease (Keeney et al. 1989; Hazelbag et al. 1994).

Hemangioendothelioma

Hemangioendothelioma has become a catch-all term for vascular tumors that have biologic activity between that of hemangioma and conventional angiosarcoma. There are several subtypes, with epithelioid hemangioendothelioma being the most common. Still, these tumors are quite rare, representing less than 1% of all primary tumors of bone. They occur most commonly in the second and third decades of life. A distinct male predominance (male-to-female ratio, approximately 2:1) has been reported (Weiss and Enzinger 1982; Tsuneyoshi et al. 1986; Ignacio et al. 1999).

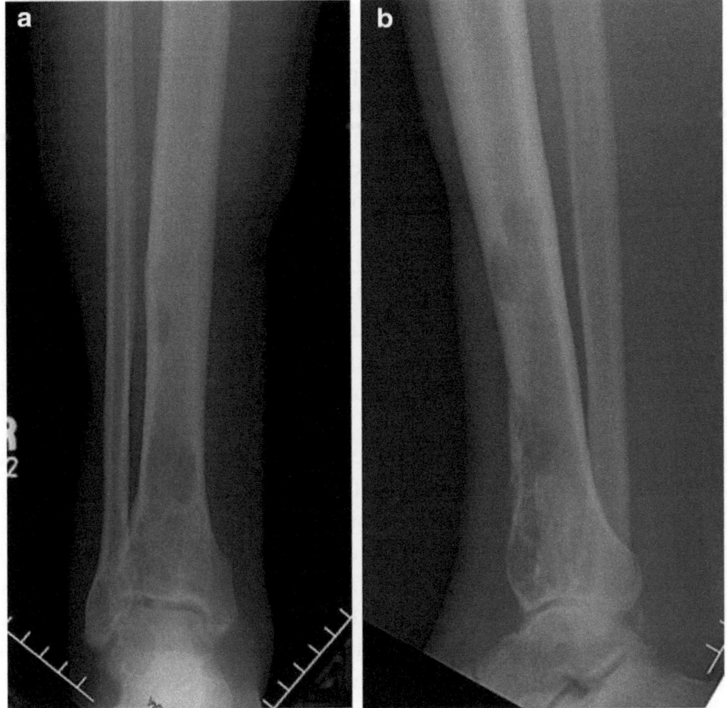

Fig. 8.5 Hemangioendothelioma of bone. (**a**) Anteroposterior and (**b**) lateral radiographs of a multifocal hemangioendothelioma. Note the multiple lesions in the tibia and talus.

Epithelioid hemangioendothelioma has been classified as an intermediate-grade lesion. These tumors can be locally aggressive, and they tend to recur locally but have a low rate of metastasis (Campanacci et al. 1980; Wold et al. 1982). They most commonly occur in the calvarium, the axial skeleton, and the long bones of the lower limbs, with the tibia and femur most frequently involved (Ignacio et al. 1999). More than 50% of cases are multifocal, and homolateral skeletal involvement is commonly noted. The lesions can also involve the lung, liver, and spleen, and as such it is recommended that patients with this diagnosis be thoroughly evaluated with CT of the chest, abdomen, and pelvis and a bone scan. If multifocal lesions are noted on the bone scan, a skeletal survey should be obtained as well.

Radiographically, the lesions classically appear as multifocal lytic lesions that tend to involve a single anatomic region or extremity (Kleer et al. 1996; Adler et al. 2005) (Fig. 8.5). A periosteal reaction is commonly seen; however, cortical destruction and cortical expansion are rare. Soft tissue masses can be seen in up to 40% of cases. In patients in their second and third decades, the differential diagnosis consists of Langerhans cell histiocytosis, giant cell tumor, fibrous dysplasia, and lymphoma; in later decades, metastatic carcinoma and myeloma disease are also considered (Tillman et al. 1997). The definitive diagnosis of epithelioid hemangio-endothelioma is often difficult to make on the basis of radiologic findings alone. Therefore, a final diagnosis requires histopathologic analysis.

Histologically, epithelioid hemangioendothelioma is typified by solid nests or cords of epithelial-like cells and prominent endothelial-lined vascular spaces surrounded by proliferating tumor cells (Wold et al. 1982). These tumors also may have intravascular papillary-like projections with epithelial or histiocyte-like cells (Tillman et al. 1997).

Epithelioid hemangioendothelioma of bone has a variable presentation and clinical course. Its clinical course can resemble those of a range of tumors, from the benign epithelioid hemangioma to the malignant angiosarcoma. Unfortunately, its behavior cannot be predicted on the basis of the radiographic and histologic features alone. However, systemic involvement appears to confer a worse prognosis (Kleer et al. 1996).

Since the presentation and clinical course of this disease are variable, the definitive treatment is not standardized; it ranges from wide resection to curettage to radiofrequency ablation. Multifocal lesions are especially amenable to curettage and/or radiofrequency ablation (Ignacio et al. 1999; Kleer et al. 1996; Gosheger et al. 2002; Rosenthal et al. 2001). Radiofrequency ablation has recently been used successfully in combination with surgical resection in order to limit the extent of surgery and spare the patient an amputation. Radiation therapy can be considered when these tumors appear in weight-bearing bones or vertebral bodies or are widely distributed in the skeleton or foot (Wold et al. 1982; Faria et al. 1985; Welles et al. 1994). The use of radiation as an adjuvant to surgery has been advocated; however, it has also been used as the sole modality in patients with unresectable lesions and/or metastatic disease. With 45–50 Gy given over 4.5–5 weeks, at least 75% of such patients can achieve symptomatic control (Faria et al. 1985). The role of chemotherapy for this disease is not clear (Haisley-Royster et al. 2002). Although vincristine was shown to be efficacious in the treatment of kaposiform hemangioendothelioma, chemotherapy is not recommended for primary epithelioid hemangioendothelioma. Whether it has a role in metastatic disease is still under investigation. Overall, because of the disease's variability, the treatment regimen for epithelioid hemangioendothelioma should be individualized.

Hemangiopericytoma

Hemangiopericytoma is a rare tumor of vascular origin that most commonly occurs in the soft tissues (Conway and Hayes 1993). Primary hemangiopericytoma of bone is very rare. It represents 0.08% of primary bone tumors and 0.1% of primary vascular bone tumors (Mirra 1989). These tumors have been reported in patients ranging from 12 to 90 years of age, with the peak incidence in the fourth and fifth decades. Hemangiopericytoma of bone can occur in any location; however, the most common sites have been the sacroiliac region, the femur, and the temporal bone.

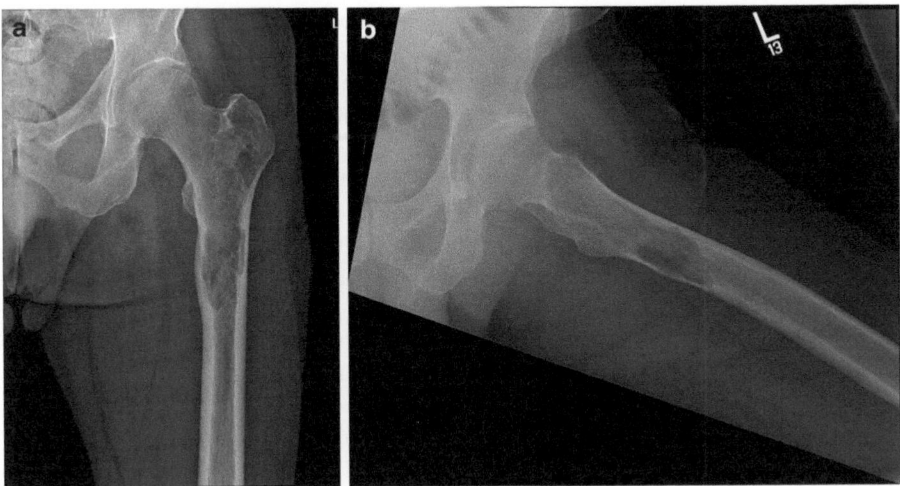

Fig. 8.6 Hemangiopericytoma of bone. (**a**) Anteroposterior and (**b**) lateral radiographs of a proximal femur. This is an osteolytic lesion, originating in the metaphyseal regions of a long bone, that marginally expands the bone but without periosteal reaction.

The presentation of hemangiopericytoma is nonspecific. The most common presenting symptoms are pain and swelling, and because osseous hemangiopericytoma is generally very slow growing, the complaints can be present for significant periods of time (even years) (Tang et al. 1988). Hypophosphatemic osteomalacia has been described in association with hemangiopericytoma of bone.

Radiographic findings of hemangiopericytomas are nonspecific. The tumors appear as osteolytic lesions originating in the metaphyseal regions of long bones. They may expand bone, but periosteal reaction and reactive sclerosis are rare (Conway and Hayes 1993) (Fig. 8.6). The radiologic differential diagnosis of the more benign-appearing tumors includes giant cell tumor, aneurysmal bone cyst, chondromyxoid fibroma, and fibrous dysplasia, while that of the more malignant-appearing tumors includes metastasis, fibrosarcoma, plasmacytoma, and angiosarcoma. In general, the radiologic diagnosis is made by exclusion.

Angiographically, hemangiopericytoma of bone has pathognomonic features: one to two feeding arteries that branch about the tumor into small and large radially arranged vessels with a "spider-shaped" appearance (Juan et al. 2000). An angiogram of the tumor reveals a well-demarcated round or oval tumor stain.

Histologically, hemangiopericytoma of bone is identical to soft tissue hemangiopericytoma. The characteristic features include: (1) sheets of spindle-like cells surrounding numerous capillaries, (2) monotonous round to oval nuclei that lack atypia, (3) indistinct cytoplasmic borders, and (4) on silver staining, a visible reticulin sheath surrounding each tumor cell outside the capillary walls (Tang et al. 1988). The histologic differential diagnosis includes mesenchymal chondrosarcoma, benign fibrous histiocytoma and MFH, and synovial sarcoma.

It has been suggested that every hemangiopericytoma of bone should be considered malignant; however, the degree of malignant potential varies from case to case. The 5-year survival rate is approximately 60% (Tang et al. 1988). The clinical behavior of hemangiopericytoma is difficult to predict; however, histologic features such as the mitotic index and the degree of cellularity, hemorrhage, and necrosis seem to correlate with the prognosis (Enzinger and Smith 1976). High-grade malignant hemangiopericytomas of bone are associated with high recurrence rates and the development of metastatic disease, while low-grade lesions have a low propensity to metastasize and thus a high survival rate. Outcome is directly related to the occurrence of metastatic disease and the adequacy of local control. Growth of the metastases may be slow or extremely rapid, with death ensuing in a matter of months. Late recurrences and distant metastases are common (Tang et al. 1988; Sahin-Akyar et al. 1997).

The definitive treatment for hemangiopericytoma of bone is primarily surgical (Tang et al. 1988; Ferigo et al. 2006; Heymans et al. 1997). The extent of the surgical treatment can be tailored to the grade of the lesion. Low-grade malignant lesions are amenable to curettage and bone grafting, while high-grade lesions are treated with wide surgical resection. When wide resection is not possible, it has been suggested that a compromise can be made between the optimal treatment for cure and the optimal treatment for function (Sahin-Akyar et al. 1997).

In inoperable cases, radiation can also be a treatment option. Adjuvant radiation therapy has been shown to have a role in the treatment of both primary and recurrent hemangiopericytoma. Radiation doses higher than 50 Gy are required for local disease control. The optimal role of chemotherapy is debatable. It may be employed in the presence of metastatic disease. Although there have only been a few relevant trials, doxorubicin alone or in combination with dacarbazine appears to be the most effective agent (Ferigo et al. 2006; Celik et al. 1997; Heymans et al. 1997).

Low-Grade Fibrosarcoma

Fibrosarcoma of bone is a rare malignant neoplasm. Since the establishment of MFH of bone as a distinct entity, the frequency of the diagnosis of fibrosarcoma has declined (Dorfman and Czerniak 1997). Essentially, the term *low-grade fibrosarcoma* refers to lesions previously or traditionally classified as grade 1 or 2 fibrosarcoma. The clinical and radiographic differential diagnosis for this tumor type includes desmoplastic fibroma, MFH, and fibroblastic osteosarcoma (Taconis and Mulder 1984; Dorfman and Czerniak 1997; Saito et al. 2003).

Plain radiographs reveal an expanding multilobular osteolytic lesion with well-defined borders. This often gives the lesion a "soap bubble" appearance. The lesions are most commonly located in the metaphysis of long bones. Periosteal reaction is rare. Soft tissue extension is common and can be associated with mineralization of the mass. The most common locations are the distal femur, proximal tibia, pelvis, proximal femur, and humerus. In the long bones, these lesions tend to be based in the metaphysis and often extend into the epiphysis. The age and sex distributions for the disease are uniform (Bertoni et al. 1984).

On gross examination, the cut surface of the tumor appears grayish white. Histologically, the tumor is composed of both cellular and hypocellular areas. The cellular areas contain a proliferation of bundles of uniform fibroblastic spindle-shaped cells with minimal cellular atypia and abundant intercellular collagen. A herringbone or storiform pattern can be observed. Pleomorphism is lacking, and rare mitotic figures can be present, but atypical ones are not seen. The hypocellular areas have myxoid features and loose bundles of collagen fibers. No osteoid formation is seen. Histologically, well-differentiated osteosarcoma and desmoplastic fibroma need to be ruled out.

The long-term prognosis for patients with low-grade fibrosarcoma is good. The definitive treatment is similar to that of other low-grade osseous sarcomas: wide surgical excision. Adjuvant chemotherapy has little role. Wide resection and reconstruction have resulted in a 10-year survival rate of 83% (Bertoni et al. 1984). In the face of disease-negative margins, the incidence of metastasis and local recurrence is low. However, as for most primary tumors of bone, long-term follow-up is warranted.

Malignant Fibrous Histiocytoma

Clinical Features

Unlike the previous entities discussed in this chapter, MFH is an aggressive, high-grade, malignant primary tumor of bone. MFH of bone is a relatively recently recognized entity that comprises less than 5% of all bone tumors. It is a distinct clinicopathologic entity from other sarcomas of bone, as well as from its soft tissue counterpart (Dahlin et al. 1977; Nishida et al. 1997).

MFH of bone is seen with fairly equal frequency in men and women; however, there seems to be a slight predominance in men. The age distribution is broad, but patients are generally older than those with osteosarcoma. MFH is more common in adults, particularly those in the fifth to seventh decades of life (Dahlin and Unni 1986; Nishida et al. 1997).

Diagnostic Workup and Staging

The most common clinical symptom of MFH of bone on presentation is pain, with or without swelling or a mass; other symptoms and signs depend on the location of the lesion and can include limping, deformity, joint stiffness, and proptosis. The lesions tend to be metaphyseal. The most common sites of involvement are the metaphyseal

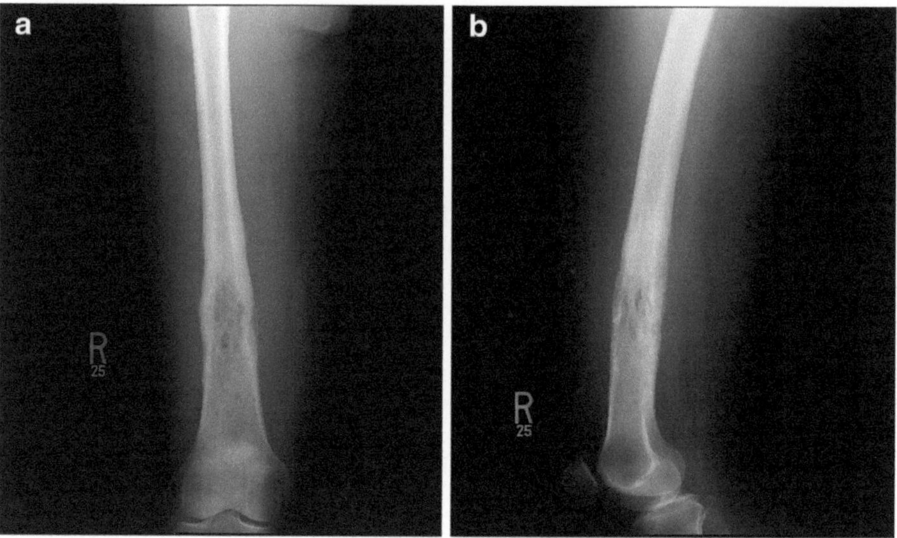

Fig. 8.7 MFH of bone. (**a**) Anteroposterior and (**b**) lateral radiographs of the distal femur. Note the permeative pattern of bone destruction, ill-defined lesion borders, and wide zone of transition from normal to abnormal bone.

regions of the distal femur, proximal tibia, and proximal femur (Nishida et al. 1997). The most common site of metastasis is the lung (82%) (Dahlin and Unni 1986).

Radiographically, the tumor appears aggressive, with a permeative pattern of bone destruction, ill-defined lesion margins, and a wide zone of transition from normal to abnormal bone (Capanna et al. 1984; Huvos et al. 1985; Nishida et al. 1997) (Fig. 8.7). Extensive destruction of the cortical bone is often seen on the radiographs. Periosteal reactions are irregular, and matrix calcifications are rarely present.

Many authors have described MFH of bone occurring in preexisting bone lesions. Up to 20% of MFHs are secondary, occurring in patients with preexisting benign conditions such as bone infarcts, Paget disease, and fibrous dysplasia (Huvos et al. 1985; Schuh et al. 2004). In addition, in several cases, MFH of bone has developed at the site of an endoprosthesis (Troop et al. 1990; Cole et al. 1997; Schuh et al. 2004), and a review of the literature revealed that 20–28% of MFHs of bone occur after radiation therapy (Mirra et al. 1974; Capanna et al. 1984; Huvos et al. 1985).

Not infrequently, MFH of bone appears to constitute the high-grade component of a dedifferentiated chondrosarcoma. In addition, MFH can often be a component of osteosarcomas. Histologically, this entity shows striking resemblance to MFH arising in soft tissues. MFH is a poorly differentiated neoplasm with often strongly pleomorphic and hyperchromatic nuclei. This basic tumor cell most likely derives from primitive mesenchymal cells such as fibroblast precursor cells. It has areas of fibrogenic differentiation (often in a storiform pattern) or areas of histiocytes and anaplastic giant cells (Dahlin et al. 1977; Capanna et al. 1984; Huvos et al. 1985; Bertoni et al. 1985). It can usually be classified as either storiform-pleomorphic or histiocytic based on the predominance of one of the patterns; these patterns were seen in 63% and 19%, respectively, of 81 patients in a study at the Mayo Clinic (Nishida et al. 1997).

Histologically, it may be difficult to distinguish MFH of bone from fibroblastic osteosarcoma. The only major difference between the two is the presence or absence of osteoid, with osteoid tumor formation favoring the diagnosis of osteosarcoma. Therefore, MFH of bone may well be part of a spectrum of osteosarcomas, in which the spindle cells do not produce osteoid visible by light microscopy but have the capability to do so at some time in the future. Cases have been documented in which the initial biopsy and the final surgical specimen were believed to be MFH, but the metastatic disease that developed later unequivocally demonstrated osteoid, lending credence to the hypothesis that MFH of bone may indeed be a variant of fibroblastic osteosarcoma. Interestingly enough, the natural histories of these two entities, including their overall survival rates, seem comparable.

Like osteosarcoma, MFH of bone also exhibits a lung-dominant metastatic pattern. The staging studies for suspected MFH are therefore identical to those described for osteosarcoma in Chap. 5.

Treatment

MFH of bone is managed under the same guiding principles as those used for osteosarcoma. Patients are therefore treated with primary chemotherapy (four cycles) followed by surgical resection and postoperative chemotherapy based on the amount of necrosis observed in response to the preoperative therapy.

Most patients described in the literature have been treated surgically, either with wide excision or amputation (Capanna et al. 1984; Bacci et al. 1997; Nishida et al. 1997; Picci et al. 1997). The prognosis is best for tumors treated with chemotherapy and wide resection with negative margins. In the Mayo Clinic study described above, the 1-, 5-, and 10-year disease-free survival rates were 72.8%, 66.5%, and 60.9%, respectively, if adequate margins were taken, compared with 59.8%, 48.3%, and 26.4% if the margins were positive for disease (Nishida et al. 1997). As for most high-grade lesions of bone, the extent and type of resection and reconstruction are predicated on the location of the tumor and its response to chemotherapy. However, since wide margins are the goal of surgical treatment, curettage has no role in the treatment of MFH.

Initially, radiation therapy was thought to marginally improve the prognosis for patients with tumors excised with inadequate margins. However, the role of radiation therapy has since been minimized because of lack of supporting data.

Without chemotherapy, the prognosis of bone MFH is poor, with a 5-year survival rate of 15% (Dunham and Wilborn 1979). With the addition of neoadjuvant chemotherapy, selected series have shown significantly improved disease-free survival rates (Bacci et al. 1997; Picci et al. 1997; Bielack et al. 1999). Outcomes reported by three groups are described below.

The MD Anderson Experience

Comparing surgery plus postoperative adjuvant chemotherapy ($n=24$) with surgery alone ($n=36$, historical controls), investigators from our institution found a statistically significant advantage in continuous disease-free survival (CDFS) with chemotherapy (median 24 months vs. 8 months, $P=0.001$, unpublished data). We have since reviewed our experience with preoperative doxorubicin and cisplatin in patients with localized MFH. Approximately 50% of patients achieved necrosis of at least 90% of tumor. Survival data computed based on Kaplan–Meier life table analysis revealed that the median CDFS duration for all patients was 19 months and the median overall survival was 23 months. The median CDFS for patients with at least 90% tumor necrosis (43 months) was superior to that of patients with less than 90% necrosis (7 months). This difference is statistically significant ($P<0.05$, one-sided log-rank test). The median overall survival for the group with at least 90% necrosis was 66 months, while that for the group with less than 90% necrosis was 20 months (unpublished data).

The Rizzoli Institute Experience

Investigators at the Rizzoli Institute reported their experience in 65 patients with MFH of extremity (bone) treated between 1983 and 1994 on 1 of 4 different protocols utilizing various combinations of the standard chemotherapy drugs for osteosarcomas, including doxorubicin, cisplatin, methotrexate, and ifosfamide (Bacci et al. 1998). Twenty-five percent of patients achieved at least 90% tumor necrosis, and 89% had a limb-sparing operation. At a median follow-up of 7 years, 69% remained continuously disease-free. The CDFS rate of patients with at least 90% tumor necrosis (94%) was higher than that of patients with less than 90% tumor necrosis (61%).

The European Osteosarcoma Intergroup Experience

In a European Osteosarcoma Intergroup study, 41 patients with primary bone MFH in the extremity were treated with doxorubicin (75 mg/m^2) and cisplatin (100 mg/m^2) for three cycles preoperatively and three additional cycles postoperatively (Bramwell et al. 1999). Fifty-six percent of patients completed all six cycles. Forty-two percent of patients achieved 90% or greater tumor necrosis, and 80% underwent limb-sparing surgery. The median time to progression was 56 months. The 5-year progression-free survival and overall survival rates were 56% and 59%, respectively. Patients with a good histologic response had a longer time to progression and overall survival than did poor responders.

Key Practice Points

- The lesions discussed in this chapter have variable presentations and clinical courses.
- Wide resection and reconstruction offer the best prognosis for the treatment of these primary lesions of bone.
- For the low-grade tumors, adjuvant therapy in the form of radiation or chemotherapy is generally relegated to the treatment of recurrent or metastatic disease.
- Chordomas, which favor the sacrum or sphenoocciput, present formidable surgical challenges and often require the collaborative efforts of multiple surgical specialists for safe excision with wide margins.
- Adamantinomas are keratin-positive, sometimes multilocular tumors of the tibia that are usually amenable to limb-sparing wide surgical excision.
- Hemangioendothelioma is a term that encompasses a spectrum of vascular tumors with varying degrees of biological aggressiveness; they are treated with a variety of different modalities.
- Low-grade fibrosarcomas are composed of fibroblast-like cells and are treated by surgery alone.
- MFH is an aggressive, high-grade tumor considered by some to be a variant of fibrosarcoma or fibroblastic osteosarcoma. Treatment consists of preoperative chemotherapy followed by surgical resection and postoperative chemotherapy based on the treatment response.

Suggested Readings

Adler B, Naheedy J, Yeager N, et al. Multifocal epithelioid hemangioendothelioma in a 16-year-old boy. Pediatr Radiol. 2005;35:1014–8.

Bacci G, Ferrari S, Bertoni F, et al. Neoadjuvant chemotherapy for osseous malignant fibrous histiocytoma of the extremity: results in 18 cases and comparison with 112 contemporary osteosarcoma patients treated with the same chemotherapy regimen. J Chemother. 1997;9:293–9.

Bacci G, Picci P, Mercuri M, Bertoni F, Ferrari S. Neoadjuvant chemotherapy for high grade malignant fibrous histiocytoma of bone. Clin Orthop Relat Res. 1998;346:178–89.

Bergh P, Kindblom LG, Gunterberg B, Remotti F, Ryd W, Meis-Kindblom JM. Prognostic factors in chordoma of the sacrum and mobile spine: a study of 39 patients. Cancer. 2000;88:2122–34.

Bertoni F, Capanna R, Biagini R, et al. Malignant fibrous histiocytoma of soft tissue. An analysis of 78 cases located and deeply seated in the extremities. Cancer. 1985;56:356–67.

Bertoni F, Capanna R, Calderoni P, et al. Primary central (medullary) fibrosarcoma of bone. Semin Diagn Pathol. 1984;1:185–98.

Bielack SS, Schroeders A, Fuchs N, et al. Malignant fibrous histiocytoma of bone: a retrospective EMSOS study of 125 cases. European Musculo-Skeletal Oncology Society. Acta Orthop Scand. 1999;70:353–60.

Bohinski RJ, Rhines LD. Principles and techniques of en bloc vertebrectomy for bone tumors of the thoracolumbar spine: an overview. Neurosurg Focus. 2003;15:E7.

Boriani S, Bandiera S, Biagini R, et al. Chordoma of the mobile spine: fifty years of experience. Spine. 2006;31:493–503.

Boriani S, Biagini R, De Iure F, et al. En bloc resections of bone tumors of the thoracolumbar spine. A preliminary report on 29 patients. Spine. 1996;21:1927–31.

Boriani S, De Iure F, Bandiera S, et al. Chondrosarcoma of the mobile spine: report on 22 cases. Spine. 2000;25:804–12.

Boriani S, Weinstein JN, Biagini R. Primary bone tumors of the spine. Terminology and surgical staging. Spine. 1997;22:1036–44.

Bramwell VH, Steward WP, Nooij M, et al. Neoadjuvant chemotherapy with doxorubicin and cisplatin in malignant fibrous histiocytoma of bone: a European Osteosarcoma Intergroup study. J Clin Oncol. 1999;17:3260–9.

Campanacci M, Boriani S, Giunti A. Hemangioendothelioma of bone. Cancer. 1980;46:804–14.

Campanacci M, Giunti A, Bertoni F, et al. Adamantinoma of the long bones. The experience at the Istituto Ortopedico Rizzoli. Am J Surg Pathol. 1981;5:533–42.

Capanna R, Bertoni F, Bacchini P, et al. Malignant fibrous histiocytoma of bone. The experience at the Rizzoli Institute: report of 90 cases. Cancer. 1984;54:177–87.

Celik I, Bascil N, Yalcin S, et al. Ifosfamide-based chemotherapy for recurrent or metastatic hemangiopericytoma. Acta Oncol. 1997;36:348.

Cole BJ, Schultz E, Smilari TF, et al. Malignant fibrous histiocytoma at the site of a total hip replacement: review of the literature and case report. Skeletal Radiol. 1997;26:559–63.

Conway WF, Hayes CW. Miscellaneous lesions of bone. Radiol Clin North Am. 1993;31:339–58.

Dahlin DC, Unni KK. Bone tumors. 4th ed. Springfield: Charles C. Thomas; 1986. p. 357–65.

Dahlin DC, Unni KK, Matsuno T. Malignant (fibrous) histiocytoma of bone—fact or fancy? Cancer. 1977;39:1508–16.

Debus J, Schulz-Ertner D, Schad L, et al. Stereotactic fractionated radiotherapy for chordomas and chondrosarcomas of the skull base. Int J Radiat Oncol Biol Phys. 2000;47:591–6.

Dorfman HD, Czerniak B. Bone tumors. St. Louis: Mosby; 1997.

Dunham WK, Wilborn WH. Malignant fibrous histiocytoma of bone. Report of two cases and review of the literature. J Bone Joint Surg Am. 1979;61:939–42.

Enneking WF. A system of staging musculoskeletal neoplasms. Clin Orthop Relat Res. 1986;204:9–24.

Enneking WF, Spanier SS, Goodman MA. A system for the surgical staging of musculoskeletal sarcoma. Clin Orthop. 1980;153:106–20.

Enzinger FM, Smith BH. Hemangiopericytoma. An analysis of 106 cases. Hum Pathol. 1976;7:61–82.

Faria SL, Schlupp WR, Chiminazzo H. Radiotherapy in the treatment of vertebral hemangiomas. Int J Radiat Oncol Biol Phys. 1985;1:387–90.

Ferigo N, Cottalorda J, Allard D, et al. Successful treatment via chemotherapy and surgical resection of a femoral hemangiopericytoma with pulmonary metastasis. J Pediatr Hematol Oncol. 2006;28:237–40.

Fourney DR, Rhines LD, Hentschel SJ, et al. En bloc resection of primary sacral tumors: classification of surgical approaches and outcome. J Neurosurg Spine. 2005;3:111–22.

Gebhardt MC, Lord FC, Rosenberg AE, et al. The treatment of adamantinoma of the tibia by wide resection and allograft bone transplantation. J Bone Joint Surg Am. 1987;69:1177–88.

Gosheger G, Hardes J, Ozaki T, et al. The multicentric epitheloid hemangioendothelioma of bone: a case example and review of the literature. J Cancer Res Clin Oncol. 2002;128:11–8.

Haisley-Royster C, Enjolras O, Frieden IJ, et al. Kasabach–Merritt phenomenon: a retrospective study of treatment with vincristine. J Pediatr Hematol Oncol. 2002;24:459–62.

Hazelbag HM, Taminiau AH, Fleuren GJ, et al. Adamantinoma of the long bones. A clinicopathological study of thirty-two patients with emphasis on histological subtype, precursor lesion, and biological behavior. J Bone Joint Surg Am. 1994;76:1482–99.

Healey JH, Lane JM. Chordoma: a critical review of diagnosis and treatment. Orthop Clin North Am. 1989;20:417–26.

Heymans O, Gebhart M, Larsimont D, et al. Malignant hemangiopericytoma of the pelvis: treatment using internal hemipelvectomy. Acta Orthop Belg. 1997;63:40–2.

Hug EB, Fitzek MM, Liebsch NJ, et al. Locally challenging osteo- and chondrogenic tumors of the axial skeleton: results of combined proton and photon radiation therapy using three-dimensional treatment planning. Int J Radiat Oncol Biol Phys. 1995;31:467–76.

Huvos AG, Heilweil M, Bretsky SS. The pathology of malignant fibrous histiocytoma of bone: a study of 130 patients. Am J Surg Pathol. 1985;9:853–71.

Igaki H, Tokuuye K, Okumura T, et al. Clinical results of proton beam therapy for skull base chordoma. Int J Radiat Oncol Biol Phys. 2004;60:1120–6.

Ignacio EA, Palmer KM, Mathur SC, et al. Epithelioid hemangioendothelioma of the lower extremity. Radiographics. 1999;19:531–7.

Juan CJ, Huang GS, Hsueh CJ, et al. Primary hemangiopericytoma of the tibia: MR and angiographic correlation. Skeletal Radiol. 2000;29:49–53.

Keeney GL, Unni KK, Beabout JW, et al. Adamantinoma of long bones. A clinicopathologic study of 85 cases. Cancer. 1989;64:730–7.

Kleer CG, Unni KK, McLeod RA. Epithelioid hemangioendothelioma of bone. Am J Surg Pathol. 1996;20:1301–11.

Marmor E, Rhines LD, Weinberg JS, et al. Total en bloc lumbar spondylectomy. Case report. J Neurosurg. 2001;95 suppl 2:264–9.

Mirra JM. Hemangiopericytoma. In: Mirra JM, Picci P, Gold RH, editors. Bone tumors: diagnosis and treatment. Philadelphia: Lea & Febiger; 1989. p. 1436–53.

Mirra JM, Bullough PG, Marcove RC, et al. Malignant fibrous histiocytoma and osteosarcoma in association with bone infarcts; report of four cases, two in caisson workers. J Bone Joint Surg Am. 1974;56:932–40.

Moon NF, Mori H. Adamantinoma of the appendicular skeleton—updated. Clin Orthop Relat Res. 1986;204:215–37.

Mori H, Shima R, Nakanishi H, et al. Adamantinoma of the tibia—a case report and a statistical review of reported cases. Acta Pathol Jpn. 1981;31:701–9.

Nishida J, Sim FH, Wenger DE, et al. Malignant fibrous histiocytoma of bone. A clinicopathologic study of 81 patients. Cancer. 1997;79:482–93.

Noel G, Feuvret L, Calugaru V, et al. Chordomas of the base of the skull and upper cervical spine. One hundred patients irradiated by a 3D conformal technique combining photon and proton beams. Acta Oncol. 2005;44:700–8.

Park L, Delaney TF, Liebsch NJ, et al. Sacral chordomas: Impact of high-dose proton/photon-beam radiation therapy combined with or without surgery for primary versus recurrent tumor. Int J Radiat Oncol Biol Phys. 2006;65:1514–21.

Picci P, Bacci G, Ferrari S, et al. Neoadjuvant chemotherapy in malignant fibrous histiocytoma of bone and in osteosarcoma located in the extremities: analogies and differences between the two tumors. Ann Oncol. 1997;8:1107–15.

Qureshi AA, Shott S, Mallin BA, et al. Current trends in the management of adamantinoma of long bones. An international study. J Bone Joint Surg Am. 2000;82:1122–31.

Rich TA, Schiller A, Suit HD, et al. Clinical and pathologic review of 48 cases of chordoma. Cancer. 1985;56:182–7.

Rosenthal DI, Treat ME, Mankin HJ, et al. Treatment of epithelioid hemangioendothelioma of bone using a novel combined approach. Skeletal Radiol. 2001;30:219–22.

Sahin-Akyar G, Fitoz S, Akpolat I, et al. Primary hemangiopericytoma of bone located in the tibia. Skeletal Radiol. 1997;26:47–50.

Saito T, Oda Y, Tanaka K, et al. Low-grade fibrosarcoma of the proximal humerus. Pathol Int. 2003;53:115–20.

Schuh A, Zeiler G, Holzwarth U, et al. Malignant fibrous histiocytoma at the site of a total hip arthroplasty. Clin Orthop Relat Res. 2004;425:218–22.

Sundaresan N, Rosen G, Boriani S. Primary malignant tumors of the spine. Orthop Clin North Am. 2009;40:21–36, v.

Taconis WK, Mulder JD. Fibrosarcoma and malignant fibrous histiocytoma of long bones: radiographic features and grading. Skeletal Radiol. 1984;11:237–45.

Tang JS, Gold RH, Mirra JM, et al. Hemangiopericytoma of bone. Cancer. 1988;62:848–59.

Tillman RM, Choong PF, Beabout JW, et al. Epithelioid hemangioendothelioma of bone. Orthopedics. 1997;20:177–80.

Tomita K, Kawahara N, Baba H, et al. Total en bloc spondylectomy. A new surgical technique for primary malignant vertebral tumors. Spine. 1997;22:324–33.

Troop JK, Mallory TH, Fisher DA, et al. Malignant fibrous histiocytoma after total hip arthroplasty. A case report. Clin Orthop Relat Res. 1990;253:297–300.

Tsuneyoshi M, Dorfman HD, Bauer TW. Epithelioid hemangioendothelioma of bone. A clinicopathologic, ultrastructural, and immunohistochemical study. Am J Surg Pathol. 1986;10:754–64.

Unni KK. Dahlin's bone tumors: general aspects and data on 11,087 cases. 5th ed. New York: Lippincott-Raven; 1996.

Weber DC, Rutz HP, Pedroni ES, et al. Results of spot-scanning proton radiation therapy for chordoma and chondrosarcoma of the skull base: the Paul Scherrer Institut experience. Int J Radiat Oncol Biol Phys. 2005;63:401–9.

Weiss SW, Enzinger FM. Epithelioid hemangioendothelioma: a vascular tumor often mistaken for a carcinoma. Cancer. 1982;50:970–81.

Welles L, Dorfman H, Valentine ES, et al. Low grade malignant hemangioendothelioma of bone: a disease potentially curable with radiotherapy. Med Pediatr Oncol. 1994;23:144–8.

Wold LE, Unni KK, Beabout JW, et al. Hemangioendothelial sarcoma of bone. Am J Surg Pathol. 1982;6:59–70.

York JE, Kaczaraj A, Abi-Said D, et al. Sacral chordoma: 40-year experience at a major cancer center. Neurosurgery. 1999;44:74–9 [discussion 79–80].

Chapter 9
Skeletal Reconstruction After Bone Sarcoma Resection

Christopher P. Cannon and David W. Chang

Contents

Chapter Overview The majority of patients with sarcomas of bone can be treated successfully with a limb-sparing surgery. Amputations are relatively uncommon. In most patients, a functional limb can be restored with a careful reconstruction. A variety of reconstructive options are now available. These include endoprostheses, allografts, allograft–prosthesis composite reconstructions, and autografts. The most effective use of the different techniques takes into account a number of factors, including the anatomic site, patient characteristics, and individual patient needs.

C.P. Cannon (✉)
The Polyclinic, 904 7th Avenue, Seattle, WA 98104, USA
e-mail: Christopher.CannonM.D@polyclinic.com

D.W. Chang (✉)
Department of Plastic Surgery, Unit 1488, Division of Surgery, The University of Texas
MD Anderson Cancer Center, 1400 Pressler Street, Houston, TX 77030, USA
e-mail: dchang@mdanderson.org

P.P. Lin and S. Patel (eds.), *Bone Sarcoma*, MD Anderson Cancer Care Series,
DOI 10.1007/978-1-4614-5194-5_9,
© The University of Texas M. D. Anderson Cancer Center 2013

Introduction

Definitive management of all bone sarcomas requires a wide resection of the primary tumor. In most cases, extremities can be reconstructed with limb-sparing surgery. Even in cases with significant soft tissue involvement, wound coverage after wide excision can usually be provided by muscle and skin flaps. Vessels involved by tumor can be resected and reconstructed with bypass grafts. Similarly, peripheral nerves can be resected and the limb spared, with nerve grafting or tendon transfers in selected cases; an isolated peripheral-nerve resection will usually result in a more functional limb than will an amputation.

Each specific anatomic site has its own unique issues with regard to reconstruction. Joint involvement, tendon attachments, and adjacent soft tissue and neurovascular structures play critical roles in selection of the type of reconstruction and in the ultimate functional outcome. This chapter describes the general reconstructive options and specific considerations for each anatomic site.

Reconstructive Options

Endoprosthesis

An endoprosthetic reconstruction (also known as segmental arthroplasty or megaprosthetic reconstruction) employs an artificial (typically metallic) device to reconstruct the resected portion of the bone and joint (Fig. 9.1). Endoprostheses have been used routinely for the past 25 years with generally good results. Early versions were custom made, but manufacturers now produce modular systems, which allow for maximal intraoperative flexibility. Defects of virtually any length can be reconstructed. Also, implants are available in multiple sizes that allow use in all patient sizes. Most implants are fixed with bone cement (polymethyl methacrylate) for immediate stability, but uncemented designs are also in use.

Universal availability and intraoperative flexibility are significant advantages of endoprostheses over allografts. Also, unlike allografts, endoprostheses allow for immediate full-weight bearing. This property facilitates earlier postoperative mobilization, which is especially important in older, sicker patients.

A significant disadvantage of endoprostheses is the difficulty in obtaining adequate tendon attachment. At specific locations—namely, the proximal humerus, proximal femur, and proximal tibia—adequate active limb motion and strength are predicated on reestablishing tendinous insertions. Current implants rely primarily on suturing tendons to metal, which generally does not work well.

Other disadvantages of endoprostheses include the potential for aseptic loosening and failure of the mobile parts. As with all artificial joints, endoprostheses generate wear debris that can contribute to the development of eventual aseptic loosening and the need for revision surgery. Also, distal femoral and proximal tibial implants have several small components (including bushings, an axle, a tibial-bearing

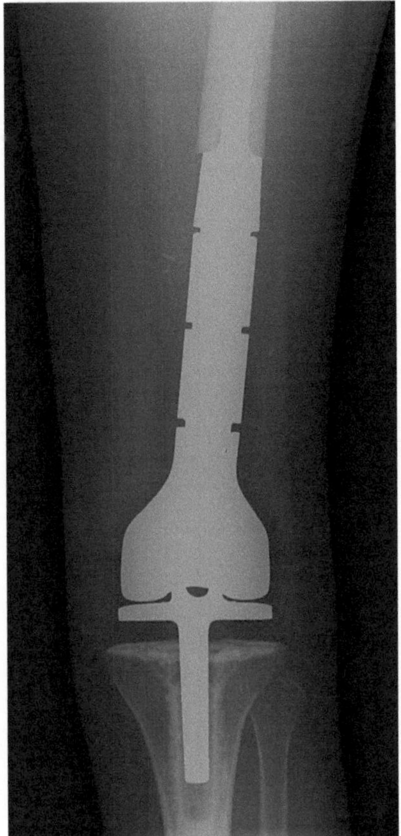

Fig. 9.1 A distal femur endoprosthesis.

component, and a bumper) that are all at risk for eventual failure, particularly in active patients. Failure of these components, though not catastrophic, necessitates a limited revision procedure.

Osteoarticular Allograft

Osteoarticular allografts are seldom used at MD Anderson Cancer Center, except in selected sites, which will be discussed later in the chapter. These allografts have the advantage of better soft tissue attachments than are possible with endoprostheses. The host tendon can be securely sutured to the allograft tendon, enabling potentially superior motor function. Also, once the allograft has healed to the host bone, the potential for the late complication of aseptic loosening is effectively eliminated.

However, osteoarticular allografts have several significant disadvantages. They are not universally available, and matching the host joint exactly can be extremely difficult. Obtaining durable joint stability, especially at the knee joint, requires careful reconstruction of the associated ligaments and is also quite difficult. There is

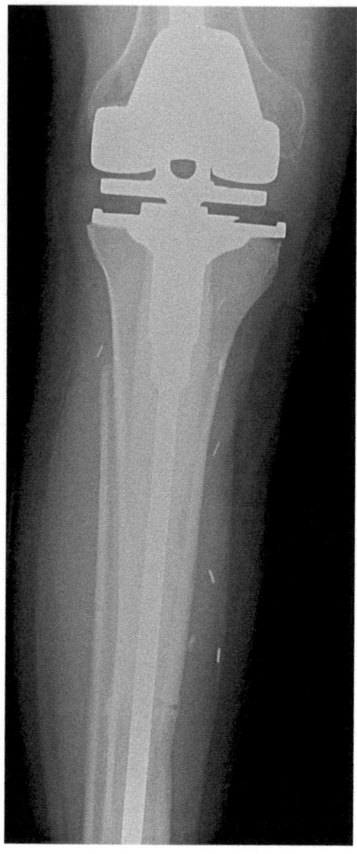

Fig. 9.2 A proximal tibia allograft–prosthesis composite (APC).

a high incidence of late instability, degenerative joint changes, and subchondral collapse. Achieving a union at the host bone–allograft junction can be problematic and frequently requires supplemental bone grafting using either an iliac crest bone graft or a bone graft substitute such as demineralized bone matrix. Finally, fracture of allografts occurs in approximately 10% of cases. Some authors have found higher infection rates for allografts than for endoprostheses; however, this issue is controversial. At MD Anderson, the infection rates have been comparable.

Allograft–Prosthesis Composite

An allograft–prosthesis composite (APC) is a reconstruction option that combines elements of both an endoprosthesis and an osteoarticular allograft (Fig. 9.2). This option has many of the best features of the other two options, without some of their individual weaknesses. Exact allograft sizing is not as critical because the joint is resurfaced. The potential for late degenerative joint changes is also eliminated. Another advantage is that joint stability at the knee can be provided by a rotating hinge much like that of an endoprosthesis. Thus, obtaining joint stability and durability is much easier and more reliable with APCs than with osteoarticular allografts. Tendon and soft tissue attachment is provided by the allograft, potentially allowing better strength and active range of motion than are obtained with an endoprosthesis alone. Also, once the host bone and allograft unite, the potential for late aseptic loosening should be diminished.

However, some of the disadvantages of other allografts still exist with APCs. Though exact sizing is not as essential, an approximate allograft match still needs to be obtained, which can delay surgery and lessen intraoperative flexibility. Achieving union at the host bone–allograft junction can still be problematic and can require supplemental bone grafting.

The best method of fixation of the allograft remains unclear. Several options exist. At our institution, the most common method of fixation involves a long-stemmed prosthesis that spans the length of the allograft and is cemented into both the host bone and the allograft. An alternative is a short-stemmed prosthesis that is cemented into the allograft and then plated to the host bone. A final option is a long-stemmed prosthesis combined with a supplemental plate to add additional strength, especially for torsion.

Segmental (Intercalary) Allograft

Segmental allografts are indicated for diaphyseal tumors without joint involvement. Because the joints above and below the tumor are spared, the potential function is quite good. Strength and active range of motion can essentially be normal. Late issues such as joint instability, degenerative joint disease, and wear debris are avoided. The main difficulty associated with segmental allografts is obtaining healing at the host bone–allograft junction sites. Diaphyseal bone typically does not heal as readily as does metaphyseal bone because of the less optimal blood supply. Primary bone grafting, usually with an iliac crest bone graft, at the time of the index procedure is generally recommended. Repeat supplemental bone grafting is performed if healing has not occurred in 6–12 months.

As with APCs, the optimal method of fixation for segmental allografts remains unclear. Potential options include an intramedullary nail, plate fixation, or a combination of both (Fig. 9.3). The method of fixation is not as important as is obtaining solid fixation, good bone contact, compression at the junction sites, and protection of the entire length of the allograft with the implant of choice. Intramedullary nails are generally stronger than plates but are more demanding technically in terms of achieving contact and compression at osteotomies. An optimally fixed plate is preferable to a poorly placed nail.

Better compression and a more intimate approximation of the bony surfaces will be obtained if the cuts are accurate. Great care must be taken while performing these cuts. We have developed an intramedullary-referenced reamer (Fig. 9.4) that works well for obtaining flat opposing surfaces after the initial cuts have been made with a standard oscillating saw. This reamer works well particularly when an intramedullary nail is used for fixation.

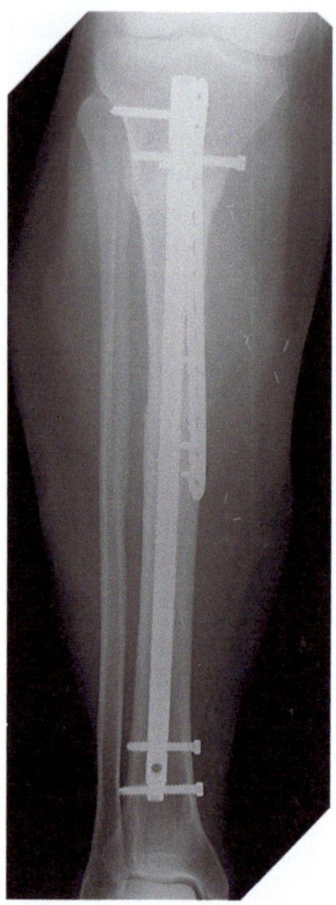

Fig. 9.3 An intercalary tibia allograft fixed with an intramedullary nail and a locking plate.

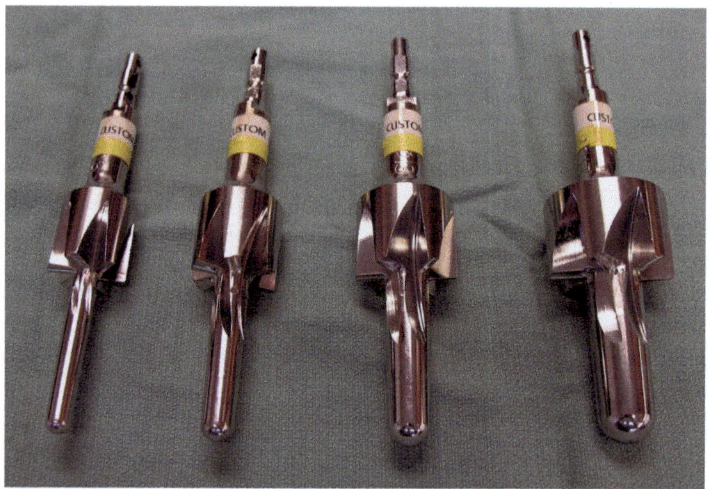

Fig. 9.4 Custom reamers designed to produce flat opposing surfaces when using a structural allograft.

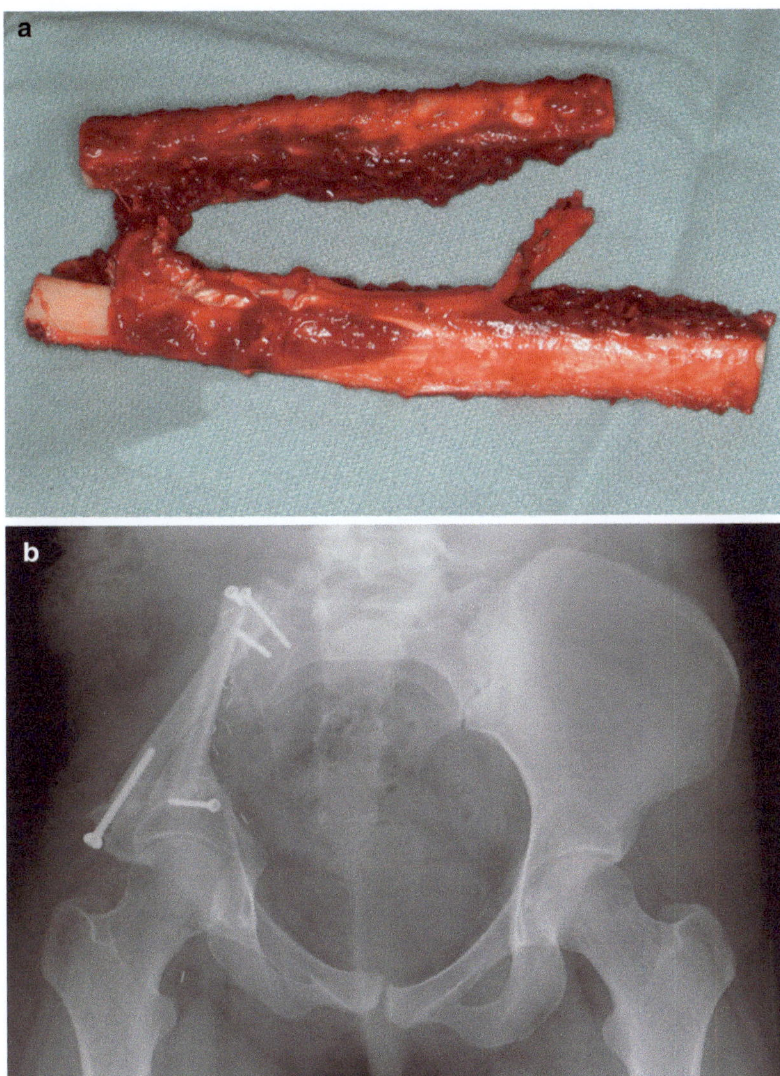

Fig. 9.5 (a) A double-barreled vascularized fibular bone flap. (b) Use of this type of flap for reconstruction of the pelvic ring after internal hemipelvectomy.

Vascularized Bone Transfer (Autologous Fibula)

Vascularized bone transfers, as exemplified by the autologous fibular bone flap, are versatile means for skeletal reconstruction. The main advantage of a vascularized bone transfer is that it does not rely on the recipient bed for revascularization and incorporation; thus, bone healing is rapid and reliable even in suboptimal conditions, leading to quicker and better return of function.

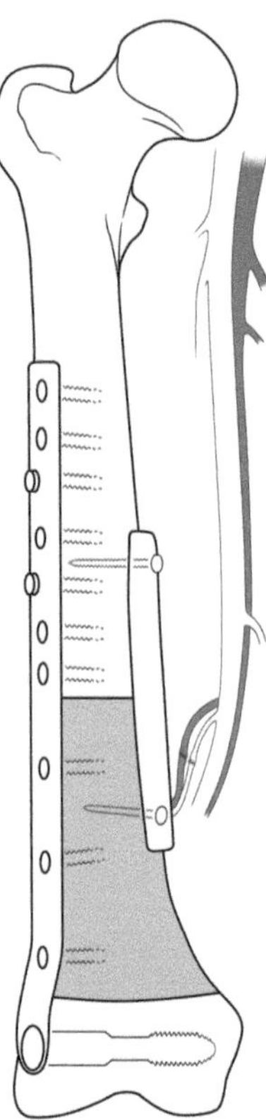

Fig. 9.6 A vascularized fibula flap placed using an onlay approach at the proximal allograft–host junction and secured with small-fragment cortical screws. Reprinted from Chang and Weber (2005) with permission.

The vascularized bone transfer can be used alone or with an allograft for skeletal reconstruction, depending on the location and the extent of the bone defect. For example, for reconstruction of the pelvic ring after internal hemipelvectomy, use of a double-barreled vascularized fibular bone flap (Fig. 9.5) provides adequate strength to allow early ambulation with normal to near-normal gait.

For difficult-to-manage allograft nonunions, the use of vascularized fibular bone flaps has promoted bone healing and allowed limb salvage (Fig. 9.6). In selected high-risk situations, such as in large diaphyseal defects in patients who require neoadjuvant and/or adjuvant chemotherapy, we often combine vascularized fibula flaps with intercalary allografts for skeletal reconstruction (Fig. 9.7). The rationale for this approach is to combine the mechanical strength of the allograft with the biological activity of the vascularized bone flap so as to enhance bone healing and minimize allograft failures.

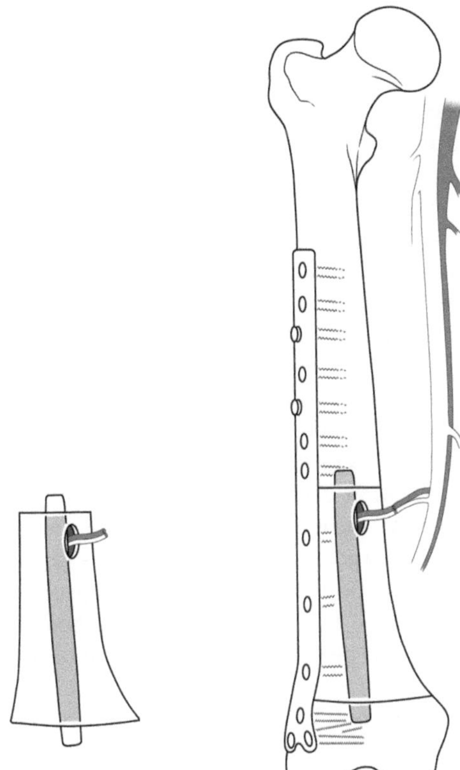

Fig. 9.7 A bone defect reconstructed with an allograft and a vascularized fibular bone flap placed into the medullary canal of the allograft. Reprinted from Chang and Weber (2005) with permission.

Specific Anatomic Sites

Major Long Bones

Proximal Humerus

One of the main challenges associated with reconstruction of the proximal humerus is restoration of rotator cuff function. Resection of the proximal humerus will disrupt the rotator cuff insertion site, which has a significant functional impact. To reestablish active range of motion at the shoulder, the rotator cuff must be either reinserted or compensated for by prosthetic design.

The brachial plexus and axillary artery are adjacent to the proximal humerus and, especially in the case of larger tumors, can be at risk during tumor resection. Some controversy exists as to whether an intra-articular or extra-articular resection should be performed and whether the deltoid can be spared. At MD Anderson, in most cases, we perform an intra-articular resection. However, direct extension into the glenohumeral joint can occur along the biceps tendon sheath or directly through the joint capsule; such extension is an indication for an extra-articular resection (described below). Close scrutiny of a high-resolution magnetic resonance imaging (MRI) scan is essential before this decision can be made. Similarly, direct extension into the deltoid requires resection of at least a portion of that muscle. However, most of the deltoid can usually be safely spared. Preservation of the deltoid and the axillary nerve allows excellent soft tissue coverage of the reconstruction as well as additional motor power for active shoulder movement.

An APC is one of our preferred reconstruction methods for the proximal humerus. This approach permits solid reconstruction of the rotator cuff and shoulder capsule. Much greater shoulder motion can be achieved than is typically realized with an endoprosthesis. For an APC, the allograft rotator cuff is securely sutured to the host rotator cuff using multiple large, nonabsorbable sutures (e.g., #2 or #5 Ethibond or FiberWire). Also, whenever possible, the allograft capsule is sutured to the host capsule in a similar fashion. A long-stemmed humeral hemiarthroplasty prosthesis is cemented into the allograft proximal humerus on the back table of the operating room, and then, this construct is cemented into the host humerus in a second stage. The long-stemmed implant protects the entire length of the allograft (Fig. 9.8). A plate is sometimes added for additional torsional strength. Because the implant stem interferes with screw placement, the use of unicortical screws through a locking plate is often necessary. As in all allograft cases, close apposition of the two bony surfaces appears to be important for bone healing. To maximize healing of the allograft–host bone junction site, bone graft material is placed around the osteotomy site. A collagen membrane or mesh may be useful to contain the bone graft around the bone.

An endoprosthesis is also a viable reconstructive option for the proximal humerus. Such implants have traditionally been used because they provide a stable, pain-free shoulder. They are also somewhat easier to implant and do not have the nonunion issues that can be seen with APCs. However, in our experience, patients are usually only able to obtain approximately 45° of abduction and forward flexion with this type of implant. Endoprostheses are definitely a reasonable option in elderly patients or those with metastatic disease and a limited life expectancy in whom early mobilization and a quicker return to activities of daily living are desirable.

In a relatively small percentage of cases, a sarcoma will frankly invade the glenohumeral joint, and an extra-articular resection will be required. In such cases, dissection is performed outside the joint capsule, and an osteotomy is made through the glenoid neck. The axillary nerve and deltoid may need to be resected as well. If so, local muscle flap coverage of the reconstruction by a plastic surgeon may be necessary. With extra-articular resections, reconstruction is performed with an endoprosthesis. The prosthesis is suspended from the distal clavicle, remaining scapula, or first rib using nonabsorbable tape. The goal is to provide a

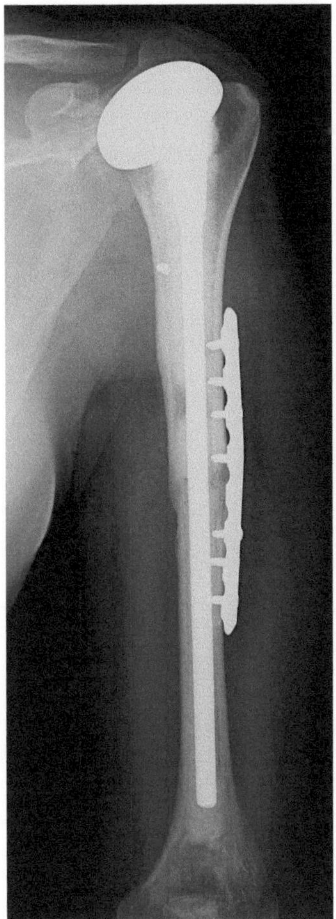

Fig. 9.8 A proximal humerus APC.

stable shoulder to support elbow and hand function. Active shoulder motion will be limited. An APC will not significantly improve function in this situation; an endoprosthesis provides equivalent function in a simple, durable construct.

Distal Humerus

In most regards, the distal humerus is easier than the proximal humerus to reconstruct. There are no significant muscle insertions on the distal humerus. Thus, this area can be resected and reconstructed without greatly compromising elbow function. The local anatomy is complex because of the close proximity of the radial, median, and ulnar nerves, as well as the brachial artery. However, with close scrutiny of a preoperative MRI scan and careful dissection, those structures can usually be preserved.

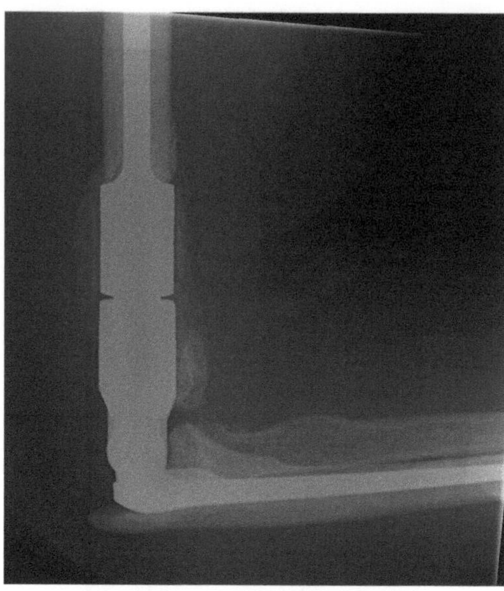

Fig. 9.9 A distal humerus endoprosthesis with a "sloppy" hinge and cemented ulnar component.

Because there are no significant muscle insertions on the distal humerus, an APC is not required, and reconstruction is usually done with an endoprosthesis (Fig. 9.9). With resection of the distal humerus, the collateral ligaments will be sacrificed, with resultant loss of elbow stability. The endoprosthesis thus has a "sloppy" hinge to provide elbow stability. The main issue with these prostheses is the potential for late loosening of the ulnar component. As with conventional total-elbow replacements, there is a relatively high surgical-revision rate for the ulnar component.

In some young patients, the best reconstructive option for a distal humerus defect is an osteoarticular allograft, both to avoid disruption of the ulnar growth plate and to delay erosion of the ulna from aseptic loosening of a metallic implant.

Proximal Femur

The main issue with reconstruction of the proximal femur, as with the proximal humerus, is repair of the tendinous insertions. The hip abductors insert on the greater trochanter, and this site is sacrificed during resection of the proximal femur, resulting in functional loss of the hip abductors. Without careful repair, patients will have marked hip abductor weakness and a Trendelenburg gait and will require assistive devices for ambulation. A second important issue is hip stability. Loss of the normal joint capsule and soft tissue can lead to a less stable construct than is typically seen with conventional hip arthroplasty.

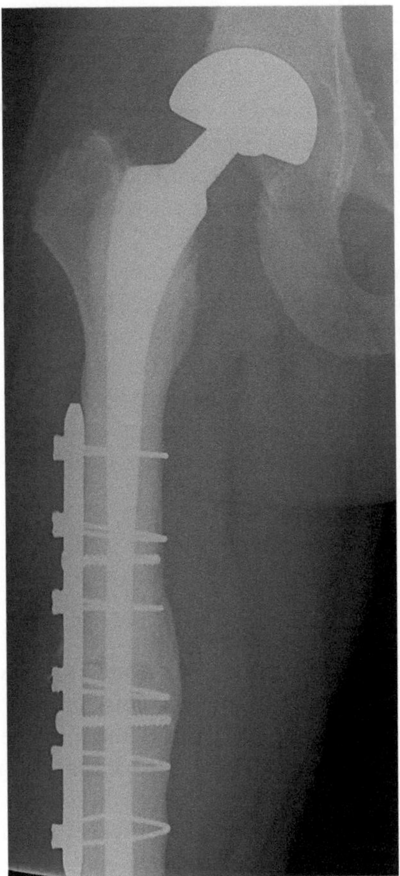

Fig. 9.10 A proximal femur APC fixed with a long-stemmed femoral component and a cable plate.

In order to maximize hip abductor function and provide optimal reconstruction of the hip capsule, at MD Anderson, we sometimes perform an APC reconstruction (Fig. 9.10). In this approach, after careful matching of the cut surfaces of the host and allograft bones, a long-stemmed hemiarthroplasty prosthesis is cemented into the allograft. This construct is then cemented into the host femur in a separate stage. A purse-string suture is placed through any residual capsule to help provide immediate stability. Also, a meticulous repair of the allograft capsule to any residual host capsule is performed. Next, a meticulous repair to attach the host hip abductor tendons to the allograft tendons is performed. This repair is done with multiple placements of suture using a #2 or #5 nonabsorbable suture such as Ethibond or FiberWire. The iliopsoas and gluteus maximus tendons are not as critical to repair; function is remarkably good even without repair. As described above, a bone graft or demineralized bone matrix is placed at the host bone–allograft junction site to help attain union. Postoperatively, the patient is placed in a hip abduction brace, which limits hip flexion to 70° and prevents hip adduction. This precaution both protects the soft tissue repair and helps prevent hip dislocation. Use of the brace is continued for 3 months. Weight bearing is limited to touchdown for at least 3 months. If no evidence of host bone–allograft union is noted by 6 months, we recommend proactive intervention with bone grafting to help facilitate union.

An endoprosthetic reconstruction is a reasonable choice for the proximal femur, especially for patients who will have difficulty with postoperative weight-bearing restrictions or who have a limited life expectancy. An endoprosthesis is a durable reconstruction that allows early weight bearing. The major disadvantage of an endoprosthesis is reduced hip abduction strength because of imperfect healing of the abductor tendons to the metallic prosthesis. Every effort must be made during repair to attach the hip abductors securely to the greater trochanteric portion of the endoprosthesis or to leave them in continuity with the soft tissue sleeve of the vastus lateralis. As with APCs, a brace is used postoperatively for 3 months to stabilize the joint and protect the abductor tendon repair.

Distal Femur

The distal femur is the osteoarticular resection site most favorable for a very functional reconstruction. There are no significant soft tissue or tendinous insertions on the distal femur. After resection and reconstruction, the extensor mechanism, consisting of the quadriceps musculature, quadriceps tendon, patella, patellar tendon, and tibial tubercle, is intact and has essentially normal function.

Since the patellar tendon insertion is usually not disturbed, an osteoarticular allograft or APC does not offer an advantage in terms of muscle strength, so most reconstructions are performed with an endoprosthesis (Fig. 9.1). Most prosthetic designs incorporate a rotating hinge that provides varus and valgus stability while dissipating forces across the prosthesis. Compared with older fixed-hinge designs, the rotating hinge significantly reduces aseptic loosening and prosthesis failure.

Two important issues with distal femoral reconstruction are obtaining equal leg lengths and ensuring proper rotation. These objectives can be accomplished by marking the femur and tibia with a small osteotome above and below, respectively, the sites of the planned osteotomies. The length should be measured and rotational alignment noted. After reconstruction, the length and rotational alignment should be accurately restored. Fine-tuning of leg lengths can be performed by varying the thickness of the polyethylene tibial tray.

Since these procedures do not involve soft tissue reconstructions that require immobility to heal, patients are encouraged to move the knee early in the postoperative period. Patients begin to work with a continuous passive motion machine in the postanesthesia care unit and continue while they are inpatients. Patients with cemented implants are also allowed to bear weight as tolerated once quadriceps function returns.

Proximal Tibia

Several issues exist that make resection and reconstruction more difficult in the proximal tibia than in the distal femur. First, the vascular structures are often quite close to the tumor. Because the popliteal artery trifurcates into the posterior tibial, peroneal, and anterior tibial arteries in this area, the vessels are tethered and cannot be as easily displaced by a growing tumor as they are in the distal femur. Fortunately, in most cases, the popliteus muscle typically protects the posterior neurovascular structures from the tumor. A second issue is that, unlike the other anatomic sites discussed in this chapter, the proximal tibia has limited soft tissue coverage to protect the reconstruction. We routinely use a gastrocnemius flap to cover the site. A final issue is that the patellar tendon attaches to the tibial tubercle on the proximal tibia. Resection of the proximal tibia thus results in loss of the tibial tubercle and the patellar tendon insertion, with significant resultant effect on active knee extension and ultimate knee function.

To maximize knee extension strength, we frequently use an APC for reconstruction in this site (Fig. 9.2). After resection of the proximal tibia, an appropriately sized allograft is selected and prepared to receive a long-stemmed rotating-hinge component. The component is then cemented into the allograft. Next, the entire construct is cemented into the remaining host tibia. At the surgeon's discretion, a plate can be added across the osteotomy site to provide additional strength, particularly rotational strength. Because a stem fills the majority of the canal, a unicortical locking plate is frequently needed. The optimal method of fixation for APCs is controversial, and alternative methods exist.

An APC reconstruction of the proximal tibia requires resection of a portion of the distal femur in order to install the rotating-hinge knee system. The distal femur is resurfaced with a stemmed component compatible with the rotating-hinge knee system. As described in the distal-femur section, the distance between osteotomy marks made above and below the sites of resection can be recorded and used to accurately restore leg length. Again, fine-tuning of the leg length can be done by varying the thickness of the polyethylene tibial tray. A bone graft or demineralized bone matrix, often held in place with a collagen membrane, is added at the junction site to aid healing. The allograft patellar tendon is carefully sutured to the host patellar tendon using multiple nonabsorbable #2 or #5 braided sutures or tape. As for the proximal tibia reconstruction, the APC is covered with a rotational gastrocnemius flap. Postoperatively, the knee is held in full extension in a locked-knee brace for a minimum of 6 weeks to aid healing of the extensor mechanism. After this period, significant physical therapy is needed to regain functional knee flexion. Adequate knee flexion of at least 90° is typically attained.

Postoperative weight bearing is limited to touchdown until radiographic evidence of union is observed. As with other allograft procedures, delayed union and the need for supplemental bone grafting are relatively common. However, once union is obtained after an APC reconstruction, the incidence of late aseptic loosening is markedly lower than the relatively common incidence after endoprosthetic proximal tibia reconstructions.

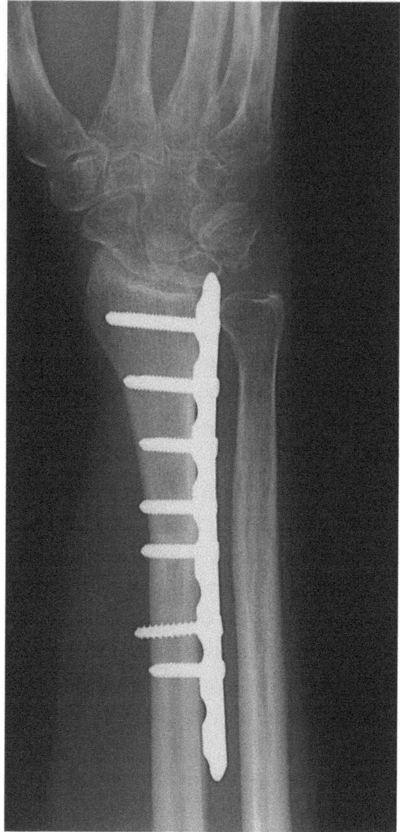

Fig. 9.11 A distal radius osteoarticular allograft fixed with a locking plate.

An endoprosthetic reconstruction is another valid option for the proximal tibia. It has the significant benefit of allowing early full-weight bearing, which is especially important in elderly patients or those with limited life expectancy. The reconstruction is somewhat simpler than that using an APC. Although function is perhaps not optimal, it is at least reasonable.

Negative aspects of an endoprosthetic reconstruction include less predictable quadriceps strength and, as mentioned above, a relatively high rate of late aseptic loosening. As with the APC reconstruction, a gastrocnemius flap is required to protect the site. Also, postoperative immobilization in a locked-knee brace is required until the patient can do a straight-leg raise without a significant extension lag.

Distal Radius

The distal radius is one of the sites in which an osteoarticular allograft can be used effectively (Fig. 9.11). Though there are no significant tendinous attachments on the distal radius, it is essential to reestablish stability at the distal radioulnar and radiocarpal joints. The osteoarticular allograft permits reconstruction of the triangular fibrocartilage complex (TFCC), joint capsule, and radiocarpal ligaments. The osteoarticular allograft is better tolerated in the upper extremity than in the lower extremity; late degenerative changes are less frequent in the upper extremity because of decreased joint forces and a limited requirement for weight bearing.

Resection of the distal radius is usually performed through a dorsal approach. After resection, multiple nonabsorbable sutures are placed in the TFCC, volar joint capsule, and radiocarpal ligaments. Placing these sutures is much easier if it is done before fixation of the allograft. After placement of these sutures, the allograft is cut to the appropriate length. The allograft should be cut to a length that will allow an ulnar-neutral wrist. The sutures should be appropriately positioned so that an anatomic reduction of the joint is possible. After the volar sutures are placed but before they are tied, the allograft is secured to the host radius using a single 3.5-mm compression or locking plate. After fixation, the volar sutures are tied through the dorsal opening of the radiocarpal joint. The remaining dorsal capsule and distal radioulnar joint repair is then performed. After completion of the soft tissue repair, the stability of the radiocarpal and distal radioulnar joints is assessed both clinically and radiographically. In particular, the stability of the distal radioulnar joint relative to wrist supination and pronation is noted. If wrist supination is required to reduce the distal ulna, the wrist will need to be immobilized in this position postoperatively. Wrist immobilization is continued for 6 weeks after the operation to allow soft tissue healing. Weight bearing is limited and the wrist further protected in a removable splint until there is radiographic evidence of healing at the osteotomy site.

A second option for reconstruction of the distal radius is an allograft arthrodesis. With this option, the host bone is denuded of cartilage, either at the proximal carpal row or, if the resection is done through the midcarpal joint, the distal carpal row. The arthrodesis site is spanned by a long compression plate. A supplemental bone graft is added. Attention must still be paid to obtaining the correct length and orientation of the wrist, though a careful soft tissue reconstruction is not needed. The benefit of an arthrodesis over an osteoarticular reconstruction is the elimination of potential late degenerative changes and wrist instability. Once the arthrodesis unites, the wrist should be quite stable and durable. The negative aspect of an arthrodesis is the obvious loss of wrist motion. At MD Anderson, we generally prefer the motion-sparing osteoarticular reconstruction when it is possible.

Whole Bone

Resection of an entire long bone is uncommon. Very occasionally, a tumor will have such extensive involvement as to mandate this procedure. More commonly, however, resection of an entire long bone occurs after revision of a previously placed endoprosthesis or APC.

With modern, modular endoprostheses, reconstruction of a whole humerus or femur is a relatively straightforward procedure. Essentially, whole-bone reconstructions combine proximal humeral and distal humeral or proximal femoral and distal femoral endoprosthetic reconstructions, which are done as described above; the endoprostheses are joined with an adapter. However, because of the involvement of two joints and the loss of soft tissue attachments, function is not as good after these procedures as it is after reconstruction for a single joint.

Expendable Bones

Clavicle

Involvement of the clavicle is managed with resection without reconstruction. The main anatomic issue at this site is protecting the underlying subclavian vessels and brachial plexus. If the tumor is large and displaces the subclavian vessels, assistance from a vascular surgeon should be considered.

Most patients have essentially no functional impairment after clavicle resection. They regain full overhead use of their arm and have minimal pain. If a soft tissue or skin defect is present after resection of the tumor, a plastic surgeon should be consulted about soft tissue coverage over the nerves and blood vessels.

Scapula

The most important component of the scapula is the glenoid. Scapular resection that preserves the glenoid usually does not require reconstruction, and in most cases, function will be good.

Tumors that require resection of the glenoid, however, result in significantly reduced function and may benefit from reconstruction. The glenoid provides the stable platform for the humeral head. Thus, loss of the glenoid significantly impairs glenohumeral joint function. At MD Anderson, the glenoid is usually reconstructed with a scapular allograft after resection. If the glenoid portion is resected and the majority of the scapular body is preserved, an allograft glenoid is secured to the host scapular body using contoured 3.5-mm reconstruction plates. If the entire scapula is resected, an entire osteoarticular scapular allograft is used for the reconstruction. In either case, the allograft joint capsule is meticulously sutured to any remaining host joint capsule using a braided, nonabsorbable suture. It is essential to cover the allograft completely with muscle before skin closure. Local muscles such as the remaining rotator cuff musculature, the rhomboids, the trapezius, and the latissimus dorsi can be used for this coverage.

Postoperatively, the patient uses a shoulder abduction sling for 4–6 weeks to allow soft tissue healing. Gentle passive and graduated active range-of-motion movements are then initiated.

Fibula

As described previously, the fibula is used at times to provide an autogenous, vascularized bone graft. With the exception of the distal portion, the fibula is an expendable bone that requires no reconstruction. The main anatomic issue at this site is preserving the peroneal nerve, which passes from behind the biceps femoris tendon and around the fibular neck. The peroneal nerve is very vulnerable to injury at the fibular neck.

With resections of the proximal fibula, a second anatomic issue is preserving the anterior tibial vessels. The vessels arise from the trifurcation of the popliteal vessels in the popliteal fossa. The anterior tibial vessels traverse the superior aspect of the intraosseous membrane, passing from the popliteal fossa to the anterior compartment of the leg. If the proximal fibula is resected, these vessels need to be either dissected free of surrounding tissues or ligated and divided.

The lateral collateral ligament (LCL) inserts on the proximal fibula. Thus, unless the ligament is reconstructed, resection of the proximal fibula will result in varus instability of the knee. Reconstruction is done by suturing the LCL to the proximal lateral tibia using a suture anchor. Postoperatively, the knee is protected from varus stresses by using a hinged-knee brace for 6 weeks.

The distal fibula forms the lateral malleolus of the ankle joint. Resection of the lateral malleolus will result in ankle instability. If such resection is required, ankle stability will need to be restored, most commonly with an ankle fusion. Vascularized proximal fibular autografts have also been used in such cases with some success.

Pelvis

The bony pelvis is a challenging area for both tumor resection and reconstruction. The anatomy in this area is quite complex. Local anatomic structures include the internal and external iliac vessels and their respective branches, the lumbar and sacral nerve roots, the colon, the ureter, the bladder, and the genitalia. Blood loss can be extensive, even in routine cases, and inadvertent vascular injury can result in dramatic bleeding. Thus, surgeons who are not familiar with working in this area should involve other surgical services as needed, to include vascular surgeons, genitourinary surgeons, gastrointestinal surgeons, and surgical oncologists.

Preoperatively, patients should undergo a bowel preparation. At MD Anderson, a ureteral stent on the operative side is routinely placed by a genitourinary surgeon at the beginning of the operation. The patient should undergo careful intraoperative monitoring with a central venous line and an arterial line. Blood products should be available. Also, careful attention should be paid to positioning the patient and padding the extremities. These are routinely long surgeries with a significant risk of development of nerve palsies or pressure ulcers if proper padding is not placed.

Pelvic resections are defined as type I (iliac), type II (periacetabular), and type III (obturator). The most important issue in regard to reconstruction of the pelvis is maintaining the function of the acetabulum. Type I and type III resections, which do

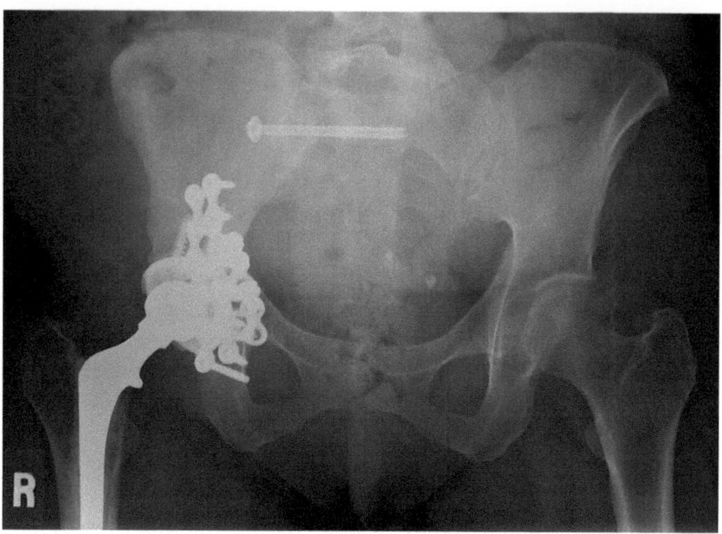

Fig. 9.12 Reconstruction after a combined type I/II pelvic resection with an allograft and total hip replacement.

not involve the acetabulum, result in much better postoperative function than do type II resections in which the acetabulum is not reconstructed.

The reconstruction for type I iliac wing resection is typically a double-barreled vascularized fibular graft (Fig. 9.5B). Single-barreled grafts are prone to fracture. The surgeon can elect to not perform reconstruction for type I resections; however, rotation of the pelvis will occur, with the development of a significant leg-length discrepancy.

The best method of reconstructing type II acetabular defects remains controversial. At MD Anderson, we sometimes utilize an allograft pelvis combined with total hip arthroplasty (Fig. 9.12). Patient selection is critical because the infection rate can be very high. Preservation of the gluteal muscles and associated nerves and vessels is important. After resection of the tumor, the allograft pelvis is carefully contoured to fit the defect. The allograft is secured to the host pelvis using contoured 3.5-mm reconstruction plates along the iliac wing and potentially along the superior pubic ramus. The plates can be augmented with intramedullary cannulated screws. For combined type I and type II internal hemipelvectomies, the allograft ilium is secured to the host sacrum using large, cannulated sacroiliac screws. A prosthetic acetabular cup is secured to the allograft using a combination of cement and screws. On the femoral side, a standard cemented or press-fit femoral stem is used. Postoperatively, to maximize hip stability and protect the soft tissue repair, a hip abduction brace is worn full time for 3 months. Weight bearing is limited to touch-down until radiographic evidence of union is observed.

A second reconstructive option is a custom pelvis prosthesis. This implant avoids the issue of potential late allograft fragmentation. However, fixation is often tenuous, and until recently, osteosynthesis at the host bone–implant interface has not been possible. At MD Anderson, custom endoprostheses have been developed with newer metal interfaces that permit bone ingrowth into the implant. Another option is the so-called "saddle" prosthesis, designed to rest on the remaining ilium. It is a viable option, particularly in patients with a limited life expectancy, as long as sufficient ilium remains to support the prosthesis. However, these prostheses have a relatively high dislocation rate, as well as a tendency to fracture and migrate through the remaining thin ilium.

A final option is to not reconstruct the hip at all but rather leave it "flail." This option does avoid many of the potential negatives of reconstruction: dislocation, infection, nonunion, and hardware failure. However, function is clearly less favorable with this option when compared with function after a successful reconstruction.

Regardless of the reconstructive option chosen, the length of hospital stay and length of recovery are often quite long after these procedures. The hospital stay is frequently 3–4 weeks. Rehabilitation to maximal recovery can take up to a year or more. Patients should be made aware of these timelines before surgery.

Spine

A true en bloc resection of a spine sarcoma is a difficult and challenging surgery and should be undertaken only by those with experience in spinal tumors. A combined anterior and posterior approach is required to gain wide exposure to all aspects of the spinal column. Clearly, the spinal cord limits a truly wide resection in most cases. However, if both the anterior and posterior approaches are used, the tumor can be removed en bloc.

Reconstruction will require both anterior and posterior instrumentation. Spinal fusion cannot be reliably counted upon given the extent of resection and frequent adjuvant use of chemotherapy and/or radiation. Thus, solid, durable anterior and posterior fixation is needed. The instrumentation must be strong enough to stand alone without the benefit of a localized spine fusion.

The sacrum is an area of frequent tumor involvement. Chondrosarcomas, chordomas, and giant cell tumors all can occur in the sacrum. The morbidity and functional outcome after resection, as well as the type of reconstruction required, depend on the level of resection. Tumors distal to the S2–S3 level can be managed with a posterior approach only. In such cases, the dorsal dissection is straightforward. The main issue is ensuring the correct operative level. An intraoperative cross-table radiograph can be quite helpful. The main anatomic issue ventrally is protecting the rectum, which is carefully mobilized away from the ventral surface of the sacrum. A chevron-shaped osteotomy is made through the dorsal cortex of the sacrum using a combination of a burr and Kerrison rongeurs. The sacral nerve roots are located. If bilateral S1, S2, and S3 can be preserved, normal continence and sexual function will be retained in most patients. If only bilateral S1 and S2 can be preserved, abnormal bowel and bladder function will result in most patients. A diamond burr is safer to use when working around the nerve roots as it does not "wrap up" soft tissue as do standard burrs. Once the dorsal osteotomy has been made, the ventral osteotomy is made through the established opening, again using a burr and Kerrison rongeurs. Also, manual manipulation of the distal sacral fragment helps create a "fatigue fracture" at the desired osteotomy level.

Sacral resections proximal to the S2 level have significantly high morbidity and also require reconstruction. After such resections, most patients will lose continence and sexual function. The spine will need to be stabilized to the bilateral ilia using pedicle screws or Galveston rods.

Key Practice Points

- Different reconstructive options exist for each anatomic site. The advantages and disadvantages of the various options must be weighed carefully for each patient.
- Endoprostheses have the advantages of relative ease of use, universal availability, early weight bearing, good durability, and a low complication rate. They are ideal for the distal femur. Soft tissue attachment, however, can be problematic.
- APCs are also durable and provide better soft tissue attachment than do endoprostheses. They should be strongly considered for the proximal humerus, proximal femur, and proximal tibia. Nonunion between the host bone and allograft is a common problem; supplemental bone grafting may be required to obtain union.
- Long-term follow-up of all reconstructions is essential to monitor for local recurrence, aseptic loosening, allograft fragmentation, and implant failure.

Suggested Readings

Asavamongkolkul A, Eckardt JJ, Eilber FR, et al. Endoprosthetic reconstruction for malignant upper extremity tumors. Clin Orthop. 1999;360:207–20.

Athanasian EA. Aneurysmal bone cyst and giant cell tumor of bone of the hand and distal radius. Hand Clin. 2004;20:269–81.

Cannon CP, Mirza AN, Lin PP, Lewis VO, Yasko AW. Proximal femoral endoprosthesis for the treatment of metastatic disease. Orthopedics. 2008;31:361.

Cannon CP, Paraliticci GU, Lin PP, Lewis VO, Yasko AW. Functional outcome following endoprosthetic reconstruction of the proximal humerus. J Shoulder Elbow Surg. 2009;18:705–10.

Chang DW, Weber KL. Segmental femur reconstruction using an intercalary allograft with an intramedullary vascularized fibula bone flap. J Reconstr Microsurg. 2004;20:195–9.

Chang DW, Weber KL. Use of a vascularized fibula bone flap and intercalary allograft for diaphyseal reconstruction after resection of primary extremity bone sarcomas. Plast Reconstr Surg. 2005;116:1918–25.

Damron TA, Rock MG, O'Connor MI, et al. Functional laboratory assessment after oncologic shoulder joint resections. Clin Orthop. 1998;348:124–34.

Donati D, Giacomini S, Gozzi E, et al. Proximal femur reconstruction by an allograft prosthesis composite. Clin Orthop. 2002;394:192–200.

Farid Y, Lin PP, Lewis VO, et al. Endoprosthetic and allograft-prosthetic composite reconstruction of the proximal femur for bone neoplasms. Clin Orthop. 2006;442:223–9.

Fortin AJ, Lewis VO, Oates SD, et al. Reconstruction of the os innominatum. Paper presented at 60th annual meeting of the Canadian Society of Plastic Surgeons, Quebec, 2006.

Fourney DR, Rhines LD, Hentschel SJ, et al. En bloc resection of primary sacral tumors: classification of surgical approaches and outcome. J Neurosurg Spine. 2005;3:111–22.

Frink SJ, Rutledge J, Lewis VO, et al. Favorable long-term results of prosthetic arthroplasty of the knee for distal femur neoplasms. Clin Orthop. 2005;438:65–70.

Gilbert NF, Yasko AW, Oates SD, Lewis VO, Cannon CP, Lin PP. Allograft-prosthetic composite reconstruction of the proximal part of the tibia. An analysis of the early results. J Bone Joint Surg Am. 2009;91:1646–56.

Gupta GR, Yasko AW, Lewis VO, et al. Risk of local recurrence after deltoid-sparing resection for osteosarcoma of the proximal humerus. Cancer. 2009;115:3767–73.

Hugate Jr R, Sim FH. Pelvic reconstruction techniques. Orthop Clin North Am. 2006;37:85–97.

Langlais F, Lambotte JC, Collin P, et al. Long-term results of allograft composite total hip prostheses for tumors. Clin Orthop. 2003;414:197–211.

Ng RHL, Sharma SK, Chang DW, et al. Vascularized bone transfers for the management of allograft non-union in cancer patients. Paper presented at American Society for Reconstructive Microsurgery annual meeting, Cancun, Mexico, 2002.

Pant R, Yasko AW, Lewis VO, et al. Chondrosarcoma of the scapula: long-term oncologic outcome. Cancer. 2005;104:149–58.

Simon MA, Springfield DS, editors. Surgery for bone and soft tissue tumors. Philadelphia: Lippincott-Raven; 1998.

Todd Jr LT, Yaszemski MJ, Currier BL, et al. Bowel and bladder function after major sacral resection. Clin Orthop. 2002;397:36–9.

Weber KL, Lin PP, Yasko AW. Complex segmental elbow reconstruction after tumor resection. Clin Orthop. 2003;415:31–44.

Wittig JC, Villalobos CE, Hayden BL, Choi I, Silverman AM, Malawer M. Osteosarcoma of the proximal tibia: limb-sparing resection and reconstruction with a modular segmental proximal tibia tumor prosthesis. Ann Surg Oncol. 2010;17:3021.

Zeegen EN, Aponte-Tinao LA, Hornicek FJ, et al. Survivorship analysis of 141 modular metallic endoprostheses at early followup. Clin Orthop. 2004;420:239–50.

Chapter 10
Soft Tissue Reconstruction After Bone Sarcoma Resection

Scott D. Oates

Contents

Chapter Overview The successful outcome of bony tumor resection followed by prosthetic reconstruction can often be improved by the addition of appropriate soft tissue reconstruction using muscle or skin flaps of various types. Such flaps are particularly useful for areas likely to encounter wound-healing problems. The benefits of flap reconstruction are seen particularly in high-risk areas such as the ankle and foot, the tibial and knee region, the distal forearm and hand, the elbow, and the shoulder. The most distal parts of the extremities usually require free-flap reconstruction because of a lack of sufficient local soft tissue; however, more proximal areas can be reconstructed with a variety of local pedicled flaps, simplifying the procedures. Fillet flaps can also be used to aid in soft tissue closure if the extremity cannot be salvaged. Flap selection for specific areas is based on the size of the defect, type of coverage required (i.e., skin versus muscle), patient position, tissue availability, and surgeon preference. Proper preoperative planning and coordination between the plastic and orthopedic surgeons are critical.

S.D. Oates (✉)
Department of Plastic Surgery, Unit 1488, Division of Surgery,
The University of Texas MD Anderson Cancer Center,
1400 Pressler Street, Houston, TX 77030, USA
e-mail: soates@mdanderson.org

P.P. Lin and S. Patel (eds.), *Bone Sarcoma*, MD Anderson Cancer Care Series,
DOI 10.1007/978-1-4614-5194-5_10,
© The University of Texas M. D. Anderson Cancer Center 2013

Introduction

Malignant bone tumors often require major bone and joint resections. The need for soft tissue coverage after resection is obvious when there is a large extraosseous tumor and the skin is compromised. In other cases, the value of soft tissue reconstruction with muscle and skin flaps is not so apparent. However, even when tumors are largely confined to the bone and minimally invade surrounding soft tissues, flap reconstruction is sometimes indicated. The mere ability to achieve primary closure of skin does not necessarily preclude the benefit of soft tissue repair.

Prevention of wound dehiscence is one of the primary goals of soft tissue reconstruction. Dehiscence with subsequent infection can be a disastrous complication for patients with large prosthetic and allograft implants. Such a complication often results in interruption of chemotherapy, reconstructive failure, and, in extreme cases, loss of limb. Certain anatomical locations, such as the tibial region, are known to be prone to wound dehiscence and therefore benefit from planned soft tissue reconstruction. The susceptibility to wound dehiscence may be increased in some patients by preoperative chemotherapy, which compromises the patients' nutritional status and resistance to infection. Pediatric patients, especially under the age of 12 years, tolerate wound complications poorly, and every effort should be made to minimize the possibility of repeated dressing changes, immobility, hospitalization, and reoperation in these patients.

At MD Anderson Cancer Center, soft tissue repair is performed frequently after major resections of bone tumors. The bone and joint reconstructions are complex and typically involve large allograft and prosthetic replacements. Coverage of vulnerable implants with well-vascularized soft tissue is an essential part of our surgical philosophy. Additional indications for flap reconstruction include intraoperative and postoperative swelling and mismatches between host bone and implanted materials. The most commonly used soft tissue reconstruction technique involves pedicled muscle flaps with skin grafts. Free-tissue transfer is utilized when defects are larger and more distal in the extremities.

Wound Defects That Require Soft Tissue Repair

Skin and soft tissue resections are frequently a necessary part of removing bone sarcomas. Large tumors may cause thinning of the overlying skin, which may be susceptible to necrosis during resection. For tumors with close proximity to skin or direct skin invasion, varying degrees of cutaneous resection may be required to obtain adequate margins.

Certain watershed regions are at higher risk of soft tissue loss due to poor perfusion, and these areas are more likely to require reconstruction. These sites include the ankle and foot, the tibial and knee region, the distal forearm and hand, the elbow, and the shoulder. Loss of skin in these areas results in more tension on the surgical closure and increases the likelihood of postoperative wound complications. Even minimal skin resection in these areas may precipitate the need for reconstruction because there is little available skin laxity and vital structures are easily exposed.

Resection of a sarcoma with subsequent bone and joint reconstruction is typically a lengthy procedure, requiring 8 h or more in some cases. The resultant soft tissue swelling during these long procedures may result in the inability to primarily close the surgical site without tension. Such an occurrence is difficult to predict preoperatively, apart from knowing which anatomic locations are at higher risk. Tension on the operative closure can lead to skin-edge ischemia and possible wound dehiscence. This situation is especially worrisome in areas with little or no muscle coverage over the implant, such as the tibial region, elbow, and ankle.

At MD Anderson, patients with tumors in areas deemed at high risk obtain plastic surgery consultation before their tumor resections. This consultation allows preoperative discussion with the patient about possible soft tissue reconstructive options, obviating the need for most intraoperative consultations when wound closure difficulties arise. This practice avoids problems associated with plastic surgeon availability, adequacy of informed consent, and other preparations for the case.

Finally, it is worth noting that the size of the implant has an impact on the size of the wound defect. Allografts tend to be more bulky and less predictable than metallic prostheses, and thus extra care must be exercised in the selection of allografts. Comparison of the donor allograft X-ray to the host X-ray with internal size markers is essential to verifying a good match. A larger-than-expected allograft may result in a bulkier implant and may increase the tension on the soft tissue repair. In some cases, a larger flap or a free flap may become necessary. This situation is particularly likely in the proximal tibial region, which is frequently reconstructed with allograft–prosthetic composites. In areas at high risk for wound complications, there is little room for error with the soft tissues, especially in the setting of intraoperative edema.

Types of Soft Tissue Coverage

Rotation (Pedicled) Flaps

The mainstay of flap coverage for bone sarcomas is the pedicled muscle flap. Although local skin flaps can sometimes be used for smaller defects, they often fall short of complete coverage of the implants used for bone reconstruction. Muscle flaps are more durable and robust. They are available in most anatomic sites, are relatively quick to harvest, and provide excellent vascular coverage for the implants. A skin graft is usually combined with the muscle flap to achieve closure of the wound.

Gastrocnemius Flap

One of the most common pedicled flaps is the gastrocnemius muscle flap (Figs. 10.1 and 10.2). It is a robust flap, is relatively easy to raise, and provides coverage for the

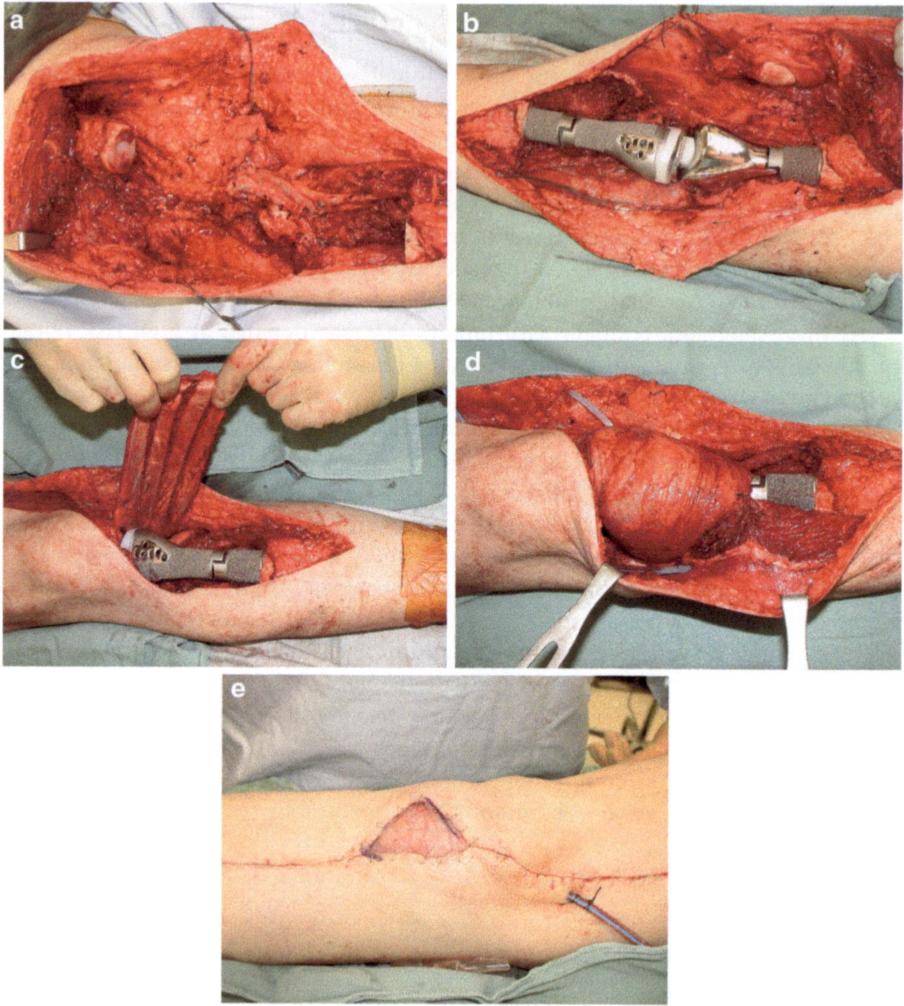

Fig. 10.1 Gastrocnemius muscle flap coverage of a prosthesis after resection of a tibial neoplasm. (**a**) The bony defect after sarcoma resection. The femur is seen at left, the tibia at right. (**b**) The prosthesis in place. (**c**) The gastrocnemius muscle flap elevated. Note that the fascia has been scored to allow a greater area of muscle coverage. (**d**) The flap in place, covering a majority of the prosthesis. (**e**) The closed wound, incorporating a split-thickness graft.

lower knee and upper third of the tibia. This area is particularly prone to wound-healing problems because of the thinness of the skin that overlies the tibia. Furthermore, our practice of using allograft–prosthesis composites for reconstruction of the proximal tibia demands a very high success rate for wound healing.

The medial head of the gastrocnemius muscle is utilized for reconstructive flaps much more frequently than the lateral head. The medial head is longer than the lateral head in most patients and can be harvested and inset without dissection or

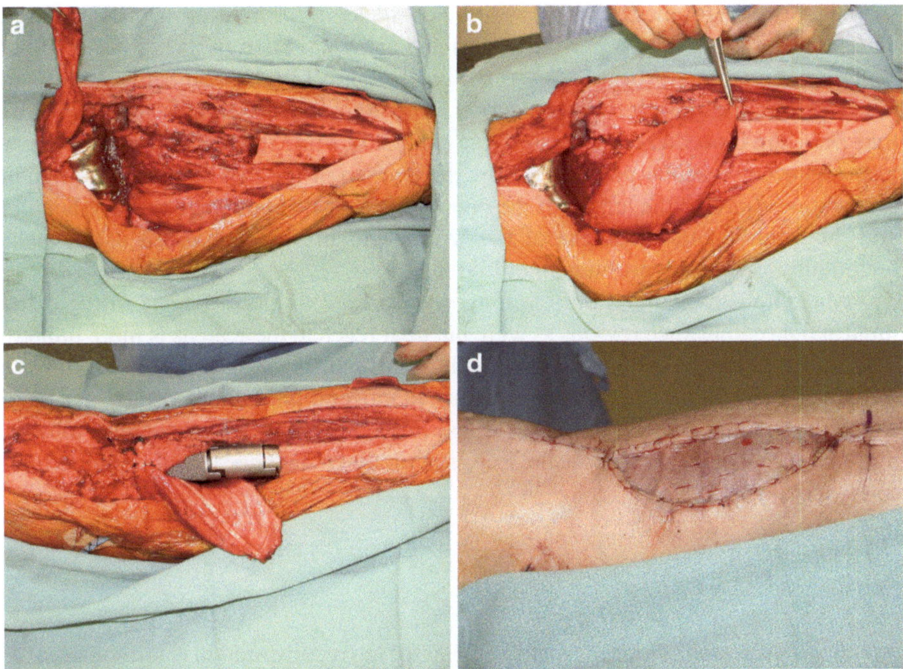

Fig. 10.2 Elevation of a gastrocnemius muscle flap prior to final placement of a prosthesis and subsequent inset of the flap. (**a**) The bony defect after sarcoma resection. The tibia is seen at right. (**b, c**) A gastrocnemius flap raised to cover the prosthesis. (**d**) The closed wound, incorporating a split-thickness graft.

exposure of the peroneal nerve near the fibular head. The lateral head of the muscle can be used for defects on the same side of the leg, but its arc of rotation is limited by the head of the fibula. Also, postoperative peroneal nerve palsies have occurred with lateral head use, likely from postoperative swelling of the soft tissues near the nerve. If this complication occurs, it may take several months to resolve, especially if postoperative radiation therapy is administered to the region.

At MD Anderson, the orthopedic oncologist works closely with the plastic surgeon for these complex bony and soft tissue reconstructions. For proximal tibial lesions, for example, after the tumor has been resected and before the prosthesis has been inset, the plastic surgery team is called to evaluate the degree of edema and soft tissue defect, if any.

The gastrocnemius muscle flap is often raised through the open incision anteriorly by the plastic surgery team while the orthopedic team prepares the implant. This methodology has several advantages. First, there is no additional donor-site incision on the back of the calf. Occasionally, a small incision is made over the Achilles tendon to release the medial or lateral gastrocnemius musculotendinous junction, but this incision is much smaller than the traditional stocking-seam incision used to harvest the muscle when the host tibia or a prosthetic is in place. Second, the mobilization of the muscle is much easier when the patient is in the supine position with the distal leg flailed. Careful rotation of the leg allows for easier visualization and delineation of the two muscle bellies and aids dissection of the sural nerve out of the midline raphe. Also, the proximal dissection near the popliteal fossa toward the origin of the muscle is much easier. This approach facilitates release of the muscle origin if needed for increased flap excursion while reducing the risk of injury to the adjacent vascular pedicle. Lastly, the overlap of the flap harvest and implant preparation shortens the length of the operation. The speed of postoperative healing and the quality and hardiness of the wound closure are enhanced using these techniques to treat the problematic tibial region.

Pedicled gastrocnemius muscle flaps can be used to close defects in the distal thigh and proximal knee regions as well, but their reach to these areas is more limited. The bulk of the muscle does not reach significantly above the knee, and the narrower and less robust distal muscle at the musculotendinous junction is left to fill more proximal defects. Because of these limitations of the gastrocnemius muscle, more proximal or larger soft tissue defects at or above the knee usually require free-tissue transfer.

Soleus Flap

Another muscle that can form a pedicled flap for leg reconstruction is the soleus. This muscle can be used to cover soft tissue defects over the middle third of the tibia. This flap is useful alone for segmental defects in which allograft reconstruction is used or in combination with a gastrocnemius flap for longer areas of exposed bone. For reconstructing large defects, no more than half the normal muscle contribution to the Achilles tendon (i.e., one hemisoleus and one head of a gastrocnemius flap from the same side) should be sacrificed to maintain adequate strength for plantar flexion. If more coverage is required, a free-tissue transfer should be used.

Latissimus Dorsi Flap

Besides the tibia, another potential problematic area is the shoulder. Soft tissue coverage is preferable if a significant portion of the deltoid muscle is resected. Prominence of an implant in this area can lead to wound dehiscence and exposure if there is insufficient soft tissue beneath. The latissimus dorsi myocutaneous flap is well suited to coverage of implants in the shoulder and proximal humerus. The muscle is easy to raise, reliable, and large enough to both cover the implant and fill adjacent dead space. It is long enough to be used for both anterior and posterior defects of the shoulder. The skin paddle can usually be placed to allow insetting directly over the top of the shoulder, where maximal soft tissue padding is needed (Fig. 10.3). Often the tumor can be removed and both bony and soft tissue reconstruction can be performed with the patient in the lateral position, facilitating flap harvest and reducing operative time. Again, close communication between the orthopedic and plastic surgery teams is crucial to maximize efficiency and minimize operative time.

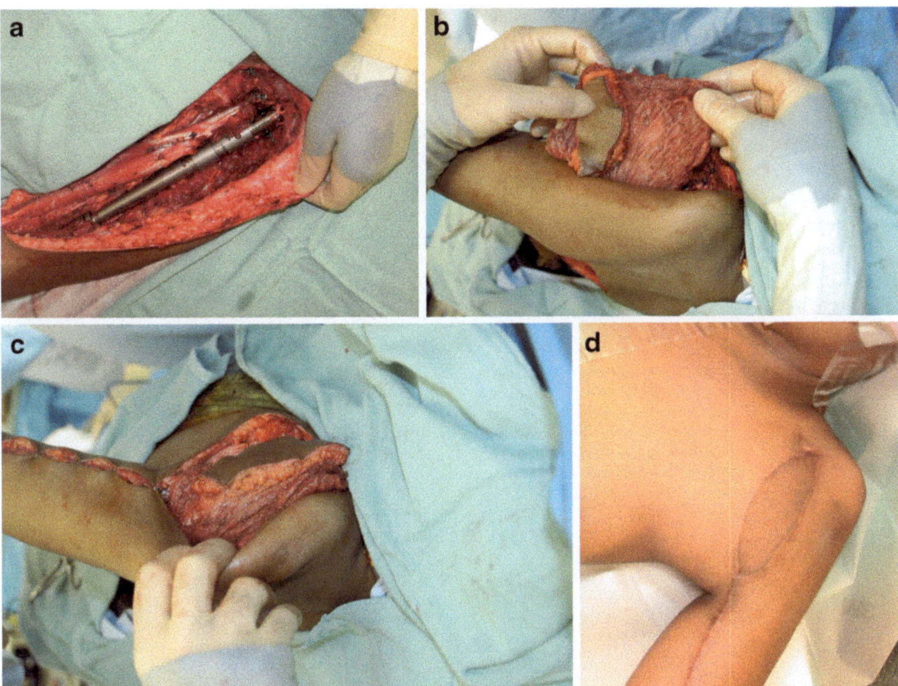

Fig. 10.3 Coverage of a humeral prosthesis with a latissimus dorsi myocutaneous flap after sarcoma resection. (**a**) A prosthesis in place after resection of an osteosarcoma of the humerus. (**b**, **c**) Placement of a latissimus dorsi myocutaneous flap to cover the prosthesis and fill the defect. The shoulder is seen on the right. (**d**) The healed flap.

Pectoralis Major Flap

The pectoralis major muscle is another option for use in reconstructing shoulder defects. Because its vascular pedicle is located anteriorly under the clavicle, the muscle is often available even if the tumor extends into the axilla and the latissimus dorsi pedicle has been compromised. The muscle itself is shorter than the latissimus dorsi, with a more restricted arc of rotation. The pectoralis major muscle is best suited to anterior defects of the shoulder, supraclavicular defects, and axillary reconstruction. For female patients who need a skin paddle, the pectoralis donor site may be cosmetically less acceptable because of possible deformation of the breast.

Radial Forearm Fasciocutaneous Flap

The elbow region is also an area in which thin skin overlying a prosthesis can be prone to healing problems. With few expendable donor muscles in the forearm, the pedicled flap of choice for elbow reconstruction is the radial forearm fasciocutaneous

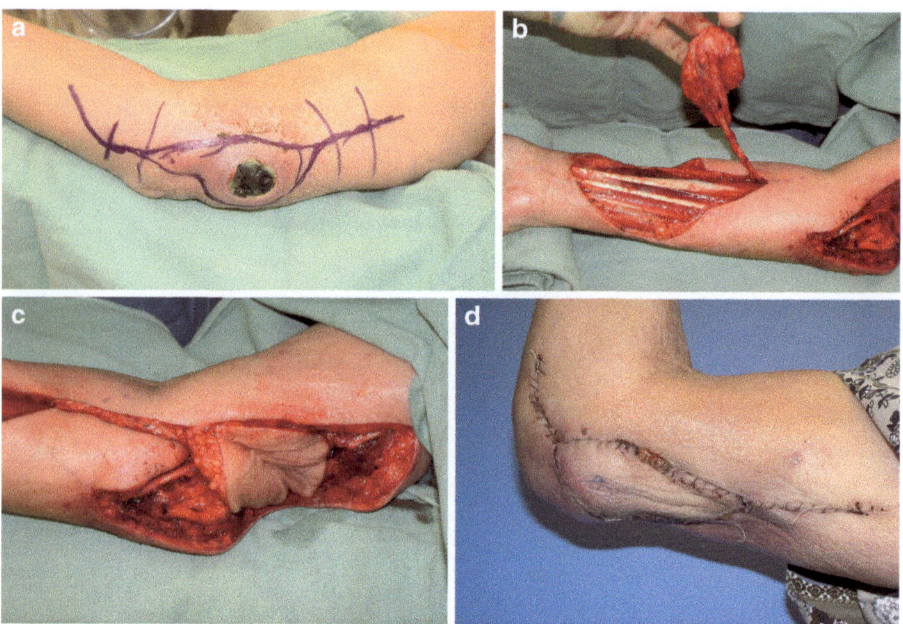

Fig. 10.4 Use of a pedicled radial forearm fasciocutaneous flap for coverage of an elbow soft tissue defect after sarcoma resection. (**a**) A large soft tissue sarcoma of the elbow. (**b**) A radial forearm fasciocutaneous flap elevated on its vascular pedicle. (**c**) The flap, prior to tunneling, shown reaching the defect. (**d**) Final closure.

flap (Fig. 10.4). It is thin but robust and large enough to cover small- to medium-sized defects of the elbow region. Its long pedicle allows it to reach medial, lateral, and dorsal defects without tension. Use of this flap does require both a skin graft for closing the donor site and sacrifice of the radial artery, but these drawbacks are well tolerated in most patients. An Allen test is used preoperatively to assess for a patent ulnar artery and vascular arch in the hand. A positive Allen test is lack of blood return to the hand after 5–6 s following release of the ulnar artery. While reassuring if the test result is negative, a positive result does not preclude the use of a radial forearm fasciocutaneous flap. Intraoperatively, vascular sufficiency on the radial side of the hand is carefully assessed before dividing the radial artery. The radial artery is explored and occluded with a vascular clamp. Then, after allowing time for equilibration, blood flow to the hand and thumb can be assessed clinically by capillary refill or handheld Doppler unit. Though rarely necessary, the radial artery can be reconstructed with a vein graft if circulatory flow to the thumb is determined to be inadequate.

Free-Tissue Transfer

Free flaps are commonly required for large soft tissue defects. In addition, moderate-sized wounds of the hand, distal forearm, distal leg, ankle, and foot often require free-tissue transfer. The elbow and knee regions may require free flaps if pedicled flaps are inadequate or unavailable, owing to the size of the defect or the loss of viable tissue (e.g., due to previous surgery or regional radiation therapy). Free-tissue transfers are significant soft tissue reconstructions and add considerable time and complexity to the operation. Nevertheless, a high success rate can be achieved when a skilled microsurgery team is combined with excellent nursing and support personnel.

In most instances, a muscle is utilized for the free flap, and it is covered with a split-thickness skin graft. Donor muscles include the rectus abdominis, latissimus dorsi, gracilis, and serratus anterior muscles. The choice of donor muscle depends on several factors: the size of the defect, type of coverage required, patient position, muscle availability, and surgeon preference.

Small- to medium-sized defects in the extremities can be covered with a rectus abdominis or gracilis muscle flap. These flaps can be harvested with the patient in the supine position. Larger defects may require a latissimus dorsi flap, requiring an intraoperative turn of the patient, unless the resection can be performed with the patient in the lateral position.

If the patient has a recurrent tumor, and a free flap was used in the original resection, the choice of a second free flap may be limited. For example, both rectus muscles should not be sacrificed because the result would be significant abdominal wall weakness.

Certain muscles have characteristics that make them desirable for certain regions of the extremities. The gracilis muscle (Fig. 10.5) works well for ankle/foot and wrist/hand reconstruction because it covers a majority of defects in these areas, atrophies significantly, and can be harvested from the ipsilateral leg, limiting donor-site morbidity. The rectus abdominis (Fig. 10.6) is an excellent choice for moderate tibial and knee defects that cannot be accommodated by gastrocnemius flaps. The latissimus dorsi muscle is generally reserved for larger knee, distal thigh, and shoulder defects. Serratus muscle flaps have the benefit of a very long vascular pedicle while allowing preservation of a functional latissimus muscle. In patients who receive preoperative radiation, this long pedicle is used to locate the microvascular connections away from the radiated and/or reconstructed vessels in the affected portion of the extremity.

Several types of free skin and fasciocutaneous flaps are also available for reconstruction after bony tumor resection. These include the free radial forearm flap, anterolateral thigh flap, and scapular flap. Such flaps (e.g., the radial forearm flap) can be used when a thinner, less bulky flap is desired. They can also be chosen in situations dictated by positioning and/or the lack of suitable donor muscles (e.g., an anterolateral thigh flap might be used for a patient in the supine position who does not have available abdominal muscles). Free skin and fasciocutaneous flaps have

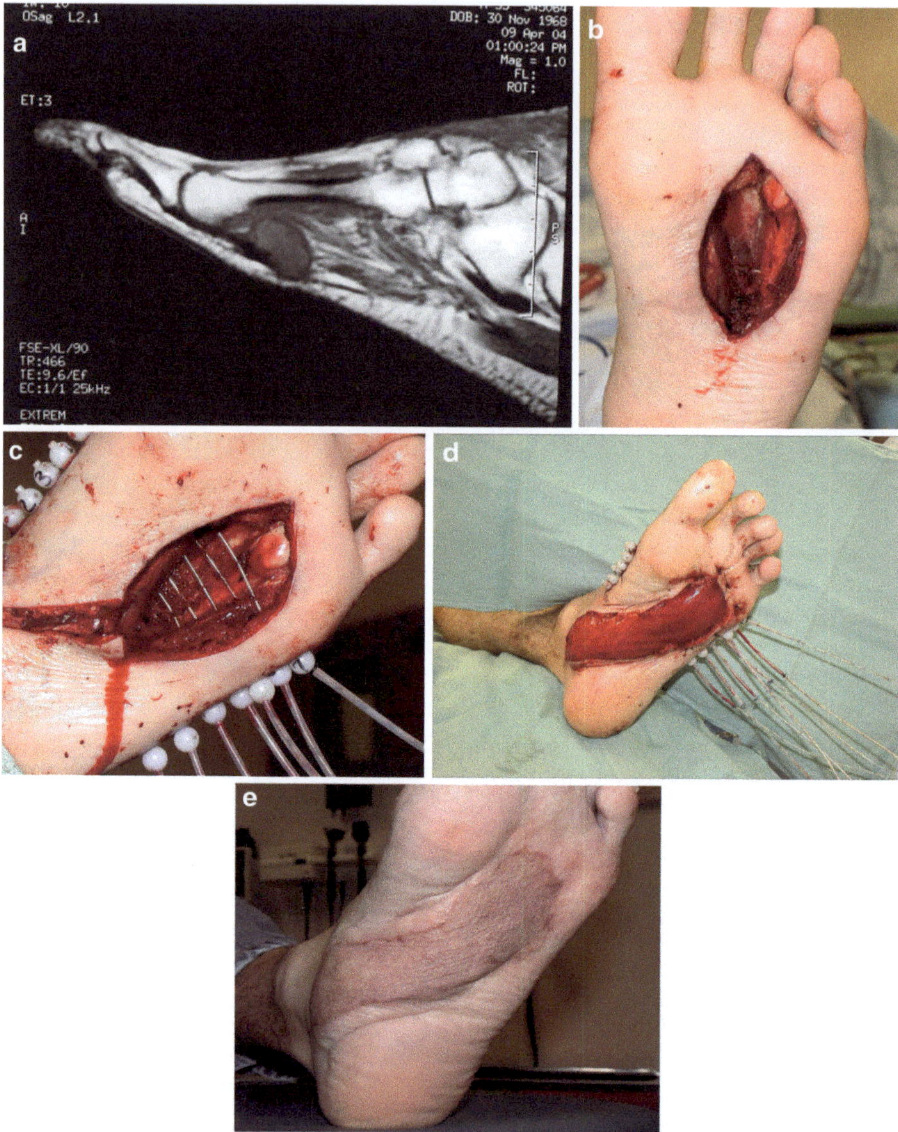

Fig. 10.5 Use of a free gracilis muscle flap for reconstruction of a plantar foot defect after tumor resection and brachytherapy catheter placement. (**a**) A recurrent sarcoma in the plantar foot. (**b**) The composite defect after excision. (**c**) Brachytherapy catheters in place. (**d**) Placement of a free gracilis muscle flap to close the wound and cover the catheters. (**e**) The healed flap several weeks after surgery.

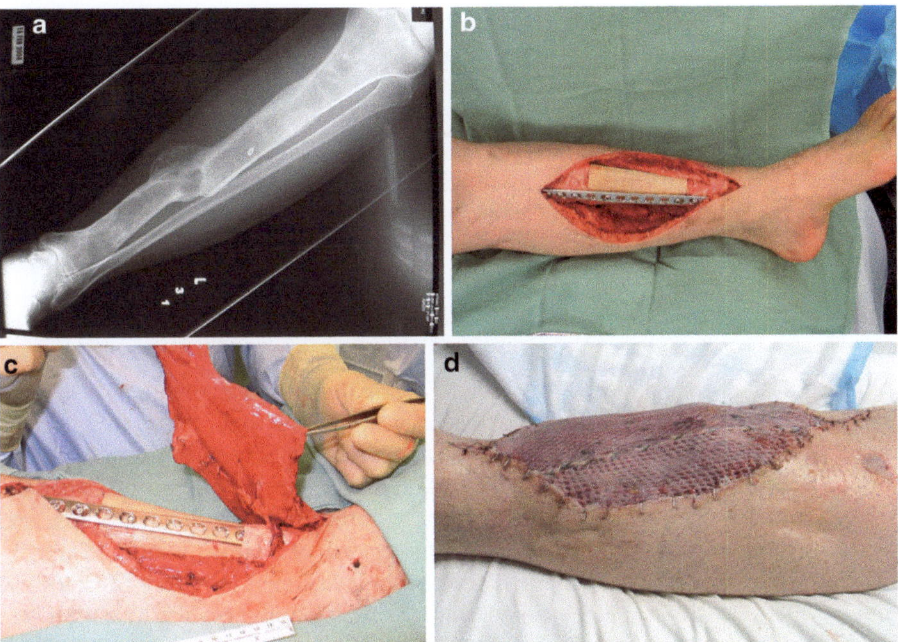

Fig. 10.6 Coverage with a free rectus abdominis muscle flap after segmental tibia resection and reconstruction for adamantinoma. (**a**) A recurrent adamantinoma in the tibia. (**b**) Tibial reconstruction with an interpositional allograft. (**c**) Use of a free rectus abdominis flap for coverage. (**d**) Early postoperative result. A skin graft has been used for closure.

the advantage of allowing primary closure of the recipient site (in most cases), but a skin graft may be required to close the donor site.

To save time, flap harvest can sometimes be performed concurrently with the resection. This timing is not always possible for a variety of reasons. First, the extent of the defect is often difficult to determine accurately before surgery. Second, the plastic surgery team may not have access to the donor site until the specimen is removed. Finally, positioning of the patient sometimes precludes access to the donor site during the resection.

When free-tissue transfers are utilized on the lower extremity, the ambulatory status of the patient will be restricted compared to that after standard prosthetic placement without flap coverage. During the patient's hospitalization, this restriction is necessary to allow initial healing of the flap and/or graft. Later, restricted ambulation and compression are used to encourage softening and atrophy of the flap, gradually increasing the time the leg is allowed in the dependent position. This regimen usually lasts 6–8 weeks after the patient is discharged, with eventual return to unlimited dependent positioning of the lower extremity.

Specialized operating room equipment and instruments and postoperative monitoring are important to achieve successful outcomes with microsurgical free-tissue transfers, and these capabilities should be in place before such reconstructions are attempted.

Regardless of the type of flap utilized, free-tissue transfers offer the ultimate in choice of donor tissue and variability of insetting options. In certain circumstances, they are the only alternative to amputation. The trade-offs are increased operative time, greater surgical complexity, potential donor-site morbidity, and prolonged rehabilitation. The increased effort on the surgeon's part and the greater need for forbearance on the patient's part are relatively small prices to pay if major complications, such as wound dehiscence and infection of the implant, are avoided.

Fillet Flap

A fillet flap is a flap taken from a portion of a limb that is being amputated. The fillet flap offers the desirable combination of a large amount of donor tissue and, usually, large-caliber vessels for vascular anastomosis (if the flap is used as a free flap). It is an excellent choice for radical amputations at the hip and shoulder girdles when the typical flaps for primary closure have been compromised by tumor, radiation, and previous surgery. In many of these situations, growth of a large tumor in the proximal portion of the extremity will have resulted in invasion of the major neurological and vascular structures, thereby rendering the limb unsalvageable. The fillet flap spares the patient the pain and morbidity of using an additional donor site. It utilizes normal tissue from the distal limb that would otherwise be lost.

Care must be exercised in determining whether a patient is a satisfactory candidate for a fillet flap. The main relative contraindication is acute or chronic lymphedema in the extremity, which can make harvest and manipulation of the soft tissues problematic.

In most cases, the fillet flap is employed as a free-tissue transfer. Pedicled fillet flaps are not often utilized because the proximal vessels are usually compromised by the tumor or by the resection. The exceptions may be where short segments of soft tissue are required (not true axial pattern flaps) or, in the hand, where the defect size is usually smaller and can be covered by one or more filleted digits.

Free-tissue transfer of fillet flaps routinely yields large amounts of tissue for reconstruction, which may be a critical advantage for massive wounds of the pelvis or chest wall. Both muscles and skin are often available, obviating the need for skin grafts (though if required, they can sometimes be harvested from another part of the amputated limb). Adequate donor vessels can usually be located because of the exposure of major vessels at the amputation site.

When amputation is deemed a possibility or is planned as part of tumor resection, the possibility of using the involved extremity to obtain a fillet flap for soft tissue coverage should always be planned in advance. The harvest of the flap must be carefully coordinated with the surgeons who perform the resection of the main tumor. These operations are often massive undertakings with large volumes of blood loss. Time is a crucial factor for success. Minimizing ischemic time for the flap and overall operative time for the patient are essential goals for the surgical team.

Key Practice Points

- After tumor resection and bony reconstruction, operative sites can benefit from closure using well-vascularized muscle or skin flaps, especially in vulnerable areas such as the proximal tibia.
- The gastrocnemius muscle flap is an excellent choice for coverage of most proximal tibial and knee reconstructions. Another pedicled flap that can be used in the leg is the soleus for central tibial defects. Both flaps can also be used together.
- For shoulder reconstruction, the latissimus dorsi or pectoralis major muscles can be used as pedicled flaps.
- The radial forearm fasciocutaneous flap can be used for reconstruction of the elbow.
- Use of free flaps may be necessary to achieve successful soft tissue reconstruction but add significant complexity to the overall operation.
- With careful planning and coordination, a fillet flap can be harvested from an unsalvageable limb and used for reconstruction.
- Close cooperation between the orthopedic and plastic surgery teams can reduce operative time and possibly patient morbidity.

Suggested Readings

Behnam AB, Chen CM, Pusic AL, et al. The pedicled latissimus dorsi flap for shoulder reconstruction after sarcoma resection. Ann Surg Oncol. 2007;14:1591–5.

Grotting JC. Prevention of complications and correction of postoperative problems in microsurgery of the lower extremity. Clin Plast Surg. 1991;18:485–9.

Horowitz SM, Lane JM, Healey JH. Soft-tissue management with prosthetic replacement for sarcomas around the knee. Clin Orthop. 1992;275:226–31.

Jones NF, Jarrahy R, Kaufman MR. Pedicled and free radial forearm flaps for reconstruction of the elbow, wrist, and hand. Plast Reconstr Surg. 2008;121:887–98.

Mathes S, Nahai F, editors. Clinical applications for muscle and musculocutaneous flaps. St Louis: Mosby; 1982.

Strauch B, Vasconez LO, Hall-Findlay EJ, Lee BT. Grabb's encyclopedia of flaps. 3rd ed. Philadelphia: Lippincott Williams and Wilkins; 2008.

Chapter 11
Bone Sarcomas in the Growing Child

Valerae O. Lewis and David W. Chang

Contents

Chapter Overview The most common primary tumors of bone occur most often in the skeletally immature patient. Historically, amputation was the procedure of choice, but improved oncologic outcomes and surgical advances have made limb-salvage therapy a feasible and valuable treatment option. However, the skeletally immature patient presents a unique group of surgical considerations. Not only may the size of the medullary canal be too small to accommodate a durable prosthesis, but also resection can create a limb-length discrepancy and gait abnormalities.

This chapter is adapted from Lewis VO, "Limb salvage in the skeletally immature patient," *Curr Oncol Rep* 2005;7:285–292 (© 2005 by Current Science Inc.), with kind permission from Current Medicine Group LLC.

V.O. Lewis (✉)
Department of Orthopaedic Oncology, Unit 1448, Division of Surgery,
The University of Texas MD Anderson Cancer Center, P.O. Box 301402,
Houston, TX 77230, USA
e-mail: volewis@mdanderson.org

D.W. Chang
Department of Plastic Surgery, Unit 1488, Division of Surgery,
The University of Texas MD Anderson Cancer Center, 1400 Pressler Street,
Houston, TX 77030, USA
e-mail: dchang@mdanderson.org

P.P. Lin and S. Patel (eds.), *Bone Sarcoma*, MD Anderson Cancer Care Series,
DOI 10.1007/978-1-4614-5194-5_11,
© The University of Texas M. D. Anderson Cancer Center 2013

Limb-salvage options available for the skeletally immature patient with a segmental long-bone defect include reconstruction with an expandable prosthesis or an intercalary autograft. A vascularized fibular transfer can preserve a limb's growing potential. Amputations and rotationplasties can result in excellent function for appropriately chosen patients.

Introduction

Osteosarcoma and Ewing sarcoma are the most common tumors of bone. Most commonly found in children, these lesions tend to occur in the metaphyses of long bones. Most of the growth of the lower extremity is contributed by the physes around the knee. The distal femur physis contributes 38% of growth, and the proximal tibia physis contributes 28% of growth (Anderson et al. 1963). Although improved oncologic outcomes and surgical advances have made limb-salvage therapy a feasible and valuable treatment option in the skeletally immature patient, resection of a sarcoma of bone can create a limb-length discrepancy and gait abnormalities (Rosen et al. 1983; Simon et al. 1986; Whelan 1997).

Although technical advances in implant design have improved limb-salvage options, procedures that rely on endoprostheses or allografts present unique challenges in the growing child. These challenges include the small size of the pediatric skeleton, the growth potential of the patient, the anticipated final length of the unaffected limb, the need for correction of the ensuing limb-length discrepancy, and the need for durable reconstruction. In particular, the small size of the childhood skeleton can limit the prosthetic options. The diameter of the intramedullary canal in small children or in children younger than 5 years is prohibitive to a durable prosthesis stem. Thus, some believe that in young children, amputation is the best option.

Growth Considerations

There are many variables that contribute to limb-length discrepancy in children who undergo treatment for sarcomas of bone. These variables include systemic chemotherapy, slowed growth of the preserved growth plate in the affected joint, muscle atrophy, muscle loss, and overgrowth of the contralateral limb. Each of these variables must be considered when estimating the final growth of a patient and the final limb-length discrepancy. Dominkus et al., in their series of 15 children who underwent tumor resection and endoprosthetic reconstruction with extendable prostheses, found that they underestimated the elongation needed to achieve equal leg lengths (Dominkus et al. 2001). They attributed their underestimation to reduced growth of the physis across the joint of the affected limb and to overgrowth of the contralateral limb.

Many methods exist for estimating the final height at skeletal maturity. The Green–Anderson growth-remaining charts (Anderson et al. 1963), the Moseley straight-line graph (Moseley 1977, 1978), and the Menelaus chronological age growth-remaining method (Menelaus 1966, 1981; Little et al. 1996) are all reliable ways of determining the final height of a child. By some or all of these methods, the length of the unaffected limb and hence the projected leg-length discrepancy can be estimated.

Limb-length inequalities are divided into three groups: less than 2 cm, 2 cm, and greater than 2 cm. Final limb-length discrepancies less than 2 cm rarely have functional or clinical significance. They can easily be corrected with shoe lifts. In addition, discrepancies of 1–2 cm after limb-salvage surgery can be beneficial if the extensor mechanism or the neurovascular bundle is compromised during resection and reconstruction. A limb that is 1–2 cm shorter than the contralateral side affords room for foot clearance if a nerve palsy or inefficient extensor mechanism is expected. However, discrepancies greater than 2 cm do not offer the same benefit. Such discrepancies are associated with gait abnormalities (Kaufman et al. 1996). Thus, when limb-length discrepancies greater than 2 cm are expected, surgical intervention is recommended.

Anticipated discrepancies between 2 and 4 cm can be addressed by epiphysiodesis of the contralateral physis or distraction osteogenesis of the shortened limb (Horton and Olney 1996; Dominkus et al. 2001). Contralateral epiphysiodesis is straightforward and can be performed percutaneously with minimal morbidity to the patient. Postoperative serial scanograms will allow the surgeon to select the proper time and date of the epiphysiodesis. However, in a young child who has undergone resection of a long-bone sarcoma, the estimated limb-length discrepancy can be quite large, and epiphysiodesis of the contralateral limb or limb lengthening of the affected limb may not achieve the length correction needed. Thus, several surgical and reconstructive procedures have been developed to reconstruct large skeletal defects and simultaneously address the ensuing leg-length discrepancies. Each reconstructive option has advantages and disadvantages, which, along with the patient's age, location of the sarcoma, lesion size, resection level, and disease stage, need to be taken into account before a reconstructive procedure is chosen.

Reconstructive Options

Expandable Prostheses

Endoprosthetic reconstruction of skeletal defects is an excellent option for the adult sarcoma patient. However, for the reasons discussed above, reconstruction with a standard static prosthesis is not a good functional option for the skeletally immature patient. Special expandable prostheses have been developed for children with a substantial amount of growth remaining. At MD Anderson Cancer Center, expandable prostheses have become the preferred reconstructive option for young patients with segmental bone loss that includes a major physis, such as the distal femur.

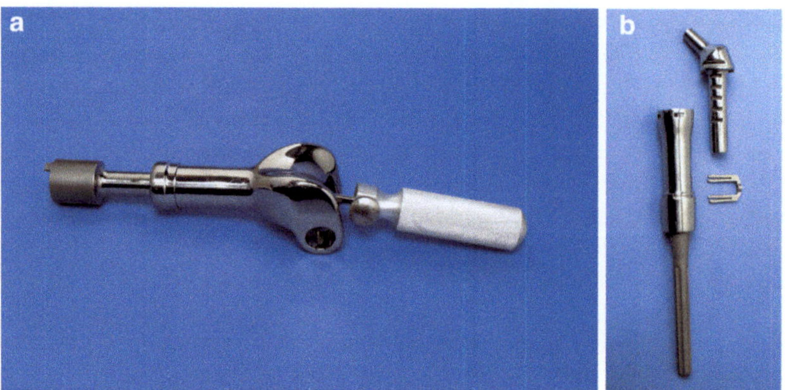

Fig. 11.1 Examples of expandable prostheses. Note the different expansion mechanisms. (**a**) The distal femoral prosthesis is approached in parallel with the prosthesis. A screwdriver is used to crank out the prosthesis. (**b**) The proximal femoral prosthesis is approached perpendicularly to the prosthesis and lengthened by insertion of a spacer and locking clip.

Scales and colleagues were the first to design a marketable expandable prosthesis (Scales et al. 1987). The Mark I prosthesis was an expandable spacer. The component did not recreate the joint but simply rested on the opposing articular surface of the joint. Although limb lengthening was possible, the functional outcome was poor. In attempts to improve the functional outcome and to decrease the complication rate, there have been many modifications of this first expandable prosthesis. Many investigators and companies have developed their own expandable prostheses (Kenan et al. 1991; Eckardt et al. 1993), and these efforts have resulted in modular, self-actuating, and self-expanding prostheses.

Each expansion of a modular prosthesis usually requires a surgical procedure and a general anesthetic. The modular expandable prosthesis is based on four segments: an articular segment, an intercalary expandable segment, exchangeable graduated segments, and an intercalary segment. Expansion takes place in the intercalary segment. In some prostheses, once the component is expanded, a spacer is inserted, and a locking clip is then secured into the spacer to prevent disassociation and collapse. In other prostheses, once the component is expanded, it is locked internally in place. The expansion process is repeated throughout the patient's growth until the desired length is achieved. Once the intercalary segment is maximally expanded, it can be exchanged for another larger intercalary segment that incorporates the length that has already been achieved. This modularity affords the prosthesis infinite expansion capabilities. Depending on the prosthesis used, the expansion mechanism is approached perpendicularly (through a lateral approach) or in parallel with the prosthesis (through the knee) (Fig. 11.1).

Generally, components are lengthened in 1- to 2-cm increments. To facilitate the lengthening process, many authors advocate either partial or complete removal of the pseudocapsule that surrounds the prosthesis (Eckardt et al. 1993, 2000; Ward et al. 1996). The limiting factor in the lengthening process is the soft tissue. If the surrounding muscles become taut, knee flexion or extension becomes restricted. If the neurovascular bundle becomes taut, a nerve palsy may develop. Thus, expansion of the prosthesis should be stopped before the neurovascular structures and surrounding muscles become tightly stretched. Taking the joint through its range of motion after lengthening will allow the surgeon to assess the degree of lengthening and the effect on the soft tissues.

Postoperatively, the patient generally remains in the hospital for 2–4 days. Physical therapy starts immediately, and the patient begins continuous passive motion (CPM) therapy. The patient is allowed to bear weight as tolerated with an assistive device.

The complication rate for expandable prostheses remains high. The most common complications are related to infection, failure of the expansion mechanism, aseptic loosening, and stem migration. In 1993, Eckardt et al. reported a complication rate of 67% in their series of patients who received a Lewis expandable adjustable prosthesis (LEAP) (Eckardt et al. 1993). The failures were due to collapse of the prosthesis, failure of the expansion mechanism, rotation of the limb, excessive wear debris, and infection. In 2000, Eckardt et al. reviewed their 14-year experience with expandable prostheses. Nineteen (59%) of the 32 patients had survived, with a median follow-up of 105 months (range, 54–156 months). Sixteen (50%) of the 32 patients underwent a total of 32 procedures expanding the prostheses to a maximum of 9 cm, without any infections. Eighteen (56%) of the 32 patients had a total of 27 complications, including aseptic loosening, collapse of the prosthesis, temporary nerve palsy, mechanical failure of the prosthesis, fatigue fracture, knee flexion contracture, and wound dehiscence. The authors concluded that the LEAP prosthesis probably should be reserved for very young patients (age 5–8 years) and that modular systems should be used for large preadolescent and adolescent children. In addition, this study reinforced that rehabilitation of the knee in very young patients (5–8 years) remains problematic and that careful selection of the patient and family is necessary.

In 1997, Dominkus et al. reported on 23 patients with expandable prostheses. Six patients had long-term follow-up, and of these patients, three had had deep infections (Dominkus et al. 1997). The authors attributed the high infection rate to the multiple operations needed for expansion. The total number of operations that a patient endures depends not only on the age and size of the patient but also on the number of complications that occur during the period of skeletal growth. It has been estimated that 10–15 operative procedures per patient may be required during the expansion period. The benefit of self-actuating and noninvasively expanding prostheses is that they eliminate the need for reoperation and thus eliminate the repeated risk of infection with each surgical intervention.

To circumvent the mechanical and surgical difficulties encountered with standard expandable prostheses, an expandable prosthesis that does not require operative intervention was developed: the Repiphysis (Wright Medical Technology Inc., Arlington, TN) (Fig. 11.2). The Repiphysis prosthesis uses energy stored in a spring that is held in place with a locking mechanism. Controlled release of the locking mechanism via an external electromagnetic field allows the prosthesis to expand. Once the component has reached full expansion, the surgeon revises the prosthesis.

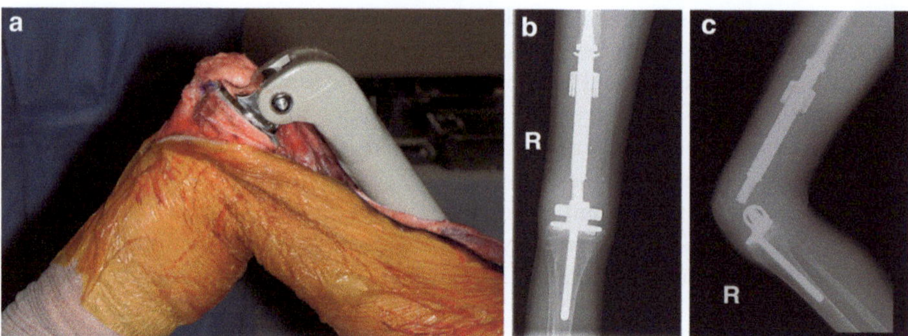

Fig. 11.2 The Repiphysis prosthesis. (**a**) Intraoperative picture. (**b**) Anteroposterior radiograph of the implanted prosthesis. (**c**) Lateral radiograph of the implanted prosthesis.

Several surgeons have reported excellent functional results with the Repiphysis (Wilkins and Soubeiran 2001; Gitelis et al. 2003). Although complications such as infection and component fracture were cited, in each case the prosthesis was salvageable. The Repiphysis offers a good option for limb salvage and noninvasive lengthening in the skeletally immature patient.

Stanmore Implants (Elstree, United Kingdom) has also developed an expandable prosthesis. It is lengthened using electromagnetic induction. Functional results have been good, and its design seems to combat some of the issues seen with the Repiphysis.

Careful patient selection is very important when considering an expandable prosthesis. Whichever model is chosen, the use of such a prosthesis is a large undertaking, not only for the surgeon but also for the patient, family, and medical oncologist. Diligent and close follow-up is necessary. Both the patient and the family have to be committed to the procedure and the long rehabilitation process. Failure to participate in rehabilitation can lead to fixed flexion contractures and poor functional results. Although excellent flexion may be achieved in the immediate postoperative period, flexion contractures of up to 20–30° can develop in as few as 2 weeks, and correction of such contractures often requires operative intervention. Physical therapy can cause discomfort to the patient, but it is necessary to achieve good functional outcome and prevent additional surgery. It is very important for the family to be supportive and enthusiastic during the rehabilitation process.

Not all children are good candidates for an expandable prosthesis. The size, age, and potential growth of the patient need to be carefully considered. It will be difficult to obtain equal leg lengths in patients who have a significant amount of growth remaining; these include the very young child (less than 5 years old) and the small child who has tall parents and thus significant potential growth remaining. If the potential growth is too much to be corrected, an alternative means of reconstruction of the extremity should be used.

The durability of the endoprosthesis, whether modular or self-expanding, remains a challenge. The long bones of children are constantly being remodeled. This remodeling and progressive change in the shape and size of the medullary canal can lead to loosening of the prosthesis (Simon and Springfield 1998). The generation of particulate debris also contributes to loosening. Stem migration and prosthetic loosening are common occurrences in cemented prostheses in children. The majority of children who undergo endoprosthetic reconstruction will need surgical revision. Press-fit prostheses may improve prosthesis longevity by limiting stress shielding, thereby maintaining bone stock.

Amputation

The distal femur is the most common location for malignant tumors of bone in the growing child. The distal femoral physis contributes approximately 10 mm of growth per year until skeletal maturity. Endoprosthetic reconstruction may not be the best option for a patient if it will leave a significant limb-length inequality (>10 cm) and significant functional impairment at the end of growth. An expandable prosthesis also may not be an option if the patient's femur is too small to accommodate a prosthesis. For these patients, amputation and rotationplasty are viable alternatives.

Although amputation is no longer the first choice in sarcoma surgery, when performed in carefully selected patients, it can provide a good functional outcome. A residual limb long enough to accommodate a prosthesis will result in an excellent long-term outcome. Children adapt well when the procedure is performed at a young age. Their prostheses are perceived as part of them as they grow. These children will be free from the multiple surgical procedures that are in the future for patients who have undergone limb-salvage reconstruction. Whereas patients with endoprostheses are dissuaded from participating in high-impact activities and hence do not return to their preresection activity levels, patients who have undergone amputation do not have such limitations. Functionally, children tend to adapt better than adult patients to amputations.

Rotationplasty

In cases in which the residual limb may not be long enough to accommodate a prosthesis or as a means of improving functional outcome, rotationplasty is an excellent alternative. The rotationplasty was first described by Borggreve (1930) for limb shortening and knee ankylosis secondary to tuberculosis; later it was popularized by Van Nes for proximal femoral focal deficiency (Van Nes 1950). This procedure and modifications of it have been employed for reconstructing the proximal femur, distal femur, and proximal tibia after sarcoma resection.

A rotationplasty transforms what would be an above-the-knee amputation into a below-the-knee amputation. Although individual surgical techniques vary depending on which bones are resected and what needs to be reconstructed, generally, segments of the distal femur and proximal tibia are excised while the neurovascular bundle is left intact. The distal portion of the limb is externally rotated 180° and attached to the proximal portion. Fixation of the proximal and distal segments is performed with a plate and screws or an intramedullary rod. The rotation of the distal segment allows the ankle to function as a knee. As time progresses, ankle motion and strength increase, and the toes on the foot atrophy. The presence of a "knee joint" adds power, stability, and control to the patient's gait.

The functional advantages of a rotationplasty include a functional knee joint, a longer lever arm to support the prosthesis, and a terminal end of the limb (i.e., the foot) that tolerates the socket load better than does an above-the-knee amputation stump. It is these anatomic advantages that explain why patients who undergo rotationplasty perform significantly better than above-the-knee amputees with respect to functional outcome and energy cost. Although a prosthesis is required for bipedal ambulation, patients who have undergone rotationplasty have been documented to have functional and psychological advantages over amputees (Murray et al. 1985; McClenaghan et al. 1989; Kenan et al. 1991; Steenhoff et al. 1993; Hoffman et al. 1998; Winkelmann 2000). They are able to walk for longer periods of time, and they are able to participate in vigorous sports activities (Cammisa et al. 1990; Gottsauner-Wolf et al. 1991). Psychologically, despite the shortened and unusual appearance of the limb, patients do quite well after rotationplasty. They tend to adjust quickly to the limb appearance and do not view themselves as amputees (Kotz and Salzer 1982; Hillmann et al. 2001). Similar results are found when comparing patients who have undergone rotationplasty to patients who have undergone endoprosthetic reconstruction. Through quality-of-life questionnaires, it was found that patients who had undergone rotationplasty could participate in daily weight-bearing activities and sports activities to a significantly greater degree than patients who had undergone limb-salvage surgery (Kotz and Salzer 1982). However, despite the potential for a superior outcome in many cases, rotationplasty is rarely the first-choice procedure in the USA. Cultural stigmas, the evolution of limb-salvage surgery, and the availability of expandable endoprosthetic components have made rotationplasty less desirable for patients and their families, and, unfortunately, rotationplasty is often relegated to use as a salvage procedure.

Intercalary Autografts and Vascularized Growth Plate Transfer

An autogenous strut bone graft is another reconstructive option for diaphyseal defects. Vascularized fibular reconstruction for segmental bone defects has been used in lower and upper extremity reconstructions. Although some authors advocate vascularized fibular reconstruction for tibia defects in children, because of the small diameter of the fibula and lack of structural integrity, vascularized fibulas may be better suited for upper extremity reconstructions. When used alone in the lower extremity, unless the extremity is protected, the incidence of fracture is significant.

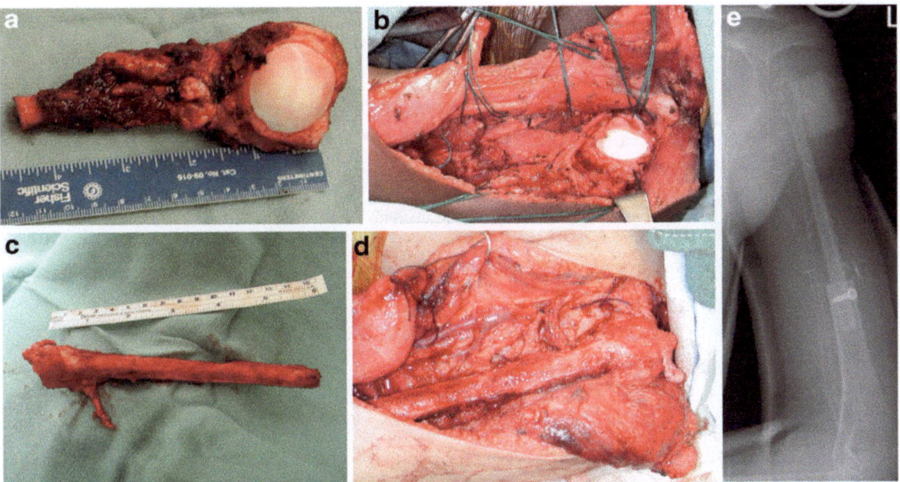

Fig. 11.3 Reconstruction using vascularized fibular head transfer. (**a**) The resected proximal humerus and humeral head. (**b**) The defect. (**c**) A vascularized fibular head and fibula bone flap. (**d**) Reconstruction of the defect with a vascularized fibular head transfer. (**e**) Postoperative radiograph.

In pediatric patients who have not reached their growth maturity, tumors involving a growth plate pose a special problem. One way to restore the ability for axial skeletal growth in these young and growing patients is to replace the resected growth plate with a vascularized growth plate transfer.

At our institution, the most commonly used vascularized growth plate transfer occurs with the transfer of the fibular head. Harvest and relocation of the vascularized fibula with its proximal physis and epiphysis can serve to transplant an active growth plate and thereby recreate a growing bone and a functional joint. The use of fibular growth plate transfer has been demonstrated to be effective in providing mean growth of more than 1 cm a year (Innocenti et al. 1998).

The advantage of using the fibular head transfer is that it not only helps restore the growth potential but also serves to reconstruct both the affected joint and the skeletal defect. For example, following resection of the humeral head and the proximal humerus, the fibular head and the proximal portion of the fibula can be used to reconstruct the bone defect and the shoulder joint (Fig. 11.3).

Similarly, defects involving the growth plates of the ulna and the radius can be reconstructed using vascularized fibular head transfer. Such a procedure has been utilized successfully in children younger than 10 years who had metaepiphyseal defects due to the resection of malignant bone tumors located in the upper limb (distal radius and proximal humerus) (Innocenti et al. 1998, 2004).

Key Practice Points

- Many reconstructive options are available for the skeletally immature patient with segmental bone loss.
- Limb-length discrepancies can be a major problem, especially when reconstruction is performed in very young patients.
- If the physis and the joint can be spared, excellent functional outcome can be achieved with an intercalary graft, often employing a vascularized fibula.
- In patients in whom the physis and joint are resected, the reconstructive option used should be chosen carefully.
- The emphasis at MD Anderson has been on expandable prostheses and vascularized fibular transfers (to recreate growing physes).
- Amputations and rotationplasties can result in excellent function for appropriately chosen patients.

Suggested Readings

Anderson MS, Green WT, Messner MB. Growth and predictions of growth in the lower extremities. J Bone Joint Surg Am. 1963;45-A:1–14.

Beebe K, Benevenia J, Kaushal N, Uglialoro A, Patel N, Patterson F. Evaluation of a noninvasive expandable prosthesis in musculoskeletal oncology patients for the upper and lower limb. Orthopedics. 2010;33:396.

Borggreve J. Kniegelenssersatz durch das in der Beinlngsachse um 180° gedrehte Fussgelenk. Arch Orthop Unfall-Chir. 1930;28:175–8.

Cammisa Jr FP, Glasser DB, Otis JC, et al. The Van Nes tibial rotationplasty. A functionally viable reconstructive procedure in children who have a tumor of the distal end of the femur. J Bone Joint Surg Am. 1990;72:1541–7.

Dominkus M, Windhager R, Kotz R. Treatment of malignant bone tumors in young children: complications and revisions. Acta Orthop Scand Suppl. 1997;276:4.

Dominkus M, Krepler P, Schwameis E, et al. Growth prediction in extendable tumor prostheses in children. Clin Orthop. 2001;390:212–20.

Eckardt JJ, Safran MR, Eilber FR, et al. Expandable endoprosthetic reconstruction of the skeletally immature after malignant bone tumor resection. Clin Orthop. 1993;297:188–202.

Eckardt JJ, Kabo JM, Kelley CM, et al. Expandable endoprosthesis reconstruction in skeletally immature patients with tumors. Clin Orthop. 2000;373:51–61.

Gitelis S, Neel MD, Wilkins RM, et al. The use of a closed expandable prosthesis for pediatric sarcomas. Chir Organi Mov. 2003;88:327–33.

Gottsauner-Wolf F, Kotz R, Knahr K, et al. Rotationplasty for limb salvage in the treatment of malignant tumors at the knee. A follow-up study of seventy patients. J Bone Joint Surg Am. 1991;73:1365–75.

Gupta A, Meswania J, Pollock R, et al. Non-invasive distal femoral expandable endoprosthesis for limb-salvage surgery in paediatric tumours. J Bone Joint Surg Br. 2006;88:649–54.

Hillmann A, Rosenbaum D, Gosheger G, et al. Rotationplasty type B IIIa according to Winkelmann: electromyography and gait analysis. Clin Orthop. 2001;384:224–31.

Hoffman C, Hillmann A, Krakau H, et al. Functional results and quality of life measurements in patients with multimodal treatment of a primary bone tumor located in the distal femur. Rotationplasty versus endoprosthetic replacement. Med Pediatr Oncol. 1998;31:202–3.

Horton G, Olney B. Epiphysiodesis of the lower extremity: results of percutaneous technique. J Pediatr Orthop. 1996;16:180–2.

Innocenti M, Ceruso M, Manfrini M, et al. Free vascularized growth-plate transfer after bone tumor resection in children. J Reconstr Microsurg. 1998;14:137–43.

Innocenti M, Delcroix L, Manfrini M, et al. Vascularized proximal fibular epiphyseal transfer for distal radial reconstruction. J Bone Joint Surg Am. 2004;86-A:1504–11.

Kaufman K, Miller L, Sutherland D. Gait asymmetry in patients with limb-length inequality. J Pediatr Orthop. 1996;16:144–50.

Kenan S, Bloom N, Lewis MM. Limb-sparing surgery in skeletally immature patients with osteosarcoma. The use of an expandable prosthesis. Clin Orthop. 1991;270:223–30.

Kotz R, Salzer M. Rotation-plasty for childhood osteosarcoma of the distal part of the femur. J Bone Joint Surg Am. 1982;64:959–69.

Little D, Nigo L, Aiona M. Deficiencies of current methods for timing of epiphysiodesis. J Pediatr Orthop. 1996;16:173–9.

McClenaghan BA, Krajbich JI, Pirone AM, et al. Comparative assessment of gait after limb-salvage procedures. J Bone Joint Surg Am. 1989;71:1178–82.

Menelaus MB. Correction of leg length discrepancy by epiphysial arrest. J Bone Joint Surg Br. 1966;48:336–9.

Menelaus M. The Anstey Giles lecture. Opening and closing the growth plate. Aust N Z J Surg. 1981;51:518–27.

Moseley CF. A straight-line graph for leg-length discrepancies. J Bone Joint Surg Am. 1977;59:174–9.

Moseley CF. A straight line graph for leg length discrepancies. Clin Orthop. 1978;136:33–40.

Murray MP, Jacobs PA, Gore DR, et al. Functional performance after tibial rotationplasty. J Bone Joint Surg Am. 1985;67-A:392–9.

Rosen G, Marcove RC, Huvos AG, et al. Primary osteogenic sarcoma: eight-year experience with adjuvant chemotherapy. J Cancer Res Clin Oncol. 1983;106(suppl):55–67.

Scales JT, Sneath RS, Wright KWJ. Design and clinical use of extending prosthesis. In: Enneking WF, editor. Limb salvage in musculoskeletal oncology. New York: Churchill Livingstone; 1987. p. 52–61.

Selber JC, Treadway C, Lopez A, Lewis VO, Chang DW. The use of free flap for limb salvage in children with tumors of the extremities. J Pediatr Surg. 2011;46:736–44.

Simon MA, Springfield DS, editors. Surgery for bone and soft tissue sarcomas, vol. 1. New York: Lippincott Williams and Wilkins; 1998. p. 756.

Simon MA, Aschliman MA, Thomas N, et al. Limb-salvage treatment versus amputation for osteosarcoma of the distal end of the femur. J Bone Joint Surg Am. 1986;68:1331–7.

Steenhoff JR, Daanen HA, Taminiau AH. Functional analysis of patients who have had a modified Van Nes rotationplasty. J Bone Joint Surg Am. 1993;75:1451–6.

Taylor GI, Wilson KR, Rees MD, et al. The anterior tibial vessels and their role in epiphyseal and diaphyseal transfer of the fibula: experimental study and clinical applications. Br J Plast Surg. 1988;41:451–69.

Van Nes CP. Rotation-plasty for congenital defects of the femur. Making use of the ankle of the shortened limb to control the knee joint of a prosthesis. J Bone Joint Surg Am. 1950;32-B:12–6.

Ward Sr WG, Yang RS, Eckardt JJ. Endoprosthetic bone reconstruction following malignant tumor resection in skeletally immature patients. Orthop Clin North Am. 1996;27:493–502.

Whelan JS. Osteosarcoma. Eur J Cancer. 1997;33:1611–8 [discussion 1618–9].

Wilkins RM, Soubeiran A. The Phenix expandable prosthesis: early American experience. Clin Orthop. 2001;382:51–8.

Winkelmann WW. Type-B-IIIa hip rotationplasty: an alternative operation for the treatment of malignant tumors of the femur in early childhood. J Bone Joint Surg Am. 2000;82:814–28.

Chapter 12
Perioperative Management of Patients with Bone Sarcomas

Janie Rutledge, Mark S. Pilarczyk, and Alan W. Yasko

Contents

Chapter Overview Bone sarcomas are associated with a host of complex and challenging issues that make perioperative management markedly different from that of the general orthopedic patient. Preoperative assessment must address cancer treatment-related comorbidities and anticipate psychosocial needs arising from the

---

Dr. Yasko died during production of this volume. Further revisions to the chapter were made by Janie Rutledge, Mark Pilarczyk, and Patrick Lin.

J. Rutledge (✉) • M.S. Pilarczyk
Department of Orthopaedic Oncology, Unit 1448, Division of Surgery,
The University of Texas MD Anderson Cancer Center, P.O. Box 301402,
Houston, TX 77230, USA
e-mail: jrutledg@mdanderson.org; mspilarc@mdanderson.org

A.W. Yasko
Department of Orthopaedic Surgery, Northwestern University,
Feinberg School of Medicine, Chicago, IL, USA

P.P. Lin and S. Patel (eds.), *Bone Sarcoma*, MD Anderson Cancer Care Series,
DOI 10.1007/978-1-4614-5194-5_12,
© The University of Texas M. D. Anderson Cancer Center 2013

sequelae of radical operations. Appropriate timing of surgery with respect to chemotherapy is crucial to avert complications such as infection, hemorrhage, and wound dehiscence. Intraoperatively, close communication is vital between the surgical and anesthesiology teams in order to prevent adverse events. Aggressive blood product and fluid resuscitation during surgery is essential for many procedures in orthopedic oncology, and this is best accomplished as a joint effort on the part of the anesthesiology and surgery teams. Postoperative management is challenging for bone sarcoma patients in a variety of ways. Postoperative pain can be difficult to control since the wound is often massive; moreover, patients may have problems with chronic skeletal pain, a high tolerance to narcotic medication, and chemotherapy-related neuropathic pain. Other postoperative concerns include proper wound care, prevention of venous thromboembolic disease, electrolyte balance, nutrition, and mobilization. Proper medical management during the perioperative period can contribute substantially to the success of the operation as well as the overall oncologic treatment of the patient.

Introduction

The sarcoma patient differs greatly from the general orthopedic patient. While most orthopedic patients in the community are healthy and active, the sarcoma patient is frequently debilitated. Even young patients who were once active and energetic become sedentary and vulnerable to a wide array of medical problems, especially after undergoing high-dose cytotoxic induction chemotherapy. Surgical treatment usually occurs after multiple cycles of chemotherapy at a point when the body is not in optimal physical condition. In general, the surgery to remove a bone sarcoma is much more complicated and extensive than a routine orthopedic operation. Oncologic surgery typically consists of a large bone and soft tissue resection, plus insertion of a large prosthesis or allograft bone. Consequently, the medical issues and perioperative concerns are of much greater magnitude. Proper measures to treat perioperative medical problems are important not only to the success of the operation but also to the overall oncologic treatment. Patients who are able to recover from surgery quickly without major complications can resume chemotherapy in a timely fashion. Adhering to a tight chemotherapy schedule and achieving the intended dose intensity of a chemotherapeutic regimen can be critical to the cure of the patient.

This chapter will focus on the key principles that underlie optimal preoperative, intraoperative, and postoperative management of the orthopedic oncology patient. Our best-practice guidelines, which have been developed over many years, will be described in detail.

Preoperative Management

The goal of preoperative treatment is to prepare the patient, physically and mentally, for surgery. Surgical planning begins at the time of diagnosis, which can be months before the actual surgery if preoperative chemotherapy is employed. Radiographic analysis, medical clearance, procurement of implants, and consultations are arranged well in advance of the operation.

Diagnostic imaging studies are reviewed to determine whether a limb-sparing surgery or amputation will be necessary. If preoperative chemotherapy or radiation is indicated, the patient is referred to the sarcoma medical oncologist or radiation oncologist. The patient is reevaluated after completion of preoperative treatment.

The reevaluation visit is scheduled to finalize the surgical plan. This visit should be scheduled before the start of the last course of preoperative chemotherapy to provide adequate time to arrange for and procure implants for reconstruction and to schedule consultations, if necessary. Cross-sectional images (computed tomography and/or magnetic resonance imaging scans) are reviewed to determine the extent of marrow and soft tissue involvement. If a limb-sparing procedure is possible, the options for reconstruction after tumor removal are evaluated.

Once the level of resection and method of reconstruction are determined, the necessary implants and equipment are ordered. The prosthesis manufacturer or a bone bank (for large segmental allografts) is contacted for procurement.

Consultation, if necessary, is arranged in advance to optimize the patient's health status before surgery. These may include the pediatric team, which can help manage fluid and electrolyte balance for young children and infants. For adults with various comorbidities, cardiologists, pulmonologists, and other specialists may be needed, depending upon the particular individual and problem.

Other consultations address the psychosocial and educational needs of the patient and family. For children and adolescents, MD Anderson's Child and Adolescent Life Program provides emotional support from the time of diagnosis throughout the patient's entire care. If limb salvage is not possible and an amputation is recommended, patient education and psychological support are provided. A prosthetist is consulted to begin discussion and answer questions related to function and use of an external prosthesis. The patient is also given an opportunity to meet with other amputees and develop a social support network. Even when amputation is not to be performed, patients can have emotional difficulty dealing with their disease and may benefit from various resources that provide psychological support.

Surgical Timing

Appropriate timing of surgery is crucial for decreasing the potential for postoperative complications. Chemotherapy and radiotherapy increase the risk of infection, hemorrhage, and wound-related problems. Because chemotherapy results in bone marrow suppression, a hematology survey is performed preoperatively to determine the patient's level of recovery. An absolute neutrophil count (ANC) of at least 1,500/µL and a platelet count of at least 70,000/µL are used as thresholds for nonemergent surgery. Preoperative radiotherapy can result in delayed wound healing; thus, surgery is not scheduled until approximately 4–6 weeks after completion of radiation.

Preoperative Visit

A preoperative evaluation is scheduled approximately 1 week prior to surgery. A complete medical history is taken, and a physical examination is performed. The patient is assessed for surgical risk factors. If the patient has significant comorbidities, a consultation with the Internal Medicine Perioperative Assessment Center is requested. If cardiotoxic agents were administered preoperatively or if the patient has risk factors for cardiac problems, a cardiac evaluation (an electrocardiogram and an echocardiogram) should be considered. A preoperative cardiology consultation is mandatory if the patient has a recent history of a major cardiac event or chronic cardiac problems.

The physical examination should include a careful inspection of the operative limb or site to ensure that there are no unanticipated problems with the area of incision. The neurological and vascular status of the limb needs to be documented thoroughly. Signs of swelling and tenderness in the leg might indicate the presence of a deep venous thrombosis and may be an indication for Doppler ultrasonography.

Preoperative radiographs of the affected limb are taken to confirm that no new occult pathological fracture or lesion has developed. Laboratory studies are obtained to ensure that blood counts are adequate, electrolyte levels are within acceptable ranges, and coagulation profiles are satisfactory. Renal function should be closely monitored since some of the chemotherapeutic agents used for sarcomas cause renal insufficiency. Blood ideally should be type-matched at least 48 h in advance. Many patients will have received transfusions during preoperative chemotherapy, and the possibility of having antibodies to red blood cells is increased in these patients.

Intraoperative Management

The goals of intraoperative medical management are to support the patient through surgery and to avoid adverse events. The anesthesiology and surgical teams communicate frequently to discuss the patient's status during surgery. The patient is monitored closely with invasive and noninvasive measures. Large-bore intravenous catheters and central lines are placed for adequate vascular access in anticipation of rapid blood product and fluid resuscitation. The rate of blood loss should be known by the surgeon and anesthesiologist at all times. The surgical team should alert the anesthesiologists when sudden blood loss is occurring. Conversely, the anesthesiology team should inform the surgeons if the patient is becoming hypotensive or showing signs of distress. Blood and fluid replacement should be performed aggressively and early. Ideally, the surgical and anesthesiology teams participate together in this process. Similarly, plasma and clotting factors should be replaced early before patients become coagulopathic.

An epidural catheter (or peripheral nerve block catheters) may be placed in the operating room to facilitate postoperative analgesia. This is typically done just prior to induction of general anesthesia so that the patient can report any pain or numbness that occurs after insertion of the catheter. Such symptoms, which are not evident if the patient is under general anesthesia, may indicate accidental nerve damage.

Prophylactic antibiotics are administered approximately 30 min before the start of the procedure. Redosing is common during long surgical procedures. A first-generation cephalosporin, such as cefazolin (Ancef), is used routinely for nonpelvic cases. For pelvic surgery, cefoxitin is administered prophylactically. However, with the emergence and increasing prevalence of methicillin-resistant strains of *Staphylococcus* and other bacteria, there is now debate about the choice of prophylactic antibiotic, particularly when a patient is to undergo placement of a large endoprosthesis or allograft. Some consideration may be given on a case-by-case basis for an antibiotic that has greater efficacy toward *Staphylococcus* than a first-generation cephalosporin. This topic is highly controversial, and definitive studies supporting or refuting the concept in orthopedic oncology are lacking. The drug sensitivity data for a given hospital may influence the decision.

Postoperative Management

The postoperative management focuses on preventing complications, providing adequate pain control, maintaining a clean wound, minimizing the risk of deep vein thrombosis (DVT), preventing nerve palsy, and mobilizing the patient as soon as possible. While most patients can recover adequately in the normal postanesthesia care unit (recovery room), some patients who have undergone massive procedures with large-volume fluid resuscitation are best managed in the surgical intensive care unit. Overnight hemodynamic monitoring and ventilatory support are common for sarcoma patients after lengthy anesthetic periods and high blood loss.

Monitoring for Anemia and Metabolic Imbalance

Metabolic and electrolyte imbalances are common in patients who were treated with preoperative chemotherapy. Serum calcium and magnesium levels are frequently low, especially in elderly patients with cardiac problems. Borderline renal insufficiency is common in patients who have undergone chemotherapy, especially those who have received cisplatin and ifosfamide, and this condition may have bearing on the choice of certain medications that can be nephrotoxic, such as vancomycin. Complete chemistry profiles and electrolyte levels are monitored daily and imbalances corrected by intravenous supplements as indicated.

Preexisting anemia and, to a lesser degree, thrombocytopenia are frequent in patients who have undergone chemotherapy. The severity may not be apparent on the preoperative blood tests, which may show only borderline low hemoglobin levels. A complete blood count is ordered in the recovery room if the intraoperative estimated blood loss is greater than 500 mL. Greater vigilance is indicated for small children, who have a lower total blood volume and may have a greater reduction in hemoglobin level for a given blood loss. Blood counts should be repeated on successive days since the magnitude of the hemoglobin drop may become manifest only with time and may continue to worsen as a result of internal hemorrhage. It may be appropriate to transfuse packed red blood cells, even if the hemoglobin level is considered adequate, if there is tachycardia, hypotension, high surgical drain output, low urine production, and other signs of distress. The goal is to maintain a blood volume and hemoglobin level adequate for end organ perfusion. Similarly, the need for transfusion of plasma and clotting factors is based just as much on clinical signs of persistent bleeding as on serum tests for coagulation.

Pain Management

Adequate pain control is essential for the patient's recovery as well as his or her optimal performance in physical therapy. Postoperative pain management can be very challenging in the orthopedic oncology patient. Radical operations that remove large segments of the bone and soft tissue are inherently painful. In addition, patients may have issues with chronic pain control as a result of long-standing osseous tumors and/or pathologic fractures. Patients who have been on narcotic pain medication may develop a degree of tolerance to the drug and need higher doses to achieve adequate pain relief. Chemotherapy-induced neuropathies can further exacerbate postoperative pain.

Intravenous patient-controlled analgesia (PCA) is the most common method of pain control. Intravenous opioids, such as morphine, hydromorphone, or fentanyl, are administered via the PCA pump. The goal is to maintain a pain level of 4 or less as measured on a visual analog scale of 1–10. The PCA is started immediately in the postanesthesia care unit. Most patients attain satisfactory pain relief with a starting demand dose of 1 mg morphine or 0.2 mg hydromorphone every 10 min. This is adjusted to a higher or lower dose or frequency on an individual basis. For patients who require much more frequent or higher dosing, a basal dose is added, but this is done with caution since there is a risk of overdose. The basal dose is set at approximately 30% of the average hourly dose. In a typical, uncomplicated case, the basal rate may be 1 mg morphine or 0.2 mg hydromorphone an hour. Patients who require a high basal rate are best managed in conjunction with a formal consultation with the Pain Service. Transition to oral analgesics begins on postoperative day 2 or 3, when the PCA is usually discontinued. The most commonly prescribed oral analgesic is hydrocodone.

Epidural PCA can be an effective modality, especially in the lower extremity. At MD Anderson, the epidural catheters and PCAs are always managed by the Anesthesia Pain Service, which maintains in-house staff on call 24 h a day. This availability is important since epidural catheters are vulnerable to interruptions in flow, which can result in severe loss of pain control. The epidural catheter remains in place until approximately postoperative day 3 or 4. Once the epidural PCA is discontinued, the patient is given intravenous PCA or oral analgesics. Because of the potential added sedation, other narcotic analgesics and sedatives are generally contraindicated in patients with epidural PCA, unless specifically approved by the Pain Service.

Similar to epidural catheters, peripheral nerve block catheters can be quite effective. The nerve block catheters are also managed by the Pain Service. They have the advantage of potentially staying in place longer than epidural catheters, and they are especially helpful with amputations. Peripheral nerve catheters have the unique benefit of not inducing any sedative effect, which is important for elderly patients, who can become disoriented with systemic opioids, and for patients with respiratory compromise, who need to maximize their inspiratory effort.

Nonsteroidal anti-inflammatory drugs (NSAIDs) are not prescribed in the immediate postoperative period without careful consideration because they have a mild anticoagulant effect. Sarcoma resections are extensive and result in large potential dead spaces that can bleed considerably. For patients with poor response to opioids and other pain modalities, ketorolac (Toradol) (60 mg as a loading dose and 30 mg every 8 h for 24 h) can be highly effective.

For amputees and other patients with neuropathic pain, it is important to start a medication such as gabapentin or pregabalin immediately. The dosage for these medications is gradually escalated to avoid neurological side effects. These medications are sometimes helpful in patients who do not exhibit signs of classic neurogenic pain and yet are not responding well to opioid analgesics.

Wound Management

Surgical-site infections can be catastrophic since they can lead to extended hospital stays, delays in resumption of adjuvant therapy, reoperations, and reconstructive failures. The orthopedic oncology patient may have numerous risk factors for impaired wound healing, including a large surgical wound, extensive soft tissue and bone dissection, substantial soft tissue dead space, long operative time, prior radiotherapy, chemotherapy, implantation of a large metallic prosthesis or allograft, and poor nutrition. The clinician must make every effort to counterbalance these negative factors. Intraoperatively, for example, meticulous wound closure and careful handling of soft tissues are of utmost importance.

Postoperatively, the value of close monitoring of the surgical wound cannot be overstated, and the operative site must be inspected at least daily. Although some surgeons still prefer traditional gauze bandages and dressings, others now prefer to close the wound with absorbable, buried sutures and seal the incision with a cyanoacrylate adhesive so as to avoid leakage of fluid, communication with the outside environment, and tape blisters. Since resection of tumors can lead to large seromas or hematomas, which can increase risk for infection and dehiscence, we typically employ surgical drains and keep them in place until the output diminishes below an acceptable level specific to the surgery performed. The drains are generally not left in place more than 2 weeks, and patients with an endoprosthesis or massive allograft are not discharged from the hospital with a wound drain. Patients with large persistent seromas and hematomas may be better managed by intermittent, percutaneous aspiration or reoperation than by an indwelling catheter beyond 2 weeks.

Muscle flaps and skin grafts are used often for reconstruction in our patients. Such procedures are typically performed by a plastic surgeon, who is a consultant on the case. The flaps provide well-perfused tissue coverage over vulnerable endoprostheses or allografts, minimizing the risk of wound-related complications and deep infections. Muscle flaps and skin grafts are monitored closely by both the orthopedic and plastic surgery teams. The vascular pedicles for free-tissue transfers are checked by Doppler assessments every 1–2 h by the nursing staff. Patients who require a muscle flap or skin graft are usually restricted to bed rest for several days after surgery to optimize perfusion and maintain viability of the flap.

Prophylactic Antibiotics

The use of prophylactic antibiotics in the postoperative setting has gradually evolved over time. Although wound-related infections are of potentially grave impact, overuse of antibiotics and development of antibiotic resistance are also concerns. Our experience with single-agent prophylactic antibiotics has been generally positive. As with intraoperative prophylaxis, postoperatively a first-generation cephalosporin is the most common antibiotic used in nonpelvic cases, and a second-generation cephalosporin is used in pelvic cases. If the patient has a penicillin allergy, clindamycin or vancomycin may be used. As stated above, with the widespread emergence of methicillin-resistant *Staphylococcus* species, there may be consideration in some cases to using antibiotics with better coverage in patients who are to receive large endoprostheses or allografts.

For patients who have undergone major resection and complex reconstruction with a massive allograft or mega-endoprosthesis, intravenous antibiotics are continued until the wound drain is removed. For less complex cases, antibiotics are discontinued after three postoperative doses.

Deep Vein Thrombosis

DVT can be catastrophic. A thrombus can embolize and result in pulmonary compromise, cardiac arrest, and sudden death. Cancer patients have long been thought to be at increased risk for DVT. One reason for this may be that release of procoagulant factors from the tumor produces a hypercoagulable state. Identification of high-risk patients is essential. Orthopedic oncology patients aged 40 years or older who undergo pelvis or lower extremity surgery are at higher risk for developing a DVT. Previous thromboembolic disease, obesity, and prolonged immobility also increase the risk for DVT. In addition, large tumors and long operative times can contribute to thrombus formation because of slower circulatory flow or endothelial damage.

Mechanical prophylaxis, such as compression stockings and sequential compression devices (SCDs), are important components of DVT prophylaxis. Our patients are routinely given mechanical prophylaxis unless contraindicated by the presence of a free flap or skin graft in the area. Early mobilization is another critical part of DVT prevention, and patients are encouraged to be out of bed on postoperative day 1 or 2 unless strict bed rest is indicated.

Chemical prophylaxis with pharmacological agents, such as low-molecular-weight heparin (LMWH) products, is used in many patients to prevent DVT at MD Anderson. In most cases, LMWH is administered on postoperative day 1 between 12 and 24 h after the end of surgery. The patient is monitored closely for signs of bleeding. The duration of chemical prophylaxis is determined on the basis of the surgical procedure as well as daily reevaluation of risk factors for both DVT and bleeding. If the immediate postoperative risk of bleeding is high, chemical prophylaxis is withheld until later in the hospital course, when the risk of bleeding has decreased. Relative contraindications to chemical prophylaxis include low platelet count (<50,000/µL), prolonged clotting time, a brain tumor, presence of an epidural catheter, or uncontrolled hypertension. Absolute contraindications to chemical prophylaxis include active bleeding and hypersensitivity to the pharmacological agent.

The risk of DVT is decreased once the patient is ambulatory. It is our current practice that patients stay on low-dose aspirin from discharge until their first postoperative evaluation unless they have a contraindication or allergy to aspirin. Alternatively, LMWH therapy may be continued after discharge if the patient is at high risk for DVT.

Nerve Palsy

Peripheral nerve palsy is an uncommon but serious complication. Fortunately, it is usually not permanent. In our experience, most palsies occur not intraoperatively but rather postoperatively. Nerve palsy can occur after prolonged compression or extensive traction on a nerve. Often, the exact cause is unclear. The most common nerve affected is the peroneal nerve. The superficial location around the fibular head may predispose the peroneal nerve to increased compression.

Several factors seem to increase patients' risk of peripheral nerve palsy. First, the orthopedic oncology patient who has been treated with chemotherapy or radiotherapy is at higher risk than the general orthopedic surgery patient. Chemotherapy- and radiotherapy-induced neuropathy predisposes the patient to nerve palsy and makes the nerve more susceptible to injury with the addition of a second insult, such as surgery.

Postoperative epidural analgesia may contribute to the risk for nerve palsy. Decreased sensation to the lower extremity can cause patients to rest their lower legs along the bed rails or orthopedic equipment such as a continuous passive motion (CPM) machine, leading to prolonged undetected pressure over the peroneal nerve. Decreased sensation may also diminish the patient's ability to sense excessive tightness of constricting bandages and splints.

A complete neurovascular assessment of the affected extremity should be completed and documented immediately after surgery once the patient is awake and able to cooperate with the examination. The neurological assessment should be repeated regularly over the next 48 h, which is typically when nerve palsies occur. Early identification of any change in neurovascular status is crucial because the potential for complete nerve recovery is greater when the palsy is identified early. Constrictive bandages must be loosened and pressure points relieved. For the lower extremity, flexion of the knee relaxes the peroneal and tibial nerves.

Mobilization and Activity Restrictions

Mobilization considerations are unique for the orthopedic oncology patient. Activity restrictions are dictated by the special type of resection and reconstruction (see also Chap. 13, "Rehabilitation in Orthopedic Oncology"). In the immediate postoperative period, the goal is to mobilize the patient as soon as possible to avoid complications associated with prolonged recumbency. Patients are generally out of bed by postoperative day 1 or 2, unless specifically contraindicated, with the assistance of crutches or a walker. The weight-bearing status depends on the type of reconstruction. For example, if an allograft is employed, patients are limited to touchdown weight bearing until there is radiographic evidence that the allograft has healed to the host bone. However, most patients with endoprosthetic reconstruction are permitted to bear weight as tolerated once the surgical pain resolves.

Certain activity restrictions in the postoperative period are particularly important to observe. Patients who undergo hip arthroplasty or proximal femoral replacement must follow hip dislocation precautions. An abduction pillow or a hip abduction brace is often used to limit certain hip motions that can lead to hip dislocation. For anterior-approach hip arthoplasty, a position of extension, adduction, or external rotation can cause dislocation. For posterior-approach hip arthroplasty, a combination of flexion, adduction, and internal rotation can result in dislocation.

In patients who undergo repair of the knee extensor mechanism, such as the patellar tendon, the leg is immobilized in a brace with the knee maintained in extension for approximately 6 weeks, followed by gradual increase in flexion over the following 6 weeks.

While the affected joint is immobilized, patients are instructed to maintain motion of the adjacent joints to prevent flexion contracture. For patients who undergo resection of the distal femur and reconstruction with an endoprosthesis or allograft–prosthesis composite, a CPM machine is often used to regain motion of the knee joint rapidly. The machine is set at 0–30° of flexion initially; flexion is increased as tolerated by about 5° every 8–12 h.

Physical and occupational therapists play an important role in the postoperative mobilization of the patient. The physical therapist instructs the patient on transfer techniques, ambulation with assistive devices, exercises to strengthen muscles, and methods to improve joint range of motion. The occupational therapist focuses on upper extremity exercises, activities of daily living, and the use of adaptive home equipment to assist with self-care and independence.

Conclusion

The perioperative management of the orthopedic oncology patient differs significantly from that of the general orthopedic surgery patient. Patients who undergo resection of bone sarcomas should be managed by clinicians with an understanding of the disease process as well as the unique issues that arise from large segmental bone loss and reconstruction. Proper medical management during the perioperative period can contribute substantially to the success of the operation as well as the overall oncologic treatment of the patient.

Key Practice Points

- Preoperative assessment includes screening for cancer treatment–related comorbidities and addressing the psychosocial and educational needs of the patient.
- Appropriate timing of surgery is crucial for decreasing postoperative complications.
- Communication between the surgical and anesthesiology team is essential in identifying potential adverse intraoperative events.
- The postoperative management goals are to optimize function and to prevent complications such as wound infection, DVT, and nerve palsy.
- Pain management can be challenging in this patient population. PCA is our most common method of pain control.

Suggested Readings

American Academy of Orthopaedic Surgeons. Guideline on the prevention of symptomatic pulmonary embolism in patients undergoing total hip or knee arthroplasty. Rosemont: American Academy of Orthopaedic Surgeons. 2007. http://www.aaos.org/news/bulletin/jul07/clinical3. asp. Accessed 1 Oct 2011.

Dellon L. Postarthroplasty palsy and systemic neuropathy: a peripheral nerve management algorithm. Ann Plast Surg. 2005;55:638–42.

Lin PP, Graham D, Hann L, Boland PJ, Healey JH. Deep venous thrombosis after orthopedic surgery in adult cancer patients. J Surg Oncol. 1998;68:41–7.

Lyman GH, Khorana AA, Falanga A, et al. American Society of Clinical Oncology guideline: recommendations for venous thromboembolism prophylaxis and treatment in patients with cancer. J Clin Oncol. 2007;25:5490–505.

Morris CD, Sepkowitz K, Fonshell C, et al. Prospective identification of risk factors for wound infection after lower extremity oncologic surgery. Ann Surg Oncol. 2003;10:778–82.

Nathan SS, Simmons KA, Lin PP, et al. Proximal deep vein thrombosis after hip replacement for oncologic indications. J Bone Joint Surg Am. 2006;5:1066–70.

Nercessian O, Ugwonali OFC, Park S. Peroneal nerve palsy after total knee arthroplasty. J Arthroplasty. 2005;20:1068–73.

Chapter 13
Rehabilitation in Orthopedic Oncology

Benedict Konzen and Christopher P. Cannon

Contents

B. Konzen(✉)
Department of Palliative Care and Rehabilitation Medicine, Unit 1414,
Division of Cancer Medicine, The University of Texas MD Anderson Cancer Center,
1515 Holcombe Boulevard, Houston, TX 77030, USA
e-mail: bkonzen@mdanderson.org

C.P. Cannon
The Polyclinic, 904 7th Avenue, Seattle, WA 98104, USA
e-mail: Christopher.CannonM.D@polyclinic.com

P.P. Lin and S. Patel (eds.), *Bone Sarcoma*, MD Anderson Cancer Care Series,
DOI 10.1007/978-1-4614-5194-5_13,
© The University of Texas M. D. Anderson Cancer Center 2013

Chapter Overview Rehabilitation of the orthopedic oncology patient poses some unique challenges. The goal of rehabilitation is to return the patient to the level of his or her highest premorbid function. Meeting this goal can be difficult since considerable musculoskeletal deficits may result from the resection of large segments of the skeletal system. For different regions of the body, rehabilitative efforts focus on specific goals. In addition, other aspects of the patient's overall well-being should be addressed. Patient education, nutrition, skin care, wound care, lymphedema, psychosocial issues, and sexuality all are important components of rehabilitative medicine. These needs may be complicated by the psychological burden of carrying a cancer diagnosis, as well as by the need for additional treatments such as chemotherapy and radiation therapy after surgery.

Introduction

The goal of rehabilitation is the restoration of function to the highest level attainable by the patient. This goal presents a challenge to physicians, nurses, and physical/occupational therapists. In the arena of general orthopedics, surgical interventions are usually effective in treating degenerative and traumatic conditions. Although recovery may be prolonged, a relatively straightforward rehabilitative plan may be anticipated, and the end result is a return to the prior level of normal function. In the field of oncology, however, the difficulties of rehabilitation are compounded by the underlying cancer. Patients with sarcomas of bone, in particular, have special needs that must be recognized. In addition to the medical and psychological impact of the underlying disorder, malignancies often create major musculoskeletal deficits that are much more severe than those encountered in general orthopedics.

Rehabilitation goals that are pertinent to the sarcoma patient include restoring the function of the affected limb, educating the patient and family about the disease and rehabilitation, providing adequate nutritional intake, maintaining skin integrity, ensuring optimal wound care, and managing lymphedema. The management of pain—both musculoskeletal and neuropathic—is critical. Other psychosocial and sexual issues may need to be addressed. Collaboration with oncologists is also an integral part of care; protocols for osteosarcoma and Ewing sarcoma require a timely resumption of chemotherapy after surgery, and thus the allotted time for postoperative rehabilitation can be limited. This chapter addresses these general rehabilitation concerns, as well as those specific to particular body sites.

Goals of Rehabilitation

Function

Function is one of the most fundamental aspects of rehabilitation, but defining function is not an easy task. Function may pertain to the specific anatomic site or limb that is affected by the tumor. Function may also be employed as a broad term that includes all aspects of a patient's health. Not surprisingly, there are multiple ways of defining both function and loss of function.

The World Health Organization has categorized types of functional loss as follows:

- *Impairment*: Loss of function, whether from an alteration in anatomic structure, a physiologic state, or psychological changes.
- *Disability*: Impairment that hinders the ability to perform an activity that is considered to be a normal human activity.
- *Handicap*: The societal disadvantage that results from the impairment or disability.

It is important to note that although these terms for functional loss are often used interchangeably in informal language, the definitions carry important distinctions in meaning. Rehabilitation specialists may use these concepts to clarify the exact goal of a particular intervention.

In oncology, the term "function" carries a rather broad connotation that encompasses all activities that a person performs. Two widely used tools for the assessment of overall function (in terms of activity level) in cancer patients are the Karnofsky and Eastern Cooperative Oncology Group (ECOG) ratings (see Chap. 14, "Follow-up Evaluation and Surveillance after Treatment of Bone Sarcomas"). Although the scores are somewhat subjective in nature, they provide a good indication of patients' general performance status. These metrics are employed most often in determining whether patients are viable candidates for chemotherapy and other treatments. Since many sarcoma patients continue to receive chemotherapy after surgical treatment, monitoring these scores may be an important part of rehabilitation.

Other evaluation tools combine physical functional assessment with quality-of-life and/or psychological function. There are multiple dimensions to function in addition to overall performance status, and it is important to assess individual components of function as well as the overall score. Furthermore, an assessment tool measures one moment in time, typically in the hospital or clinic setting. Learned skills in the rehabilitation center may not be carried over successfully without reinforcement in the home and community. Thus, repeated assessment during follow-up is important.

Patient Education

The patient's perception of the disease is an important aspect of treatment. The patient's understanding may be limited or erroneous at times. Furthermore, the patient's goals may be quite different from the physician's priorities. As a result, the patient and physician may not always be striving toward the same objectives, which can lead to difficulties with treatment.

Unrealistic expectations on the part of patients and family members are frequent barriers to successful rehabilitation. The average American life span has now reached the late seventies, and projections suggest a continued increase over time. As medical advances improve the length and quality of life, many people no longer accept debility as a natural part of aging and disease. Even with cancer, individuals often expect to be cured and to return to normal, premorbid function.

Communication with the patient and education of the patient are vital components of rehabilitation. An assessment of the patient's understanding should be performed early in the course of rehabilitation. Although physicians generally assume that patients are familiar with their disease, such is not always the case. A clear, concise explanation of the diagnosis is absolutely essential. It needs to be conveyed to both the patient and the designated family member. In many instances, the patient and the family are overwhelmed by the general concept of "cancer," which can adversely affect the ability to retain medical information. The education of the patient may require multiple conversations, reiteration of essential points, and an interactive rapport between individuals. The conversations should address in simple terms a number of basic themes: what the tumor is, how the tumor typically behaves, how pain will be controlled, how various symptoms—e.g., cachexia, anorexia, nausea, constipation—will be treated, the rehabilitative goals, and finally, the time frame in which the patient is expected to attain his or her projected level of function.

Nutrition

Promoting nutritional intake is an important goal, particularly for postoperative patients, who require extra energy for the physical exertion of rehabilitation. These patients typically have sizable wounds, which require large amounts of nutritional intake to heal promptly. In order to optimize patients' recovery, caloric intake should be between 115% and 130% of the resting energy expenditure. Protein needs typically range from 1.5 to 2.5 g/kg/day.

There are many impediments to adequate nutritional intake. In the postsurgical setting, the use of narcotic pain medication and the resumption of chemotherapy are frequent causes of nausea, so aggressive treatment of nausea is essential. The traditional antiemetics have included phenothiazines (e.g., prochlorperazine, promethazine) and selective 5-hydroxytryptamine (5-HT3) receptor antagonists (e.g., ondansetron). Newer antiemetics, such as aprepitant (Emend), may be employed when the other medications are not effective.

Anorexic syndromes may be the result of increased levels of cytokines such as tumor necrosis factor/cachectin and interleukin-1. On rare occasions, appetite stimulants such as megestrol and dronabinol may prove useful for such syndromes.

Skin Integrity and Wound Care

After surgery, skin and wound care is a high priority of postoperative care. Wound healing may be affected by a host of variables, including inadequate nutrition, swelling, prior radiation, adjuvant chemotherapy, infection, and increased pressure over bony prominences in the bed-bound patient. Diminished mobilization in the perioperative period may exacerbate some of the above-mentioned factors as well as contribute to decubitus ulcers. Meticulous attention to skin and wound care is critically important to preventing the complications of wound dehiscence and ulcers. Elevation of the affected extremity, frequent changes of body position to avoid prolonged pressure, low-air-loss mattresses, regular dressing changes, and antibiotics are helpful measures. Sensitive regions that have been affected by prior irradiation may benefit from emollient creams, such as Biafine or Aquaphor, to retain a necessary moisture barrier.

Lymphedema

Controlling swelling and lymphedema can be challenging. Although some degree of swelling is normal after any surgical intervention, oncologic treatments that include radiation and lymph node dissection can result in marked lymphedema. The lymphatic system is a delicate network of lymphatic capillaries and lymph nodes. Once this network is interrupted by either surgery or radiation, lymph flow can be severely altered, leading to impaired mobilization of lymph fluid and protein. The net effect is protein deposition in the soft tissues, followed by fibrosis of lymphatic channels. Without aggressive manual decongestive techniques, compressive bandaging, and elastic sleeve garment wear, disability may indeed follow. Despite intact nervous and vascular systems, motor function can be severely compromised by the disproportionate limb or body region.

Psychosocial Issues

Although rehabilitation and physical medicine have traditionally dealt with physical incapacities of patients, psychosocial issues are increasingly being recognized as a critical aspect of patients' overall care and thus an important component of rehabilitation. Adjusting to the life-altering event of a sarcoma diagnosis and its treatment will require assistance from family, friends, social supports, and medical professionals.

The psychological impact of a malignancy is profound. Patients are faced with a potentially fatal illness. The fear of surgery and of alteration of the body can lead to feelings of uncertainty and anxiety. Depression may be manifested by a constellation of symptoms, including anorexia, insomnia, fatigue, weight loss, dysphoria, hopelessness, self-debasement, guilt, and suicidal ideation. As patients are forced to confront their mortality and potential disability, psychological stress becomes an increasingly difficult problem, one that is often not discussed with physicians. In one study, 45% of patients demonstrated at least one psychiatric disorder (Weddington et al. 1986). Furthermore, 15% of patients concurrently had an affective disorder complicated by alcoholism.

Interventions may include the use of serotonin reuptake inhibitors, antidepressants, and psychostimulants, such as methylphenidate. Concurrent supportive psychotherapy should also be considered; such therapy may include behavioral modification, relaxation techniques, guided imagery, therapeutic touch, massage, and hypnosis.

From a social perspective, the patient may be concerned with adaptation to new patterns of living. This adaptation involves, on one level, basic issues with mobility. Adjustments in household layout and remodeling of the home may be necessary. The patient may require placement of assistive equipment, such as a wheelchair, walker, sling lift, tub bench, and 3-in-1 commode chair.

Socioeconomically, there may be important changes in relationships with other people. There may be a reversal of hierarchical roles in terms of who supports the family financially, assumes control of bill paying, and serves as the spokesperson for the family. The patient may become dependent on other family members or friends for assistance with ongoing medical and nursing care needs. In many households, financial constraints are likely to affect both the patient and the entire family. Medical caregivers must be sensitive to these issues and attempt to provide, when possible, social and counseling services to assist with these difficulties.

Sexuality

The sarcoma patient is faced not only with the reality of cancer and its treatment but also with changes in physical appearance. Because most patients undergo major operations to remove their primary tumors, many experience disfigurement to varying degrees. The surgery may have, at least initially, a marked effect on the patient's psychological state, which in turn can affect sexual function.

Sexuality may also be affected physiologically. Surgery in the spine and pelvic regions can inflict neurological damage and reduce the mobility needed to engage in intercourse. Radiation-induced changes in the pelvis and lumbosacral plexus can have a similar effect. Chemotherapy may affect the reproductive organs and cause neuropathies.

In men, sexual problems may include erectile dysfunction, altered spermatogenesis, and decreased testosterone production. In women, loss of estrogen may lead to vaginal atrophy, dryness, and dyspareunia. For both sexes, physical disfigurement, fatigue, weight change, hair loss, and difficulties in positioning all contribute to an impairment of sexual function. When compounded by the psychological barriers of grief, guilt, and fear of disease recurrence, the problem can become severe.

Frank discussion with the patient is perhaps the first and foremost aspect of helping with these sensitive issues. It is incumbent upon the medical and rehabilitation teams to try to address the problem because patients are often too embarrassed to broach the topic. Counseling and supportive interventions should be provided. From a therapeutic standpoint, the use of lubricants, medications, hormone therapy, vaginal dilatation, modification in sexual positioning or practice, and surgical reconstruction of an affected area may be required. Consultation with urologists, gynecologists, and/or mental health professionals is likely to be beneficial for many patients.

Collaborative Efforts

The physical medicine and rehabilitation team attempts to address all aspects of a patient's impairment. The team involves not only the physician, who specializes in physical medicine, but also nurse specialists, physical therapists, occupational therapists, orthotists, prosthetists, social workers, case managers, psychologists, and chaplains. Collaboration among the various components of the team is essential, and frequent multidisciplinary conferences to assess objectives and progress are an important part of the rehabilitative program.

The medical professionals involved in rehabilitation must also collaborate with the surgical, radiation, and medical oncologists. The rehabilitative goals for each sarcoma patient are modulated by the specific type of tumor, stage of disease, location of the neoplasm, and medical therapies received.

In cases of advanced disease and late-stage sarcomas, the goals of rehabilitation may be modest. Just getting the patient mobile, with either a walker or a wheelchair, is a worthy achievement. The hope for these patients is that they can access their homes once again and possibly be independent with hygiene and basic activities of daily living. Patients with aggressive tumors may require treatments to address pain, relieve symptoms, and maximize function. Palliative radiation is an important modality for pain management. Surgical intervention may reduce the pain of pathologic fractures or bone metastases. Systemic treatment in the form of bisphosphonates, steroids, and even chemotherapy may also have a valuable palliative effect.

In cases of early-stage disease, prolonged survival or outright cure may be feasible. With the advent of newer protocols and treatments, long-term survival is becoming a possibility for an increasing proportion of patients. The rehabilitative goals for such patients may include not just home independence and community access but also a return to higher levels of function. Patients often desire or need to return to work, which may require accommodations on the part of the patient and employer. Vocational rehabilitation may be needed, and job retraining may sometimes be necessary. Evaluation for both short- and long-term disability may be crucial for patients to receive proper medical and financial benefits.

Rehabilitation for Specific Anatomic Sites

Shoulder and Upper Extremity

Upper extremity functional deficits depend on the location of tumor, the amount of tissue resection, the type of reconstruction performed, and the use of adjuvant treatment modalities such as radiation therapy. Patients may have difficulties related to deficits in innervation, strength, sensation, and mobilization. The patient's extremity dominance, if affected, may have to be relearned to maximize the ability to write, eat, groom, dress, and perform personal hygiene.

With current chemotherapy, radiation, and surgical techniques, the great majority of sarcomas, including those in the upper extremity, can be treated with limb-sparing surgery. The proximal humerus is a common site for bony sarcomas and requires resection of the affected portion of the bone. Reconstruction is typically performed with an endoprosthesis, allograft–prosthesis composite (APC), or osteoarticular allograft. If an extra-articular resection is required with removal of the entire glenohumeral joint, shoulder function is severely compromised. After reconstruction with an endoprosthesis, the goal is for the shoulder to provide a stable platform for normal elbow and hand function (Fig. 13.1). Thus, physical therapy focuses on elbow and hand strengthening and range of motion, with immobilization of the shoulder for 2–6 weeks to allow healing. The range of motion of the shoulder is not emphasized.

If an intra-articular resection of the proximal humerus is performed with preservation of the glenoid and deltoid musculature, shoulder function after endoprosthetic reconstruction is somewhat better than that after an extra-articular resection, though patients still typically obtain only approximately 45° abduction and forward flexion (Fig. 13.2). Again, a shoulder immobilizer is used for 2–6 weeks after surgery. Subsequently, greater emphasis is placed on strengthening the remaining deltoid and rotator cuff. With diligent rehabilitation, a minority of patients may be able to obtain 90° shoulder elevation.

An APC or osteoarticular allograft is used to reconstruct the proximal humerus when greater shoulder range of motion is desired. In this reconstruction, the remaining rotator cuff muscles are sutured to the rotator cuff tendons on the allograft. The shoulder is then immobilized for 6 weeks after surgery to allow healing of the host tissue to the allograft. Progressive active and active-assisted range-of-motion training is then initiated. Elbow and hand motion are also emphasized. Shoulder motion of 90° or greater can be obtained by many patients.

Occasionally, a sarcoma will require resection of the diaphyseal portion of the humerus, allowing preservation of both the shoulder and elbow joints. Reconstruction is usually performed with an intercalary portion of allograft and fixation with a plate or humeral nail. Function is generally quite good after these surgeries, with near-normal shoulder and elbow motion. Postoperative immobilization is not necessary, and range-of-motion training can commence immediately after surgery.

Tumors of the distal humerus are less common. However, when they occur, resection of the distal humerus, reconstruction with an endoprosthesis, and total elbow arthroplasty are required. As there are no significant muscle or tendon insertions on the distal humerus, function is generally good after this type of reconstruction. Immobilization is not required, and active and active-assisted range-of-motion training can begin immediately following surgery. The cemented ulnar components used in these reconstructions have a relatively high incidence of aseptic loosening, so patients are encouraged to only use the affected arm for light-duty activities to protect the arm as much as possible.

For patients who undergo forequarter amputation of the shoulder girdle, the possibility of a functional prosthesis is rare. Effective suspension would require a more substantial bony/muscular framework in order to fit the prosthesis firmly along a

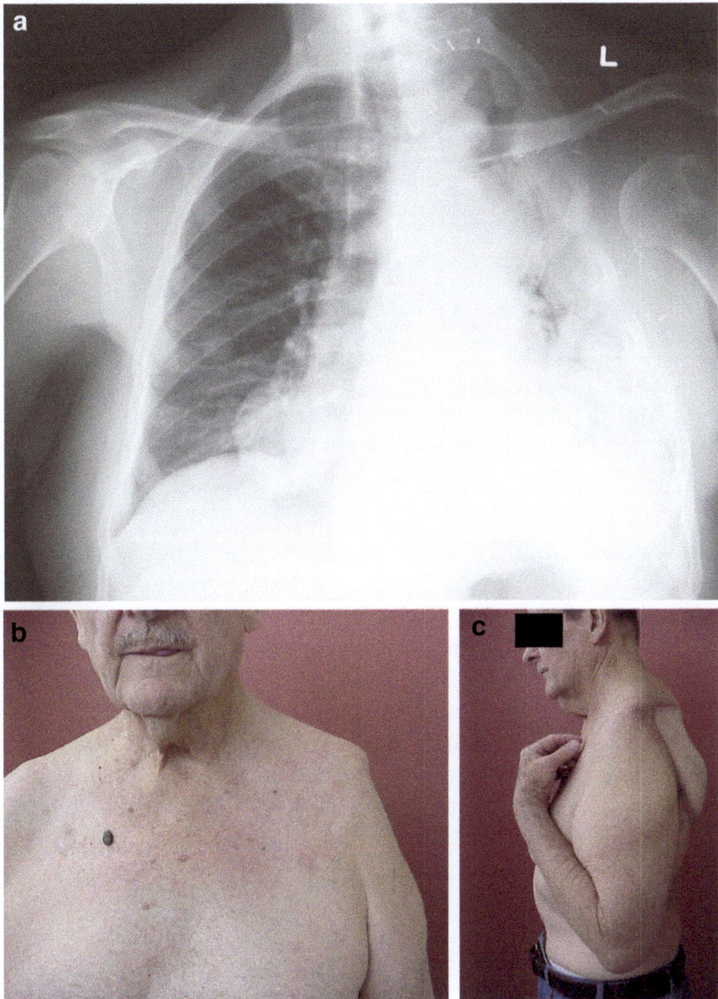

Fig. 13.1 Suspension of the proximal humerus from the clavicle after resection of the glenohumeral joint. The result is poor shoulder function but good function of the limb from elbow to hand. (**a**) A chest X-ray shows suspension of the left shoulder. The humeral head is slightly displaced medially and inferiorly compared to the normal right side. (**b**) The deltoid muscle is absent, resulting in a soft tissue concavity and change in cosmesis. (**c**) The patient has adequate flexion at the elbow, wrist, and fingers. The limb is still functional and useful.

largely curved thoracic wall. However, a lightweight shoulder cap can be fabricated for better clothing fit and to improve cosmesis. Postsurgical considerations should include changes in upper body mass, postural changes, and compensatory alteration of the spinal curvature.

Patients who require above-elbow (transhumeral) amputations can be effectively fitted with a functional prosthesis. Prostheses can either be body powered or externally

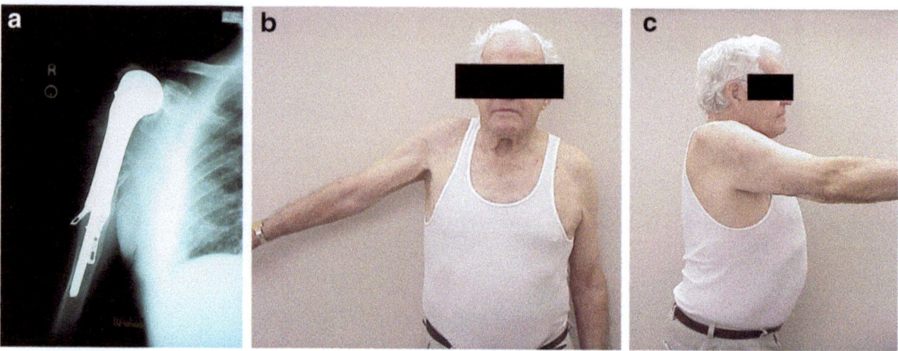

Fig. 13.2 Reconstruction of the proximal humerus with a custom endoprosthesis after resection of an osteosarcoma. (**a**) An X-ray of the affected region. (**b**, **c**) The function of the shoulder is limited in abduction (**b**) and forward flexion (**c**), but this result is better than it would be with no reconstruction.

powered (e.g., myoelectric). The most appropriate type of prosthesis depends on the lifestyle and needs of the patient. The patient should be referred to the prosthetist early in the postoperative period. Fitting immediately after wound healing has been associated with a higher likelihood of using the prosthesis. Also, close communication should be established between the physician, prosthetist, and therapists.

Patients with below-elbow amputations can also be fitted with highly functional prostheses. Because the elbow joint is preserved, function is better than that after above-elbow amputation. As with above-elbow amputations, the choice of body-powered or externally powered prosthesis is based on the needs of the individual patient.

Pelvis

Pelvic resections of bone sarcomas often result in formidable rehabilitation challenges. If the hemipelvis (or a portion thereof) is resected with preservation of the limb, the surgery is termed an "internal hemipelvectomy." If an amputation is performed, it is termed an "external hemipelvectomy" or "hindquarter amputation." The postoperative deficits vary according to the portion of the pelvis that is removed. Internal hemipelvectomies are classified as type I, II, or III resections. In a type I resection, the ilium is resected; in a type II resection, the acetabular region is resected; in a type III resection, the ischium is resected. Combinations of the resections can be performed, for example, a type I/II resection or type II/III resection. Loss of the ilium (type I resection) often produces a leg-length discrepancy due to proximal rotation of the remaining portion of the pelvis. However, if the hip joint is preserved, function is generally quite good, and mobilization can be initiated immediately following surgery. A hip-abduction brace is used for 6–8 weeks to protect the hip abductor muscle repair.

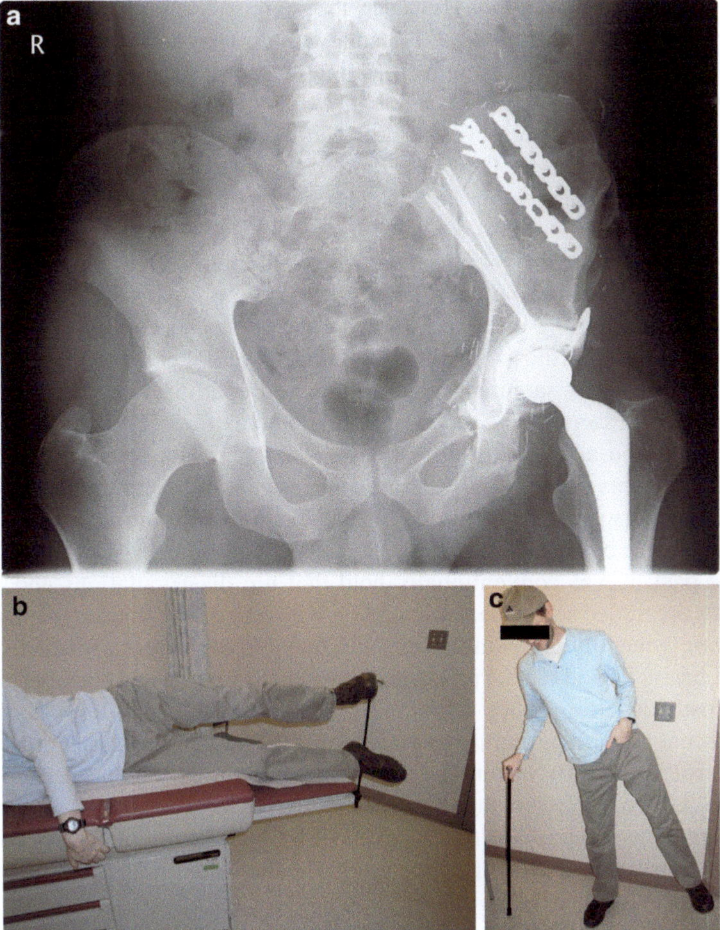

Fig. 13.3 Reconstruction of the pelvis with a large allograft after an internal hemipelvectomy. (**a**) An X-ray of the pelvis. (**b, c**) The gluteal muscles, which serve as the hip abductors, were preserved, but they were weakened, as demonstrated by side-lying abduction (**b**) and standing abduction of the hip (**c**). The patient uses a cane for ambulation to compensate for a Trendelenburg limp.

Resection of the acetabular region (type II resection) results in marked postoperative functional limitations, the extent of which depend on the type and success of the reconstruction performed. One option is to perform no reconstruction and leave the hip flail. Without an intact hip joint, mobilization and the ability to bear weight progress slowly. The remaining proximal femur eventually scars into the surrounding tissue to form a reasonably stable construct. Patients are protected in a hip-abduction brace and slowly progress from touch-down weight bearing to weight bearing as tolerated. If, on the other hand, the pelvis is reconstructed with an allograft, custom prosthesis, or saddle prosthesis, earlier initial stability is obtained (Fig. 13.3). Patients still require protection with a hip abduction brace, largely to prevent dislocation of the hip. However, they typically are able to mobilize more quickly than those with flail hips. Patients with custom and saddle prostheses are allowed to begin weight bearing as tolerated as soon as the hip abductor muscles heal, at approximately 6 weeks. Patients with allograft reconstructions are not allowed to bear weight until evidence of radiographic healing is seen, which often requires 6 months or more. The prevention of hip dislocation is imperative with all of these reconstructions, so hip flexion is limited to 70°, and adduction and internal rotation are avoided.

Loss of the ischium (type III resection) will likely affect a balanced sitting surface, though overall function tends to be very good. After surgery, the patient often experiences sitting discomfort and compensatory hip hiking. To avoid pressure ulcers, a sitting orthosis or specialized air-cell or gel cushion may be required.

Resection of pelvis sarcomas may result in neurogenic bowel and bladder function secondary to sacral nerve root or pudendal nerve injury. These tumors may also involve the lumbosacral plexus directly. Neuropathic pain may be severe, requiring neuropathic agents such as tricyclic antidepressants, duloxetine (Cymbalta), anti-epileptics such as pregabalin (Lyrica) or gabapentin (Neurontin), or celiac plexus/splanchnic nerve blocks.

In the past, it was conventionally held that hip disarticulations and hemipelvectomies precluded subsequent ambulation with prostheses. Indeed, the older prostheses were generally too cumbersome and unwieldy for most patients to use on a practical basis. The advent of prosthetics with microprocessor-controlled joints has made prosthetic fitting more attainable for patients with high-level amputations. These current prostheses require less energy for the patient to use and provide better knee control and improved stumble recovery. Nevertheless, patients need to be fairly strong to utilize such prostheses. Referral to physical therapy for generalized strengthening, as well as for improvement of balance, is important. As with upper extremity prostheses, early fitting (as soon as the incision is no longer tender) results in more predictable use by the patient.

Hip and Lower Extremity

The level of function of lower limbs after limb reconstruction varies greatly, depending on the bone and soft tissue structures involved as well as the type of prosthetic reconstruction performed after removal of the bone sarcoma. In general, rehabilitation is largely focused on gait, since the primary function of the legs is ambulation.

For soft tissue sarcomas, gluteal involvement results in impairment in hip extension during the stance phase of the gait cycle and during climbing. Altered gluteus medius function often results in a Trendelenburg gait, which may necessitate usage of a cane or walker. Psoas muscle involvement will affect gait advancement and climbing. Hip contractures may lead to excessive lordosis of the lumbar spine with resultant back pain.

Resection of the hamstring muscles or sciatic nerve may alter gait and lead to knee flexion contractures. Distally, the ankle joint may need to be stabilized. Such stabilization is often achieved using a lightweight prefabricated or custom-molded ankle-foot orthotic (AFO). Contractures of the thigh may not only result in an unstable gait but also affect the lower back. Stretching during the 12-week postoperative period is important to maintain full active knee and hip range of motion.

Knee dysfunction often results after quadriceps or femoral nerve resection. Maintenance of stance phase may require a ground-reactive AFO in order to control knee flexion. Patients with partial quadriceps loss may be able to achieve sufficient stability at the knee utilizing the residual knee extensor muscles.

After ankle and foot resections, the use of an AFO may provide a stable base of support. Additionally, patients may require customized shoe inserts and footwear aimed at stabilization of the longitudinal and transverse arches of the feet and flexibility at the metatarsophalangeal joints.

Resection of the proximal femur has a significant impact on lower extremity function due to the loss of the skeletal insertions for the hip flexors, hip extensors, and, most important, hip abductors. Reconstructions in this area can be performed with endoprostheses or APCs. With either type of reconstruction, the hip flexors and hip extensors are not typically reattached. With an endoprosthesis, the hip abductors are sutured to a beaded surface on the prosthesis. However, the ability to securely attach the muscles to the prosthesis is limited, typically resulting in hip abductor weakness, a Trendelenburg gait, and the need for an assistive device. With an APC, a better repair of the hip abductor tendon to the allograft tendon can be performed, with potentially better hip abductor function. With either reconstruction, a hip abduction brace is used for approximately 3 months, both to protect the abductor repair and to prevent hip dislocation. Vigorous hip abductor strengthening is then initiated.

Resection of diaphyseal femoral or tibial sarcomas is typically followed by placement of an intercalary allograft, much like in the humerus. The allograft is supported with an intramedullary nail or plate fixation. Because the hip and knee joints are preserved, function is generally very good. Weight bearing must be limited, however, until radiographic evidence of healing is confirmed.

Bony sarcomas of the distal femur are treated with resection and reconstruction with an endoprosthesis that has a rotating hinge mechanism. Because there are no important muscle origins or insertions on the distal femur, postoperative function is usually very good. Early active and passive range-of-motion training, as well as progressive quadriceps strengthening, can be initiated. Patients may also bear weight as tolerated. With appropriate therapy, patients can walk without a significant limp.

Conversely, sarcomas of the proximal tibia result in a more significant impact on lower extremity function due to the patellar tendon insertion at this site. Loss of the tendon insertion results in postoperative weakness in knee extension. Reconstruction can be performed with an endoprosthesis or an APC. Most, but not all, patients treated with an endoprosthesis will demonstrate an extensor lag (Fig. 13.4). Similar to considerations for the proximal humerus and proximal femur, the goal of an APC is to obtain a better patellar tendon repair to eventually allow better active knee extension. With either endoprosthetic or APC reconstruction, patients are kept

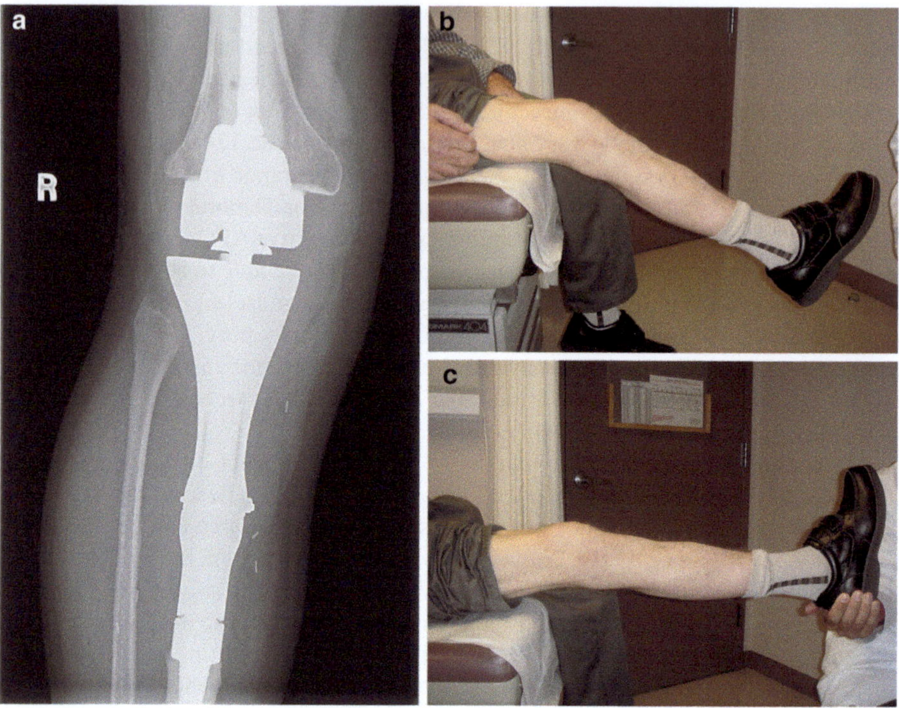

Fig. 13.4 Extensor lag of the knee. (**a**) Endoprosthetic reconstruction of the proximal tibia required attachment of the patellar tendon to the metal prosthesis. (**b, c**) As a result, the quadriceps tendon was weakened, and active extension of the knee lacks 30° (**b**) compared with full passive extension (**c**).

immobilized in a long leg brace for a minimum of 6 weeks to allow healing of the extensor mechanism. Also, a gastrocnemius flap is commonly used in the reconstruction, both to cover the allograft or prosthesis and to potentially assist with healing of the patellar tendon. Since only part of the gastrocnemius–soleus group of muscles is used, ankle plantarflexion is not impaired. Patients with allografts must limit weight bearing until evidence of healing at the allograft–host bone junction site is demonstrated radiographically.

Tumors that cannot be successfully treated with a limb-sparing surgery will require an amputation. After an above-knee (or transfemoral) amputation, the patient is typically treated with a soft compressive dressing, followed by placement of a stump shrinker for 2–4 weeks. Once the swelling decreases and the incision is no longer tender, a prosthesis is fitted. Modern knee mechanisms are quite sophisticated and allow for very good function (Fig. 13.5). As mentioned previously, energy usage is decreased with these mechanisms, and knee control and stumble recovery are improved. In the early postoperative period, avoidance of flexion contracture is imperative; the patient must lie prone several times a day. Patients typically require 3–6 months of therapy to maximize function.

Fig. 13.5 A modern prosthesis with a microprocessor-controlled knee joint, for use after above-knee amputation (C-Leg, Otto Bock HealthCare). Compared with those of the past, this prosthesis affords better control of the knee during stance phase, which decreases the likelihood of the knee collapsing and the patient falling.

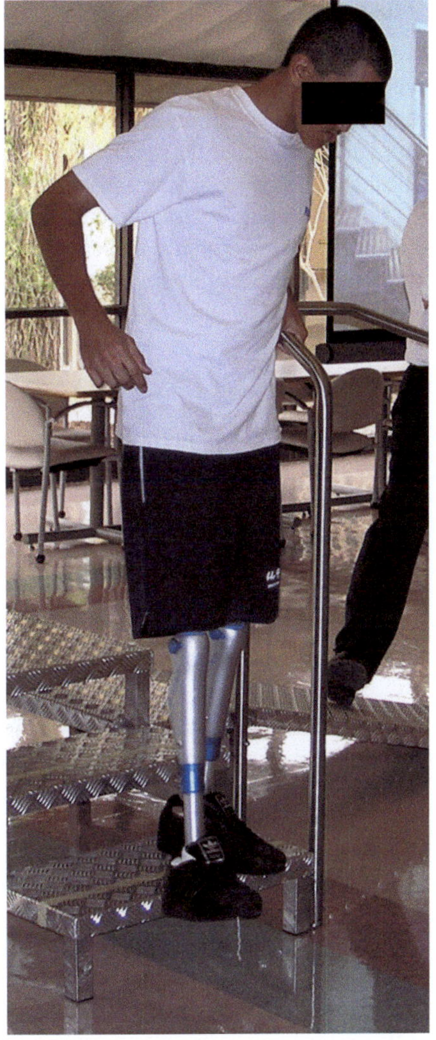

After below-knee (or transtibial) amputations, patients' residual limbs are generally placed in an immediate rigid dressing. These prostheses allow for mobilization immediately after surgery, as well as preparation of the residual limb for the definitive prosthesis. Function after below-knee amputation is usually excellent, especially with younger, healthier patients. Physical therapy with the prosthesis is typically only required for a few weeks to assist with gait training. A variety of prosthetic feet can be selected to allow participation in many different sports activities.

Thorax

Thoracic sarcomas may alter the bone and joint integrity of the ribs and scapula. Extensive sarcomatous involvement can lead to scoliosis, limit pulmonary expansion, and subsequently restrict air exchange. Pulmonary rehabilitation may include chest expansion exercises and inspiratory resistance training.

Following surgery on the scapula and chest wall, postoperative scarring or tumor-related pain may result in scapulothoracic immobility and ensuing rotator cuff impingement. Early institution of range-of-motion exercises may serve a preventative function. The goal is stretching and restoration of mobilization at the shoulder complex.

Musculoskeletal and neuropathic pain is frequently severe after surgery on the brachial plexus region and chest wall, especially if nerves are severed. Treatment for such pain often involves tricyclic antidepressants or antiepileptics, as noted above, or opiates. Nerve blocks are often beneficial. Newer modalities of transcutaneous electrical nerve stimulation and anodyne therapy may also assist in resolution of discomfort.

Spine

Sarcomatous involvement of the spine may lead to paralysis or paresis, kyphosis, scoliosis, and nociceptive or neurogenic pain. Extreme kyphosis may compromise ventilation. Spinal orthoses such as bracing, cervical collars, halos, sternal-occipital-mandibular orthoses, and thoracolumbosacral custom-molded orthoses may structurally immobilize affected segments, but they are often limited by their imposed discomfort and appearance. Surgical stabilization may optimally preserve neurologic and pulmonary function and provide pain control.

In cases of spinal cord injury secondary to metastatic involvement, the patient may experience a sudden loss of neurologic function, which could affect both motor and sensory systems. Treatment may emergently require resection of the metastasis followed by reconstructive surgery and/or radiation. Additional concerns may include issues of life expectancy, neurogenic bowel and bladder management, and future social supports. After the initial phase of treatment, patients often enter a more formalized rehabilitation phase aimed at self-care, mobilization, family teaching, and, it is hoped, community reentry and a subsequent return to the workplace.

Head and Neck

The delicate nature of the head and neck region and the societal and cosmetic implications of a surgery in this area are important to consider. Functionally, treatment of a sarcoma in the facial or neck region may affect swallowing, anatomic structures of the hard and soft palates, the pharynx, and the vocal cords. Fittings for facial, dental, or oropharyngeal prostheses may be necessary. Vestibular and cerebellar involvement may lead to audiovisual-motor difficulties. In these cases, rehabilitative techniques may mirror traditional stroke rehabilitation.

Postirradiation fibrosis may result in oral contractures. Cervical contractures can lead to ongoing disability and pain. Treatment from a rehabilitation perspective focuses on an aggressive stretching and scar mobilization program during and immediately after radiation therapy.

Surgical resection that involves the sternocleidomastoid and strap muscles, trapezii, and cervical paraspinal muscles may lead to impaired range of motion at the neck. Reestablishing normal anatomic parameters as well as using stabilization techniques at the shoulder girdle may provide benefit.

Surgeries of the head and neck sometimes result in loss of the spinal accessory nerve. This loss may lead to partial or total denervation of the trapezius and sternocleidomastoid muscles. The trapezius muscle allows for 60° of scapular motion and is involved in full-shoulder abduction while opposing the anterior pull of the serratus and pectoralis muscles. Poor scapular stability may lead to supraspinatus tendinitis/tendinopathy. The rehabilitation goals are to maintain passive range of motion and to facilitate future active-assisted motion when possible. For treating the neurapraxic injury, rehabilitative aids can include slings and scapular stabilizing orthotics.

Conclusion

Rehabilitation of the sarcoma patient encompasses a multitude of unique opportunities and challenges. Rehabilitation medicine's role in cancer makes use of general physiatric principles but has evolved to meet the demands of specific patients' needs. Like all patients, cancer patients require knowledge of their disease process. The decision to treat and the extent of that treatment are the result of complex interactions between the patient, the family, and multiple treating physicians. Once treatment is defined and implemented, patients require ongoing physical, emotional, and social support through the hospital, home environment, and community at large. The goal of oncologic and surgical intervention is no different than that of rehabilitation medicine—returning a patient to the highest possible level of premorbid function. Orthopedic intervention from an oncologic perspective requires a unique sensitivity and understanding of not only the temporal disease process but also the best way to maintain function. New surgical techniques, materials, and supportive care measures in cancer care are allowing individuals who previously had little hope of ambulatory or upper extremity function, the opportunity to once again access their environments and to reclaim their lives.

Key Practice Points

- Rehabilitation medicine is concerned with reestablishing the highest possible level of premorbid comprehensive physical and psychosocial function.
- Rehabilitation is a multidisciplinary approach involving the physician, oncologist, surgeon, nursing staff, physical/occupational therapists, speech pathologist, social worker, case manager, and psychologist.
- Supportive care measures aimed at relieving fatigue and pain lead to improved physical function and healing.
- Interactive dialogue between the patient and treating physician results in a collaborative course of treatment.
- Functional deficits depend on the location of tumor, the amount of tissue resected, reconstruction efforts, and the adjuvant treatment modalities used.
- In current practice, the great majority of sarcomas can be treated with limb-sparing surgery.
- Each body part and each surgical reconstruction have specific issues that need to be addressed; thus, the nature and extent of therapy vary among patients.
- Pelvic resections of bone sarcomas often pose formidable rehabilitation challenges, including prosthetic fitting, neurogenic bowel and bladder function, and neuropathic pain management.
- Sarcomatous involvement of the spine may result in spinal instability, paresis or paralysis, nociceptive or neuropathic pain syndromes, and neurogenic bowel and bladder.
- Prosthetic technology continues to improve, enabling improved function for many patients who undergo amputation.

Suggested Readings

Burgess J. Cancer therapy. In: Skipper A, editor. Dietitian's handbook of enteral and parenteral nutrition. Rockville: Aspen; 1989. p. 121.

Clerici CA, Ferrari A, Luksch R, et al. Clinical experience with psychological aspects in pediatric patients amputated for malignancies. Tumori. 2004;90:399–404.

Custodio CM. Barriers to rehabilitation of patients with extremity sarcomas. J Surg Oncol. 2007;95:393–9.

Gillis T, Yadav R. Rehabilitation of the patient with soft tissue sarcoma. In: Pollock RE, editor. American Cancer Society atlas of clinical oncology soft tissue sarcomas. Hamilton: BC Decker Inc; 2002. p. 395.

Hopyan S, Tan JW, Graham HK, et al. Function and upright time following limb salvage, amputation, and rotationplasty for pediatric sarcoma of bone. J Pediatr Orthop. 2006;26:405–8.

Karasek K, Constine LS, Rosier R. Sarcoma therapy: functional outcome and relationship to treatment parameters. Int J Radiat Oncol Biol Phys. 1992;24:651–6.

Lane JM, Christ GH, Khan SN, et al. Rehabilitation for limb salvage patients: kinesiological parameters and psychological assessment. Cancer. 2001;92(suppl):1013–9.

Maillet JO. The cancer patient. In: Lang CE, editor. Nutritional support in critical care. Rockville: Aspen; 1987. p. 250.

Massie MJ, Holland JC. Depression and the cancer patient. J Clin Psychiatry. 1990;51(suppl):12–7 [discussion 18–9].

Parsons JA, Davis AM. Rehabilitation and quality-of-life issues in patients with extremity soft tissue sarcoma. Curr Treat Options Oncol. 2004;5:477–88.

Refaat Y, Gunnoe J, Hornicek FJ, et al. Comparison of quality of life after amputation or limb salvage. Clin Orthop Relat Res. 2002;397:298–305.

Robinson MH, Spruce L, Eeles R, et al. Limb function following conservation treatment of adult soft tissue sarcoma. Eur J Cancer. 1991;27:1567–74.

Schover LR, Montague DK, Schain W. Sexual problems. In: Devita VT, Hellman S, Rosenberg SA, editors. Cancer: principles and practice of oncology. 4th ed. Philadelphia: JB Lippincott; 1993. p. 1464–80.

Vignaroli E, Bruera E. Multidimensional assessment in palliative care. In: Bruera EH, Ripamonti VG, editors. Textbook of palliative medicine. New York: University Press; 2006. p. 324.

Weddington Jr WW, Segraves KB, Simon MA. Psychological outcome of extremity sarcoma survivors undergoing amputation or limb salvage. J Clin Oncol. 1985;3:1393–9.

Weddington WW, Segraves KB, Simon MA. Current and lifetime incidence of psychiatric disorders among a group of extremity sarcoma survivors. J Psychosom Res. 1986;30:121–5.

World Health Organization. Classification of impairments, disabilities and handicaps. Geneva: WHO; 1980.

Zebrack BJ, Zevon MA, Turk N, et al. Psychological distress in long-term survivors of solid tumors diagnosed in childhood: a report from the childhood cancer survivor study. Pediatr Blood Cancer. 2007;49:47–51.

Chapter 14
Follow-Up Evaluation and Surveillance After Treatment of Bone Sarcomas

Colleen M. Costelloe and Patrick P. Lin

Contents

Chapter Overview Successful follow-up of patients treated for bone sarcoma requires a proactive regimen of regularly scheduled clinic visits, during which the patient receives evaluations appropriate to treatment issues that change predictably

C.M. Costelloe (✉)
Section of Musculoskeletal Imaging, Department of Diagnostic Radiology, Unit 1475, Division of Diagnostic Imaging, The University of Texas MD Anderson Cancer Center, 1400 Pressler Street, Houston, TX 77030-4009, USA
e-mail: ccostelloe@mdanderson.org

P.P. Lin
Department of Orthopaedic Oncology, Unit 1448, Division of Surgery, The University of Texas MD Anderson Cancer Center, P.O. Box 301402, Houston, TX 77230, USA
e-mail: plin@mdanderson.org

P.P. Lin and S. Patel (eds.), *Bone Sarcoma*, MD Anderson Cancer Care Series,
DOI 10.1007/978-1-4614-5194-5_14,
© The University of Texas M. D. Anderson Cancer Center 2013

with increasing time from the surgery. Early issues include wound healing and resumption of basic mobility, leading into a period of heightened surveillance for tumor recurrence, followed by long-term issues centering on the integrity of hardware and reconstructions. Abnormalities that present in each of these phases produce characteristic findings on the medical history, physical examination, and imaging studies. Imaging is an essential part of the follow-up regimen. Radiographs can reveal complications such as tumor recurrence, hardware loosening, infection, or allograft resorption. Other studies, such as computed tomography or magnetic resonance imaging, are commonly indicated when an abnormality is suspected and can be optimized for patients with metallic hardware. Outcome measures, such as performance tests, are useful for assessing many factors that affect the lives of bone sarcoma patients; these factors include mobility, function, pain, and emotional acceptance. Scheduled clinic visits and well-balanced patient assessment can optimize patient outcome.

Introduction

Upon completion of primary therapy, employment of a specific strategy for the follow-up of patients treated for bone sarcoma is essential to optimal therapeutic outcome. A regular schedule of follow-up visits, with the appropriate tests at each visit, is vital to the quality and consistency of patient care.

The follow-up visit still largely depends on the time-honored elements of the medical history, the physical examination, and radiographs. The majority of disease recurrences and reconstructive problems are detected by these three basic measures. Suspected tumor recurrence or hardware failure can be confirmed and further evaluated with cross-sectional or multiplanar imaging modalities such as computed tomography (CT) or magnetic resonance imaging (MRI). While metallic implants pose a considerable challenge for both imaging modalities, specific modifications to standard CT and MRI protocols have been developed to improve image quality and produce diagnostic-quality scans.

The follow-up of patients treated for sarcomas of bone must address a combination of oncologic and functional issues. Although recurrence of disease is of foremost concern, the functional status of the patient is also critical. Many patients undergo complex skeletal reconstructions that place limitations on their activity. Patients may also have lasting side effects from chemotherapy and radiation. Anticipation of functional problems, such as cardiomyopathy or hearing loss, should prompt specific testing for these disorders. Assessment of the overall well-being of the patient is also essential to a complete evaluation. Use of a wide variety of instruments that quantify functional outcome and quality of life is becoming an increasingly standard part of the follow-up evaluation.

Schedule for Follow-Up

The timing of scheduled follow-up visits reflects objectives that change temporally in priority and emphasis. Shortly after surgery, wound healing and resumption of basic mobility are of greatest concern. Over the next few months, attention shifts toward bone and tendon healing, which is essential to restore maximum function. During this same period and for the next several years, oncologic concerns, such as the detection of local recurrence and distant metastases, increase in priority. Years later, tumor recurrence is less likely, and implant survival and durability become the primary focus. The timeline for these objectives for any individual patient may be modified based on the grade of the tumor, the perceived likelihood of recurrence, and individual patient concerns, such as function and bone healing.

After resection, a 2-week follow-up appointment is necessary to ascertain proper wound healing and the patient's overall recovery. Such progress is critical for resumption of chemotherapy, which cannot begin in the presence of major wound complications or poor patient mobility. Initiation of formal physical therapy, if not already begun, can usually be implemented at this time.

Evaluation for functional return is performed at 6 weeks. Although maximal functional recovery is not yet expected, most patients will have made progress with regard to range of motion and motor strength. Patients who have undergone certain forms of arthroplasty, such as distal femoral replacement, must be monitored closely to avoid development of stiffness and contractures. Radiographs should be obtained at this time to ensure stability of the operative implant.

The schedule for oncologic surveillance depends upon the tumor grade and pathologic diagnosis. The National Comprehensive Cancer Network (NCCN) Clinical Practice Guidelines in Oncology provide a general outline that can be modified for particular patients and diseases (http://www.nccn.org/professionals/physician_gls/f_guidelines.asp). Patients treated for low-grade sarcomas, such as grade I chondrosarcoma, parosteal osteosarcoma, and adamantinoma, are generally monitored less frequently than patients treated for higher-grade lesions. Patients treated for less aggressive malignancies require oncologic follow-up visits every 6 months for 3–5 years, then annually until year 10.

Patients treated for high-grade sarcomas, including conventional osteosarcoma and Ewing sarcoma, are monitored more frequently. Patients are typically seen every 3 months for the first 2 years, every 4 months for the third year, every 4–6 months for the fourth year, and then every 6 months for the fifth year. At MD Anderson Cancer Center, patients are monitored on a yearly basis thereafter until year 10.

After year 10, oncologic considerations greatly diminish, except possibly in patients who have received radiation therapy (such as those with Ewing sarcoma), which increases the risk of a secondary malignancy. For this or other concerns unique to individual patients, it is reasonable to continue follow-up every 1–2 years. Certain forms of chemotherapy predispose patients to chronic medical problems, such as doxorubicin-induced cardiomyopathy. Such patients benefit from yearly cardiac assessment. Ototoxicity and hearing loss caused by cisplatin are another prevalent medical complication, and patients who have received this drug require yearly otologic evaluations. Counseling regarding exercise, diet, and weight gain is also important because patients with cardiomyopathy or extensive reconstructions are prone to obesity.

At the 10-year mark, some patients can be discharged from the clinic with orders to return as needed should any concerns arise. Nevertheless, many patients require lifelong monitoring of the skeletal reconstruction. Endoprosthetic replacements may eventually fail as a result of aseptic loosening, polyethylene wear, or fracture of the components. Patients with osteoarticular allografts develop degenerative changes in the articular cartilage and may need resurfacing or total joint replacement after 10–20 years.

History and Physical Examination

Cancer patients may develop a wide variety of medical concerns that do not relate directly to their reconstructions. Depression and other psychological problems may develop as a result of the stresses of a life-threatening illness. Inquiry and appropriate referrals may positively affect the overall well-being of the patient.

Characterization of physical pain is one of the main objectives of medical history taking. Pain can reflect tumor recurrence, implant failure, weakness of the extremity, infection, or nerve damage. The specific type of pain can suggest its etiology. Deep-seated, achy, constant pain unrelieved by rest or recumbency implies a destructive process in bone, such as tumor or infection. Groin pain that is present with weight bearing but relieved by sitting suggests degenerative changes in the acetabulum. Pain in the shaft of a long bone near the tip of a prosthetic stem is associated with loosening of the stem. Periarticular pain near tendons that is noticed with prolonged ambulation suggests chronic tendinitis, which may be secondary to chronic weakness of the muscle unit. Burning, radiating pain, and hypersensitivity of the extremity signal the possibility of neuropathic pain; such pain does not respond well to increasing the dosage of narcotics.

The physical examination can corroborate clinical suspicions uncovered by the history and can provide additional clues to the patient's status. Swelling is a very common finding. Causes of swelling that occurs shortly after surgery include seroma, hematoma, and, most commonly, simple lymphedema. Swelling of the lower limb that does not resolve with bed rest and elevation of the extremity raises the possibility of deep venous thrombosis. Unexplained swelling that occurs months or years after surgery may represent tumor recurrence, especially if a firm mass is palpable. Infection is possible but typically causes a more diffuse swelling of the limb without a focal hard mass. Erythema, warmth, and fluctuance are variably present in infections.

Neurologic and vascular examination of the extremity should be performed routinely. Compromise of motor, sensory, or vascular function that developed between follow-up visits could indicate tumor regrowth with involvement of nerves and vessels.

Motor strength has important implications for the function of the limb. For ambulation, the two most important sets of musculature to test are the hip abductors and the quadriceps. Patients who undergo hip surgery, particularly resection of the proximal femur, are likely to develop some degree of weakness of hip abduction. Hip abduction can be tested with the patient lying on the side. Weakness in abduction also correlates well with a Trendelenburg limp, which is characterized by the patient leaning toward the affected leg during the stance phase of the gait cycle.

Surgery on the proximal tibia and distal femur may result in weakness of the quadriceps. This weakness is manifested by the inability to perform a straight-leg raise without some degree of extensor lag (i.e., the patient cannot hold the knee in a completely extended and straight position without the lower leg sagging a few degrees). Weakness of the quadriceps will cause the patient to walk with a limp and is also associated with symptoms of pain and tendinitis around the knee.

In the upper or lower extremity, range of motion must also be quantified at the time of examination. Both active and passive range of motion should be tested and recorded. At the shoulder, passive forward flexion usually exceeds the active range of motion, especially after proximal humeral replacement. At the knee, passive range of motion is often limited in flexion. Defining the range of motion is critical for understanding the patient's physical limitations and for directing physical therapy.

Imaging Studies

Serial conventional radiography is the most frequently used follow-up imaging modality for patients treated for sarcoma of bone. Bone radiography is the primary means of assessing implant stability and detecting recurrence in bone, while chest radiography is the standard method of surveillance for detecting pulmonary metastases. CT, MRI, skeletal scintigraphy, ultrasonography, and other modalities are used for evaluation of suspected complications, such as tumor recurrence, hardware loosening, infection, or allograft resorption.

Radiography

Radiography is the primary imaging modality used for routine follow-up of patients treated for sarcoma of bone and is therefore often the initial study with which local tumor recurrence is detected. Each examination should include a minimum of two views [anterior–posterior (AP) and lateral] of the entire bone, because recurrence can appear a considerable distance from the site of the original tumor. The entire prosthesis, which often extends into an adjacent bone, must also be included in order to fully evaluate for impending hardware failure or tumor recurrence.

In native bone, recurrence is usually seen as areas of osteolysis (Fig. 14.1) with or without periosteal reaction. Recurrent primary tumors such as giant cell tumor of bone or metastases from tumors such as breast or renal cell carcinoma may also

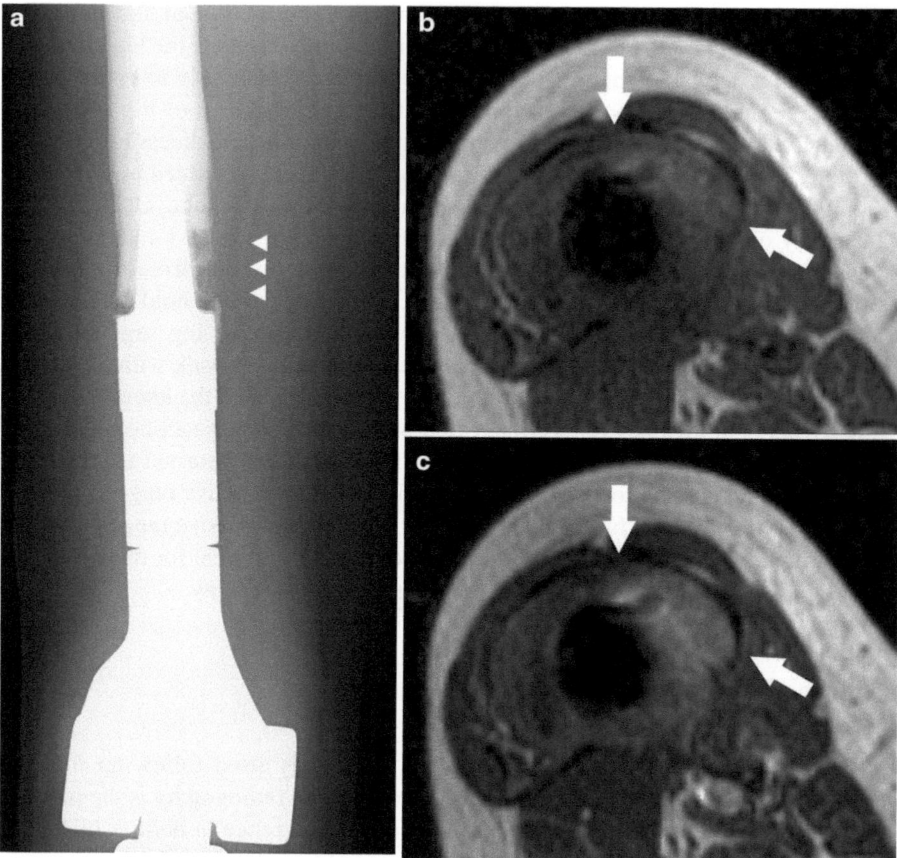

Fig. 14.1 Focal tumor recurrence in bone. Five years after resection arthroplasty of the knee for osteosarcoma of the distal right femur, the patient complained of swelling. (**a**) A frontal radiograph reveals focal lucency in the distal aspect of the medial femoral cortex (*arrowheads*). The margin is irregular, suggestive of tumor or infection. (**b**, **c**) Axial fast spin echo (FSE) T1-weighted images before (**b**) and after (**c**) the administration of intravenous gadolinium contrast reveal an enhancing mass (*arrows*). Solid enhancement excludes the possibility of abscess and mechanical loosening in this patient. The diagnosis was locally recurrent osteosarcoma.

expand the cortex. Matrix mineralization, such as the stipples and rings and arcs of chondroid matrix or the "fluffy" quality of osteoid matrix, may be seen in the recurrent nodules of these primary tumors (chondrosarcoma and osteosarcoma, respectively) and can be helpful for identification of recurrence. In contrast, allograft bone is not prone to internal tumor lysis, and recurrent disease may manifest insidiously as a focal area of surface erosion.

Tumor masses that do not involve bone are difficult to detect on radiographs unless they displace soft tissue planes or produce mineralized matrix. The presence of these radiographic abnormalities or detection of a palpable mass with "negative" radiographic findings is an indication for MRI in order to verify recurrence and evaluate the extent of disease. MRI is also recommended if radiographic signs of tumor recurrence are present (osteolysis or periosteal reaction) because the actual extent of disease is often greater than is evident on radiographs, particularly in the soft tissues or the marrow cavity. Although ultrasonography is an excellent option for the detection of superficial recurrent tumor, sound waves cannot penetrate the cortex to reveal the extent of disease in the marrow cavity. Therefore, MRI provides the most comprehensive means of evaluating the extent of locally recurrent disease.

In addition to being used for surveillance for disease recurrence, radiographs are vital to the orthopedic assessment of the patient. Limb-length determination is an important part of the routine surveillance of skeletally immature patients. Because the en bloc resection of bone sarcomas often removes one or more growth plates, actively growing patients with expandable prostheses require periodic lengthening procedures to maintain limb-length equality. Bilateral telograms with radiolucent rulers are necessary to quantify the degree of discrepancy that develops in the operated extremity as the opposite extremity grows normally.

Radiographs are the primary means of evaluating the integrity of skeletal reconstructions and the extent of bone healing. Most reconstructions involve endoprostheses, autografts, and/or allografts. Modes of failure and radiographic concerns vary for different types of reconstruction. An appreciation for the various types of surgical reconstructive techniques is essential for meaningful interpretation of the radiographs.

For endoprostheses, aseptic loosening is a major cause of failure. Aseptic loosening is most commonly seen on radiographs as a progressive radiolucent line that develops between the bone and cement or bone and metal (Fig. 14.2a). The area of lucency gradually widens and becomes more pronounced on serial follow-up examinations. These areas are of concern when they exceed 2 mm in width. In contrast, nonprogressive areas of lucency may be seen postoperatively as a result of the heat generated by polymethyl methacrylate cement as it sets during surgery.

Additional radiographic signs of loosening include migration of the stem (Fig. 14.2b), erosion through cortical bone, formation of abnormal sclerosis at stress points (as the bone attempts to reinforce those areas), and cement fracture. Aseptic loosening undermines the stability of the construct and is a common indication for revision of the prosthesis.

Comparison of follow-up and previous radiographs is essential for the detection of areas of subtle bone lucency and can provide important clues to its origin. Tumor is not necessarily confined to the bone–prosthesis interface, whereas mechanical loosening typically is. Nor is tumor confined to periarticular regions, where particle disease from prosthetic wear can form erosions, such as are commonly seen in the acetabulum (or insinuated around the prosthesis on either side of the joint). Infection can also present as widening of the bone–prosthesis interface but may progress more quickly and may or may not produce lucencies that are more irregular than those seen with aseptic loosening. While recurrent tumor and infection can be virtually indistinguishable radiographically, MRI can be used to differentiate masses with variable degrees of internal enhancement (typical of tumor) from rim-enhancing masses (typical of abscess).

Allografts are susceptible to a unique set of complications that differ from those of endoprostheses. Babyn et al. (2001) studied 37 patients with either osteosarcoma

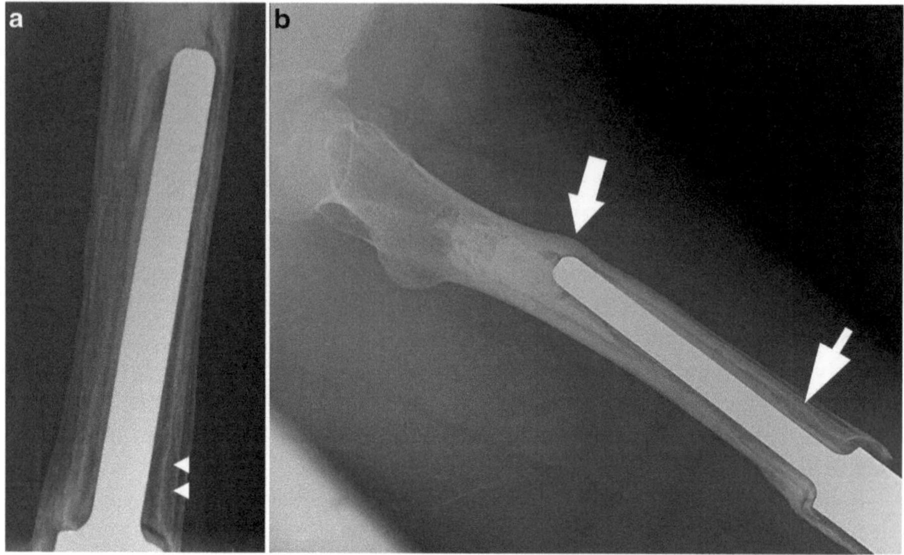

Fig. 14.2 Mechanical loosening. (**a**) A frontal radiograph of the left femur in a patient who underwent resection arthroplasty of the knee for osteosarcoma of the distal metaphysis. Three years after resection, smooth, circumferential areas of lucency had developed around the metallic stem (**a**, *arrowheads*) and bone–cement interface (**b**, *thin arrow*). Anterior migration of the proximal femoral stem had occurred (**b**), and the adjacent cortex had thickened (*thick arrow*), providing reinforcement in this area of chronic mechanical stress.

or Ewing sarcoma who had undergone limb-salvage surgery. The most common complication was fracture, particularly of allografts (Fig. 14.3). Most fractures occurred within 3–4 years of the initial surgery.

Resorption is a phenomenon that underlies many allograft complications. Commonly held theories as to the etiology of resorption involve vascular invasion or an immunologic response. Gross disappearance of bone can be particularly alarming, since it may simulate the external erosion seen with tumor recurrence (Fig. 14.4). Ultrasound imaging is well suited to evaluate superficial locations and can be simultaneously used to evaluate the cause of the radiographic lucency by guiding needle biopsy if a nodule is found.

Infection of the allograft is a feared complication that is often difficult to diagnose confidently using radiographs. Allograft bone may not be capable of producing a periosteal reaction, and the osteolysis associated with infection has no characteristic features to help distinguish it from simple resorption. Cross-sectional imaging is helpful for excluding recurrence because no discrete mass should be present when the osteolysis is due to simple resorption. As in patients with endoprostheses, a rim-enhancing mass visible on MRI in the setting of osteolysis often represents an abscess, whereas small recurrent tumor nodules often demonstrate some degree of central enhancement. Although MRI is the most comprehensive modality for evaluating extent of recurrence or infection, cystic and solid masses can also be distinguished using ultrasonography, and the latter can also facilitate

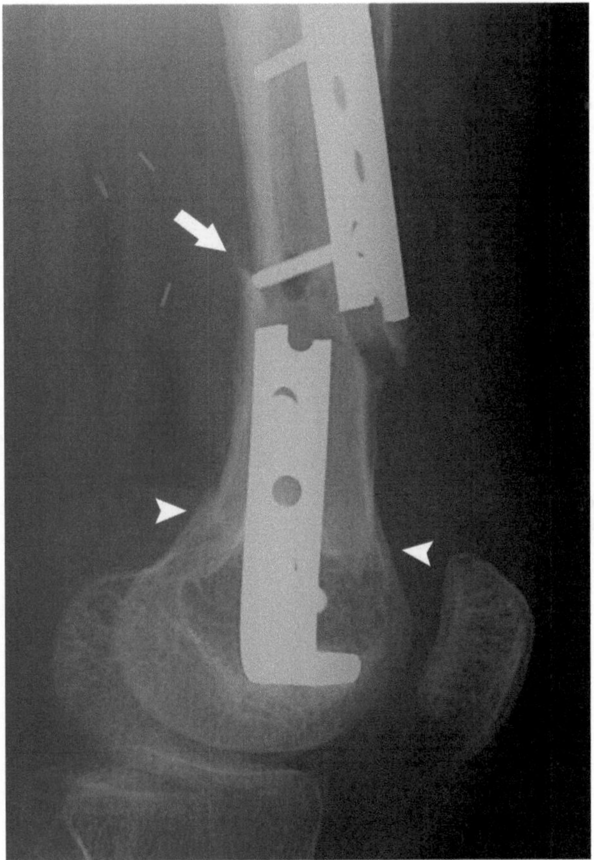

Fig. 14.3 Fracture through allograft bone. Lateral oblique radiograph of the left femur in a patient who underwent intercalary cadaveric allograft reconstruction after resection of a high-grade sarcoma of bone with malignant fibrous histiocytoma–like features. Four years after resection, an oblique fracture occurred through the distal aspect of the allograft (*arrow*), proximal to the well-healed junction with the native distal femur (*arrowheads*). The allograft is denser than the native bone, as can be seen when comparing the femoral condyles and tibia to the proximal allograft bone. The allograft fracture occurred at the site of a screw tract with concomitant fracture of the metallic side plate.

biopsy. Biopsy is often necessary to distinguish infection from recurrent tumor. Part of the specimen should always be sent for microbiologic analysis, including culture and sensitivity testing.

Healing at the osteotomy site is of primary concern in regard to the stability of allografts and vascularized fibular grafts. Slow healing is a vulnerability of allografts that is not typically seen with vascularized fibular grafts, which retain their native blood supply and usually heal more promptly. Healing is defined as the presence of bridging callus that unites the bone on both sides of the osteotomy. Complete healing, characterized by obliteration of the osteotomy line, can usually be recognized on radiographs. However, partial healing may be difficult to ascertain because of the

Fig. 14.4 Allograft resorption. (**a**) A postoperative CT scan obtained 2 weeks after resection of dedifferentiated chondrosarcoma and placement of a cadaveric left iliac allograft. Tiny air bubbles demonstrating low attenuation are incidentally seen in the intramedullary cavity of the allograft. (**b**) One year later, a follow-up CT scan shows small areas of erosion of the lateral cortex (*arrowhead*). (**c**) A T1-weighted axial MRI scan obtained at the same time reveals no tumor adjacent to the erosion. The round structures seen lateral to the allograft represent loops of bowel.

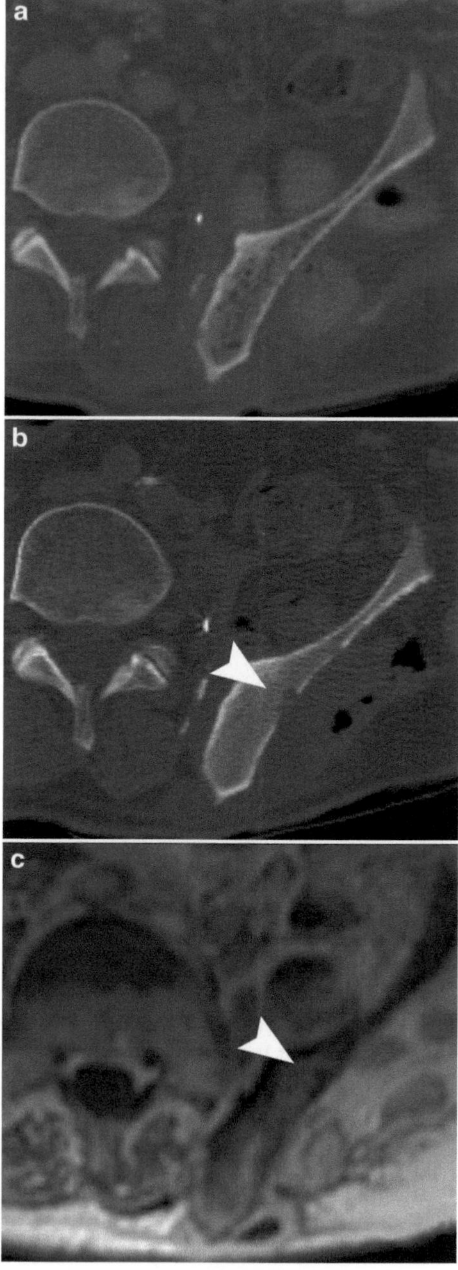

faintness of the mineralization and overlap from other structures on the image. Conversely, the degree of bridging can also be overestimated because conventional radiographs are summation images in which all spatial points in the plane overlap. Therefore, one small area of hypertrophic callus may be overrepresented on conventional radiographs. These limitations can be overcome with the help of CT.

Table 14.1 CT metal and bony bridging protocols

Protocol	Voltage (kV)	Tube current[a]	Rotation (s)	Detector configuration (mm)	Table speed (mm/rotation)	Pitch
16-Channel metal	140	360	0.5	16×0.625	13.75	1.375
16-Channel bridging	120	400	0.5	16×0.625	13.75	1.375
64-Channel metal	140	360	0.5	64×0.625	55	1.375
64-Channel bridging	120	400	0.5	64×0.625	55	1.375

[a]Can be modulated to suit patient body size, reducing radiation exposure.

Computed Tomography of the Bone

CT is exquisitely sensitive for the detection of calcium. It is particularly useful for visualization of cortex, detection of matrix mineralization, and evaluation of bone healing. Many patients with sarcoma of bone require metallic hardware for postoperative reconstruction, and metal typically produces artifacts that obscure the anatomy. Use of a specific CT metal protocol can suppress metallic artifact. CT protocols can also be modified to evaluate callus at a fracture or an osteotomy site.

Metallic artifact can be decreased on CT examinations, and bridging callus can be visualized using specific protocols that optimize the kilovoltage, collimation, and pitch. Since the higher kilovoltage or tube current utilized by the specialized CT protocols presented in this section results in greater radiation exposure, these techniques are used with reserve, particularly in young patients. At our institution, CT imaging of metal and bony bridging is performed on either 16- or 64-channel GE LightSpeed scanners. The protocols are provided in Table 14.1. The initial set of images is reconstructed at 0.625 mm using a bone algorithm with additional reconstructions at 2.5 mm using soft tissue and bone algorithms. Sagittal and coronal CT reformations are performed (Fig. 14.5). Intravenous contrast is not routinely administered for CT bone imaging at our institution.

Computed Tomography of the Body

CT of the chest is not routinely used for surveillance for pulmonary metastases but is indicated when an abnormal finding is detected on chest radiographs or when equivocal nodules were detected on a prior CT scan. Serial follow-up CT, performed at 3-month intervals for a total of 2 years, can be used to evaluate equivocal nodules. An increase in size is an indication for biopsy. CT of the abdomen and pelvis is likewise not routinely performed because metastases to the abdomen are rare in the absence of widespread metastatic disease. An exception is that CT of the pelvis is an option for the routine surveillance of patients treated for pelvic chondrosarcoma. The stippled and/or ring-and-arc matrix mineralization that is often

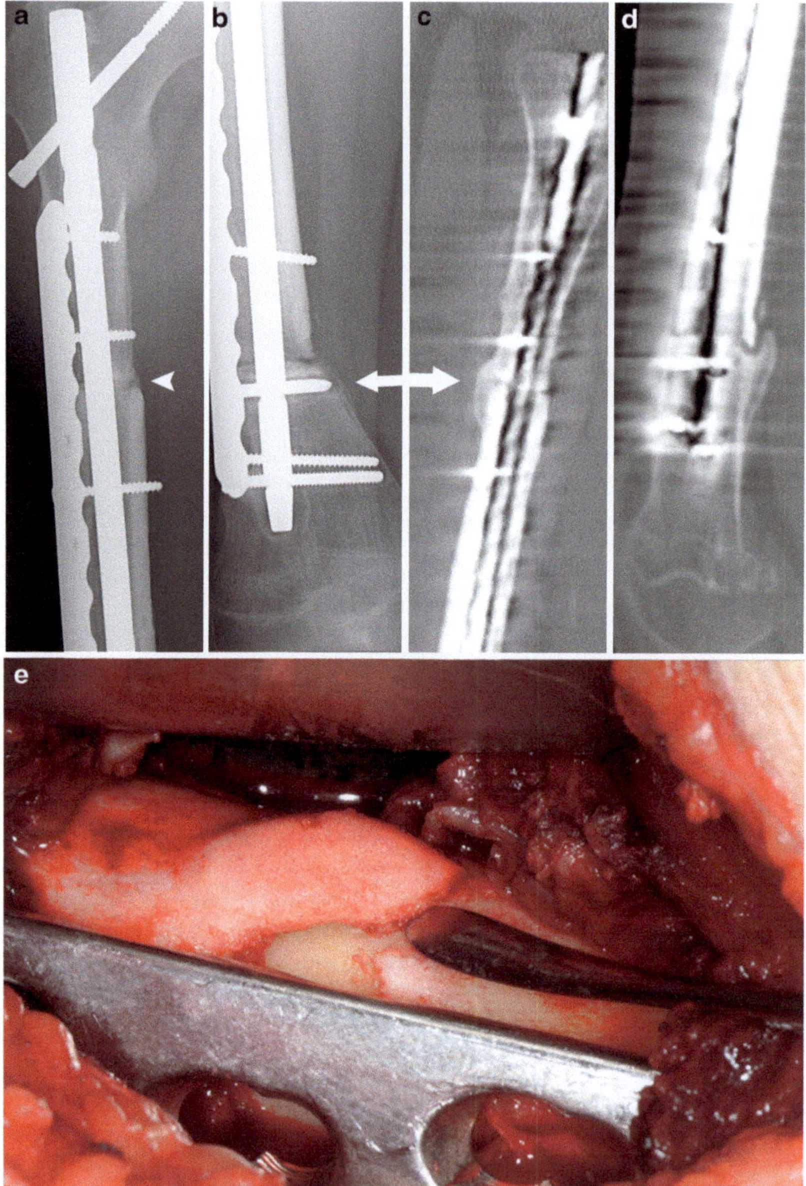

Fig. 14.5 CT for evaluation of bony bridging. (**a**) Frontal radiographs of the right femur in a patient with an intercalary diaphyseal allograft placed after resection of osteosarcoma. Blurring of the proximal osteotomy site represents bony bridging at the proximal junction (*arrowhead*). (**b**) No bridging is seen at the distal junction. The areas of lucency around the distal screws (*small arrow*) and distal aspect of the intramedullary nail indicate loosening due to lack of distal femur fixation. (**c, d**) Sagittal CT reformation confirms proximal bridging (**c**, *large arrow*) with no distal bridging (**d**). (**e**) Subsequent surgery revealed bony bridging at the proximal junction (intraoperative photograph courtesy of Alan Yasko, MD). No bridging was detected at the distal junction (not shown), and the distal aspect of the reconstruction was revised.

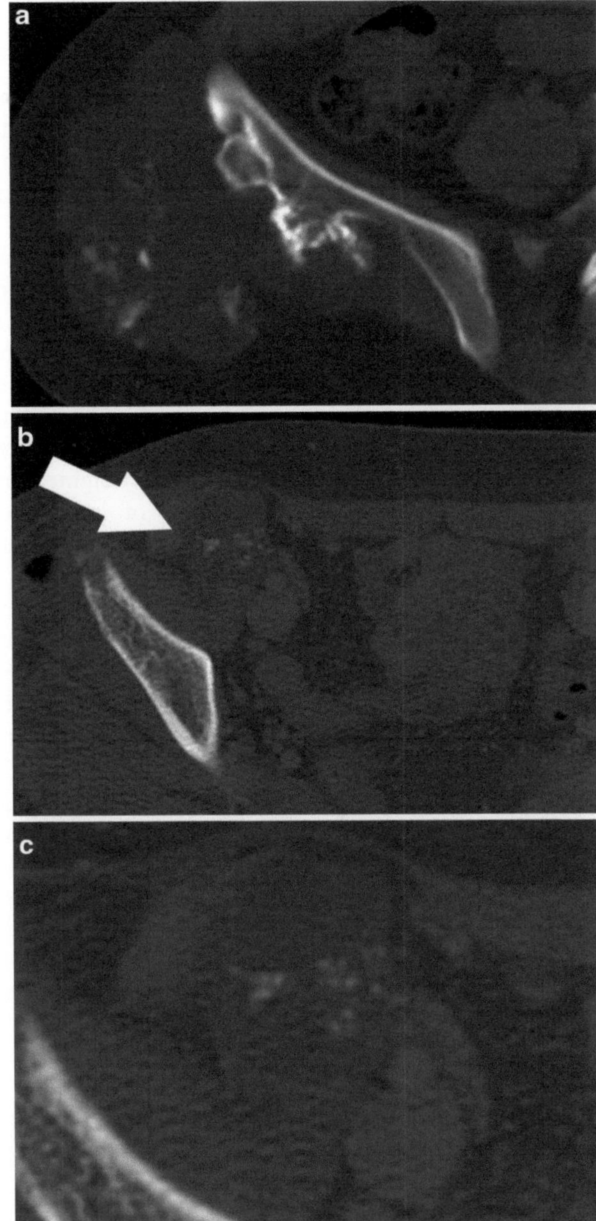

Fig. 14.6 CT of recurrent chondrosarcoma. (**a**) A preoperative axial CT scan of a chondrosarcoma arising from an osteochondroma of the right iliac wing. (**b**) The postoperative CT scan demonstrates a nodule containing cartilage matrix mineralization (*arrow*). (**c**) An enlarged image of the nodule allows better visualization of the punctate and curvilinear matrix mineralization that identifies the nodule as recurrent chondrosarcoma.

produced in recurrent chondrosarcoma nodules is better demonstrated with CT than with radiography and provides specificity regarding the origin of soft tissue nodules found on MRI (Fig. 14.6). Neither intravenous nor enteric (oral or rectal) contrast agents are recommended for CT scans performed for this indication because contrast may obscure faint matrix mineralization.

Magnetic Resonance Imaging

Because of its excellent soft tissue contrast resolution, MRI is superior to CT for evaluating soft tissues and bone marrow. MRI is the study of choice to further delineate suspected soft tissue masses, to evaluate the extent of recurrent disease, and to define the relationship of recurrent tumor to adjacent vital structures such as nerves and blood vessels.

Because of limitations such as metallic susceptibility artifact and expense, MRI is often used secondarily to further investigate abnormalities detected by physical examination or radiography. Nevertheless, MRI may be used for the primary routine imaging follow-up of resection sites located in anatomic regions where complex bone structures overlap and tend to obscure areas of recurrence, such as in the pelvis. Routine follow-up MRI can also be used in patients at high risk for local recurrence.

Most recurrent nodules demonstrate signal intensity that is classified as isointense or nearly isointense to muscle on T1-weighted images and as hyperintense on T2-weighted images. Variable degrees of internal enhancement are seen after administration of intravenous gadolinium contrast agents. Unlike the majority of soft tissue sarcomas and many other primary bone tumors that exhibit vigorous contrast enhancement, the mineralized osteoid matrix of osteosarcomas and the relatively avascular chondroid matrix of chondrosarcomas may demonstrate moderate or poor enhancement (Fig. 14.7). Contrast increases the conspicuity of the majority of recurrent nodules as a result of the weak enhancement of most normal surrounding structures. Since both unsuppressed fat and enhancing pathologic features are bright, contrast is particularly useful when fat suppression is utilized to darken the fat signal. This allows a brightly enhancing recurrent nodule to be easily seen on a dark background. Contrast also helps to differentiate recurrent tumor from fluid-filled cysts and seromas that demonstrate high T2 signal intensity but only rim enhancement. Nodular scar and granulation tissue demonstrates internal enhancement but either remains stable or decreases in size on follow-up examinations.

At our institution, the typical magnetic resonance protocols used for detecting recurrent tumor utilize fast spin echo (FSE) T1-weighted sequences, fat-saturated T2-weighted sequences with chemical fat saturation ("chem sat"), and postcontrast fat-saturated T1-weighted sequences. Typically, all three pulse sequences are obtained in the axial plane, in addition to fat-saturated T2-weighted and precontrast T1-weighted images in the coronal plane. Depending on the anatomic region, sagittal sequences may be performed in addition to coronal sequences, such as when imaging joints.

Diagnostic MRI can be performed in patients prone to artifacts. Typical predispositions to artifact in patients with sarcomas of bone include metallic hardware or pathologic features that are distant from the isocenter of the magnet, such as in the upper extremity (Fig. 14.8). The presence of orthopedic hardware is not a contraindication to MRI, and the magnetic susceptibility artifacts that can distort or obscure anatomy can be greatly reduced by utilizing a specific metal protocol. At our institution, the MRI metal protocol employs inversion recovery rather than our typical FSE T2-weighted sequence with chem sat. Chemical fat saturation is susceptible

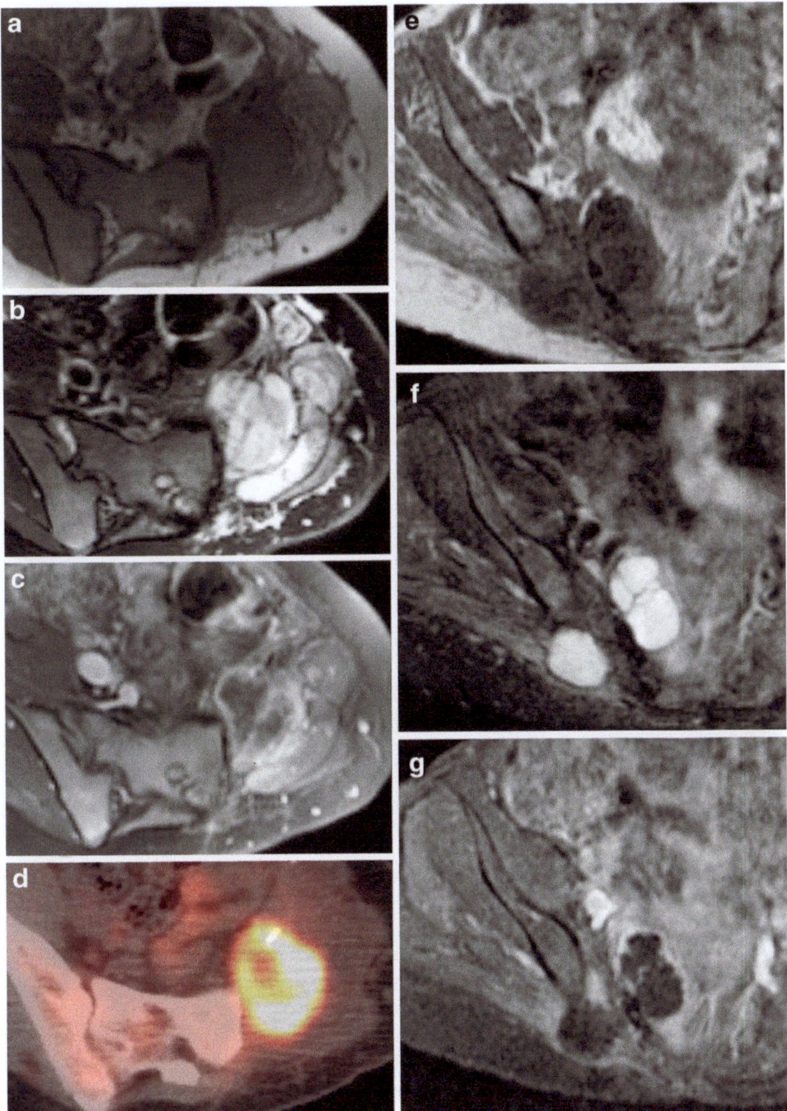

Fig. 14.7 MRI of recurrent bone sarcomas with moderate and poor enhancement. (**a–d**) Axial MRI and PET/CT of recurrent osteosarcoma of the left iliac bone. (**a**) On the T1-weighted image, the signal intensity of the nodule is similar (isointense) to muscle and is inconspicuous. (**b**) The recurrent tumor demonstrates heterogeneously high T2 signal intensity. (**c**) While enhancement is mostly peripheral in location, it is not confined to the periphery, indicating that the nodule contains soft tissue. (**d**) Tracer uptake is seen in the nodule on FDG PET/CT, indicating the presence of glucose metabolism in a recurrent tumor. (**e–g**) Axial MRI of recurrent high-grade chondrosarcoma of the sacrum 3 months after irrigation and debridement for sacral wound dehiscence and 1 year after resection of a prior recurrence. Recurrent tumor nodules have developed medial and lateral to the right iliac bone. (**e**) Chondroid stroma often has lower signal intensity than muscle on T1-weighted images. (**f**) The recurrent nodules demonstrate high T2 signal intensity and lobulated borders. (**g**) Enhancement is typically seen primarily at the rim of small chondrosarcoma nodules because of the lack of vascularity in the chondroid stroma. Therefore, the recurrent nodules can mimic simple fluid collections. A recurrence rather than a postoperative seroma should be suspected if the primary tumor was a chondrosarcoma.

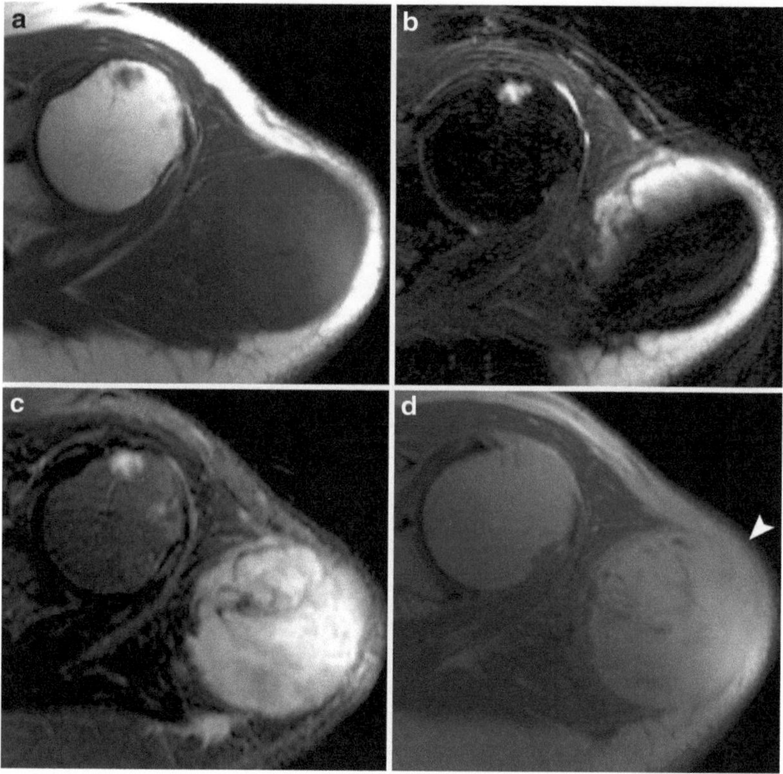

Fig. 14.8 Correction of artifact on MRI. The use of inversion recovery sequences may be preferable to chemical fat saturation in challenging situations, such as in the presence of metal or for structures that are distant from the isocenter of the magnet, e.g., in this case of a malignant fibrous histiocytoma of the left deltoid. (**a**) Axial T1-weighted FSE MRI demonstrates signal intensity that is isointense to muscle. (**b**) The tumor is largely obscured by artifact caused by failure of chemical fat saturation on the FSE T2-weighted axial sequence. (**c**) Robust fat saturation with clear delineation of the morphology of the hyperintense tumor is seen with utilization of an inversion recovery sequence. (**d**) The T1-weighted FSE sequence obtained after administration of intravenous gadolinium shows vigorous enhancement of the tumor in comparison with the precontrast T1-weighted image. The signal intensity of the enhancing tumor is similar to that of the unsuppressed subcutaneous fat (*arrowhead*). Pathologic features that enhance or demonstrate high T2 signal can be difficult to distinguish from fat, which is also bright. Meticulous comparison must be made between pre- and postcontrast T1-weighted images if fat saturation cannot be utilized. This tumor remains conspicuous because it is partially surrounded by muscle.

to artifacts and is easily disrupted by metal. Inversion recovery automatically delivers robust fat saturation but is not routinely used due to its lower signal-to-noise ratio and resultant "grainier" images as compared with FSE T2-weighted sequences. However, most tumor nodules will demonstrate a conspicuous high signal on inversion recovery sequences. The metal protocol also omits fat saturation on the gadolinium-enhanced T1-weighted postcontrast sequences. Meticulous comparison between T1-weighted images obtained before and after administration of contrast can verify internal enhancement and differentiate solid nodules from cysts.

The following are methods for decreasing metallic artifact in MRI (Costelloe et al. 2007):

1. Inversion recovery sequences rather than chemical fat saturation can be utilized to increase the uniformity of fat suppression.
2. FSE is more resistant to metallic artifacts than are spin echo or gradient recalled echo sequences. If these sequences are utilized, the echo time can be decreased.
3. The voxel size can be decreased, by decreasing the field of view, decreasing the slice thickness, and/or increasing the matrix size.
4. The receiver bandwidth can be increased.
5. The long axis of the hardware can be oriented as parallel as possible to the main magnetic field (B_0).
6. "Blooming" artifact associated with metal can be diminished by orienting the frequency-encoding direction to align with the hardware.

MRI with contrast is valuable not only for the detection of recurrence but also for the detection of postoperative soft tissue complications. Soft tissue grafts may have been placed to cover a resection site. Areas of nonenhancement in a graft may indicate necrosis and graft failure. Painful stump neuromas may form at the severed end of a nerve after amputation and can be readily distinguished from recurrent tumor with MRI visualization of the nerve leading into the mass.

Other Imaging Modalities

Ultrasonography is an inexpensive, versatile modality that can be useful for interrogating superficial soft tissues and palpable masses. It is especially helpful for delineating small tumor nodules that directly abut metallic prostheses and may be obscured by metallic artifact on MRI, even when a metal protocol is utilized. Similar to contrast-enhanced MRI, ultrasonography can also be used to distinguish fluid collections from solid tumor masses. However, no imaging modality can definitively distinguish a sterile from an infected fluid collection, particularly in the absence of phlegmon surrounding an abscess.

Skeletal scintigraphy (bone scan) is most commonly performed with technetium Tc 99m–methylenediphosphonate (MDP) and is highly sensitive for the detection of bone metastases. Some institutions perform yearly bone scans for the first 2–5 years of follow-up after treatment of sarcomas with a propensity for bone relapse, such as Ewing sarcoma. Bone scans are not routinely obtained at MD Anderson for surveillance after treatment for bone sarcomas. At our institution, such scans are typically obtained for restaging after the discovery of pulmonary metastasis or local tumor recurrence.

Whole-body MRI is an emerging imaging technique that provides the excellent soft tissue resolution of MRI throughout the body in a single imaging session. Conventional MRI is lengthy and limited to relatively small anatomic regions. The development of fast pulse sequences that are relatively resistant to artifact has enabled whole-body examinations to be completed in approximately 1 h with standard scanners (Ma et al. 2009). Whole-body MRI has been proven more sensitive than skeletal scintigraphy for the detection of osseous metastases (Eustace et al. 1997). This high sensitivity and the ability of MRI to simultaneously evaluate numerous organ systems may allow it to compete with the less expensive skeletal scintigraphy for restaging purposes.

Positron emission tomography (PET) is a form of functional imaging that most commonly employs [^{18}F]fluorodeoxyglucose (FDG). This tracer localizes to tissues that metabolize large amounts of glucose, including a wide variety of malignancies. Modern PET imaging is rarely performed without a fused CT data-set that is created using a hybrid scanner. FDG PET imaging has been shown to be advantageous in the evaluation of sarcomas of bone. For example, FDG PET/CT is able to provide prognostic information when used before and after chemotherapy for osteosarcoma (Costelloe et al. 2009) and is helpful for the detection of recurrent tumor and distant metastases in osteosarcoma and Ewing sarcoma (Völker et al. 2007). The role of PET/CT in the routine follow-up of patients with bone sarcomas remains under investigation. At present, this modality is most commonly used at our institution for initial staging, monitoring of therapeutic response, or the postoperative follow-up of high-risk patients. FDG PET has been compared with whole-body MRI. Antoch et al. (2003) compared whole-body MRI and FDG PET/CT in 98 patients with a variety of malignancies and found that whole-body MRI was more sensitive than FDG PET/CT for the detection of metastases to bone (85% vs 62%, respectively) and liver (93% vs 86%). FDG PET/CT was more sensitive than whole-body MRI for the detection of pulmonary metastases (89% vs 82%) and for nodal staging (93% vs 79%). These results suggest that whole-body MRI and FDG PET/CT may play complementary roles in the comprehensive staging of cancer patients.

Laboratory and Other Tests

Sarcomas of bone cannot be effectively monitored by serum laboratory tests. Patients may need monitoring of serum electrolytes such as calcium, magnesium, and creatinine as a result of the nephrotoxic effects of chemotherapy. Patients suspected of harboring a deep infection of a prosthesis or an allograft may benefit from tests such as a complete blood count, erythrocyte sedimentation rate, and C-reactive protein level.

Outcome Measures

In addition to the history, physical examination, and imaging studies, quantitative measures to assess functional outcome, performance status, and quality of life are important for follow-up of patients. These assessments/questionnaires are designed to evaluate treatment result with regard to function of the limb and overall patient well-being.

Musculoskeletal Tumor Society Score

The Musculoskeletal Tumor Society (MSTS) rating scale (Table 14.2) was developed as a physician-administered assessment of patients' function and outcome. It is based upon six parameters: pain, function, emotional acceptance, and three parameters specific to either the upper or lower extremity as applicable. For the lower extremity, the three additional factors are supports (e.g., crutches), walking ability (endurance), and gait (presence or absence of a limp). For the upper extremity, the factors are hand positioning, manual dexterity, and lifting ability. Each factor carries a maximum score of 5 points, and the maximum overall score is 30 points (or 100%). This straightforward test is the most widely reported measure of patient function for orthopedic oncology patients. Nevertheless, several weaknesses of the test have been identified, including the lack of patient input and poor correlation with other outcome measures.

Performance Status

Performance status testing provides a general overview of the patient's overall well-being and activity level. These scores are commonly employed as part of the inclusion criteria for chemotherapy and treatment protocols. The Karnofsky and Eastern Cooperative Oncology Group (ECOG) scales are two common measures (Tables 14.3 and 14.4). Both the ECOG and the World Health Organization (WHO) performance status scores are based upon the Zubrod scale. The Lansky score is similar to the Karnofsky score but is designed specifically for children and is the preferred measurement for young patients (ages 1–16 years).

SF-36

The Medical Outcomes Trust short-form questionnaire, commonly referred to as the SF-36 form (http://www.sf-36.org), was designed to evaluate health-related issues across age, disease, sex, and additional parameters. The 36-question survey is one of the most commonly used global measures of quality of life. Nevertheless, the SF-36 may lack sufficient depth and detail to fully evaluate patients who undergo treatment for musculoskeletal tumors. A number of similar instruments, such as the European Organisation for Research and Treatment of Cancer (EORTC) questionnaire, have been developed but have yet to be proven superior.

Table 14.2 Musculoskeletal Tumor Society scale for rating function and outcome[a]

	Shared criteria		
Score	Pain	Function	Emotional acceptance
5	No pain—no medication	No restriction	Enthused—would recommend to others
4	Intermediate	Intermediate	Intermediate
3	Modest/nondisabling—nonnarcotic analgesics	Recreational restriction	Satisfied—would do again
2	Intermediate	Intermediate	Intermediate
1	Moderate/intermittently disabling—intermittent narcotics	Partial occupational restriction	Accepts—would repeat reluctantly
0	Severe/continuously disabling—continuous narcotics	Total occupational restriction	Dislikes—would not repeat

	Lower extremity		
Score	Supports	Walking[b]	Gait
5	None	Unlimited—same as preoperative	Normal
4	Occasional use of brace	Intermediate	Intermediate
3	Brace	Limited—significantly less	Minor cosmetic
2	Occasional cane/crutch	Intermediate	Intermediate
1	One cane or crutch	Inside only	Major cosmetic—minor functional deficit
0	Two canes or crutches	Not independently—can walk only with assistance or wheelchair bound	Major handicap—major functional deficit

	Upper extremity		
Score	Hand positioning	Dexterity	Lifting ability
5	Unlimited—180° elevation	No limitations—normal dexterity and sensation	Normal—same as opposite extremity
4	Intermediate	Intermediate	Less than normal
3	Not above shoulder or no prosupination—90° elevation	Loss of fine movements or minor loss of sensitivity	Limited—minor load
2	Intermediate	Intermediate	Against gravity only
1	Not above waist—30° elevation	Cannot pinch—major sensory loss (specify)	Helping only—cannot overcome gravity
0	Flail—0° elevation	Cannot grasp—anesthetic hand	Cannot help or move

[a]Six components are measured for a maximum total score of 30 points (100%). Patients with lower extremity tumors are scored with the three shared criteria plus the three lower extremity criteria. Patients with upper extremity tumors are scored with the three shared criteria plus the three upper extremity criteria.

[b]If limitations are imposed by other considerations (cardiac, respiratory, neurological), do not consider this category.

Summarized, with permission, from Enneking et al. (1993).

Table 14.3 Karnofsky scale of performance status

Condition	%	Comments
Able to carry on normal activity and to work. No special care is needed.	100	Normal. No complaints. No evidence of disease.
	90	Able to carry on normal activity. Minor signs of symptoms of disease.
	80	Normal activity with effort. Some signs or symptoms of disease.
Unable to work. Able to live at home, care for most personal needs. A varying degree of assistance is needed.	70	Cares for self. Unable to carry on normal activity or to do active work.
	60	Requires occasional assistance, but is able to care for most personal needs.
	50	Requires considerable assistance and frequent medical care.
Unable to care for self. Requires equivalent of institutional or hospital care. Disease may be progressing rapidly.	40	Disabled. Requires special care and assistance.
	30	Severely disabled. Hospitalization is indicated although death is not imminent.
	20	Hospitalization necessary. Very sick; active supportive treatment necessary.
	10	Moribund; fatal processes progressing rapidly.
	0	Dead.

Reprinted from Karnofsky and Burchenal (1949).

Table 14.4 ECOG performance status scale

Score	Criteria
0	Fully active; able to carry on all predisease performance without restriction.
1	Restricted in physically strenuous activity but ambulatory and able to carry out work of a light or sedentary nature, e.g., light housework, office work.
2	Ambulatory and capable of all self-care but unable to carry out any work activities. Up and about more than 50% of waking hours.
3	Capable of only limited self-care; confined to bed or chair more than 50% of waking hours.
4	Completely disabled. Cannot carry on any self-care. Totally confined to bed or chair.
5	Dead.

Reprinted from http://ecog.dfci.harvard.edu/general/perf_stat.html (accessed June 19, 2012). Eastern Cooperative Oncology Group; Robert Comis, M.D., Group Chair. Originally published in Oken MM, Creech RH, Tormey DC, et al. Toxicity and response criteria of the Eastern Cooperative Oncology Group. *Am J Clin Oncol* 1982;5:649–655.

Toronto Extremity Salvage Score

The Toronto Extremity Salvage Score (TESS) (Table 14.5) was developed as a self-administered patient questionnaire that emphasizes functional activities. It addresses a shortcoming of the MSTS score by including patient participation in the assessment. The TESS involves 2 sets of approximately 30 questions, 1 set for the upper extremity and 1 for the lower extremity. Each item is rated from 1 to 5. The overall score is based upon a maximum of 100%.

Table 14.5 Toronto Extremity Salvage Score (TESS) for upper and lower extremities

Upper extremity

1. Lifting	15. Picking up small items
2. Performing heavy household duties	16. Showering
3. Participating in social activities	17. Doing up buttons
4. Putting on pants	18. Handling change
5. Gardening	19. Putting on shoes
6. Carrying	20. Working usual number of hours
7. Performing leisure activities	21. Preparing meals
8. Tying a bow or tie	22. Turning a key in a lock
9. Performing work duties	23. Shopping
10. Brushing hair	24. Performing light household duties
11. Dressing	25. Putting on socks
12. Pushing or pulling open a door	26. Shaving or putting on makeup
13. Cutting food	27. Brushing teeth
14. Writing	28. Drinking from a glass

Lower extremity

1. Kneeling	16. Shopping
2. Rising from kneeling	17. Putting on shoes
3. Gardening	18. Participating in sexual activities
4. Performing heavy household duties	19. Walking indoors
5. Walking up and down hills	20. Putting on pants
6. Performing leisure activities	21. Preparing meals
7. Walking upstairs	22. Showering
8. Bending	23. Standing
9. Getting in and out of a bathtub	24. Sitting
10. Walking downstairs	25. Performing light household duties
11. Getting in and out of a car	26. Participating in social activities
12. Working usual number of hours	27. Driving
13. Walking outdoors	27. Rising from a chair
14. Putting on socks	28. Getting in and out of a bed
15. Performing work duties	

Impossible to do 1	Extremely difficult 2	Moderately difficult 3	A little bit difficult 4	Not at all difficult 5	Does not apply to me

From Davis et al. (1996) (Table 1). Reprinted with permission from Springer Science+Business Media.

Brief Pain Inventory

The Brief Pain Inventory (BPI) (Fig. 14.9) is primarily a measure of pain and discomfort. It is useful for precise characterization of the degree of pain experienced by patients who have either ongoing disease-related pain or complications secondary to treatment.

STUDY ID #:__________   DO NOT WRITE ABOVE THIS LINE   HOSPITAL #:__________

Brief Pain Inventory (Short Form)

Date:_____/_____/_____   Time:_______

Name:_________________ ________________ _______________
              Last   First   Middle Initial

1. Throughout our lives, most of us have had pain from time to time (such as minor headaches, sprains, and toothaches). Have you had pain other than these every-day kinds of pain today?

      1.   Yes   2.   No

2. On the diagram, shade in the areas where you feel pain. Put an X on the area that hurts the most.

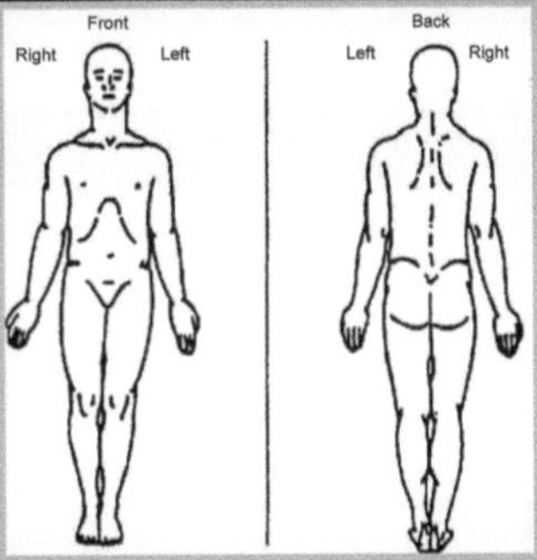

3. Please rate your pain by circling the one number that best describes your pain at its worst in the last 24 hours.

| 0 | 1 | 2 | 3 | 4 | 5 | 6 | 7 | 8 | 9 | 10 |
No   Pain as bad as
Pain   you can imagine

4. Please rate your pain by circling the one number that best describes your pain at its least in the last 24 hours.

| 0 | 1 | 2 | 3 | 4 | 5 | 6 | 7 | 8 | 9 | 10 |
No   Pain as bad as
Pain   you can imagine

5. Please rate your pain by circling the one number that best describes your pain on the average.

| 0 | 1 | 2 | 3 | 4 | 5 | 6 | 7 | 8 | 9 | 10 |
No   Pain as bad as
Pain   you can imagine

6. Please rate your pain by circling the one number that tells how much pain you have right now.

| 0 | 1 | 2 | 3 | 4 | 5 | 6 | 7 | 8 | 9 | 10 |
No   Pain as bad as
Pain   you can imagine

Page 1 of 2

Fig. 14.9 The Brief Pain Inventory (BPI). Courtesy of Charles S. Cleeland, PhD, Department of Symptom Research, MD Anderson Cancer Center.

STUDY ID #:__________   DO NOT WRITE ABOVE THIS LINE   HOSPITAL #:__________

Date:____/____/____   Time:_________

Name:_________________ _________________ _____________
           Last   First   Middle Initial

7.   What treatments or medications are you receiving for your pain?

8.   In the last 24 hours, how much relief have pain treatments or medications provided? Please circle the one percentage that most shows how much relief you have received.

0%	10%	20%	30%	40%	50%	60%	70%	80%	90%	100%
No Relief										Complete Relief

9.   Circle the one number that describes how, during the past 24 hours, pain has interfered with your:

A.   General Activity

0	1	2	3	4	5	6	7	8	9	10
Does not Interfere										Completely Interferes

B.   Mood

0	1	2	3	4	5	6	7	8	9	10
Does not Interfere										Completely Interferes

C.   Walking Ability

0	1	2	3	4	5	6	7	8	9	10
Does not Interfere										Completely Interferes

D.   Normal Work (includes both work outside the home and housework)

0	1	2	3	4	5	6	7	8	9	10
Does not Interfere										Completely Interferes

E.   Relations with other people

0	1	2	3	4	5	6	7	8	9	10
Does not Interfere										Completely Interferes

F.   Sleep

0	1	2	3	4	5	6	7	8	9	10
Does not Interfere										Completely Interferes

G.   Enjoyment of life

0	1	2	3	4	5	6	7	8	9	10
Does not Interfere										Completely Interferes

Page 2 of 2

Fig. 14.9 (continued)

Conclusions

Follow-up evaluation of patients after primary therapy for bone sarcomas includes a well-balanced combination of history taking, physical examination, imaging studies, and functional assessment. The physical and mental well-being of each patient can be safeguarded through a preplanned schedule of clinical visits that incorporate these elements at regular intervals.

<table>
<tr><td align="center">Key Practice Points</td></tr>
<tr><td>

- A well-designed schedule for the follow-up of patients with sarcoma of bone is crucial to the success of disease management.
- Patients with low-grade sarcomas require less frequent follow-up than those with high-grade sarcomas.
- Long-term follow-up is required for oncologic and reconstructive reasons. At least 10 years of follow-up is recommended.
- The medical history, physical examination, and conventional radiographs form the crux of oncologic surveillance. Advanced imaging modalities, such as CT and MRI, are used selectively.
- Metallic artifact can compromise CT and MRI image quality, but the use of metal-specific protocols typically results in diagnostic-quality images.
- Global measures of functional outcome and quality of life are recommended as part of follow-up assessment.

</td></tr>
</table>

Suggested Readings

Antoch G, Bogt F, Freudenberg L, et al. Whole-body dual-modality PET-CT and whole-body MRI for tumor staging in oncology. JAMA. 2003;290:3199–206.

Aoki J, Endo K, Watanabe H, et al. FDG-PET for evaluating musculoskeletal tumors: a review. J Orthop Sci. 2003;8:435–41.

Arush MW, Israel O, Postovsky S, et al. Positron emission tomography/computed tomography with [18]fluoro-deoxyglucose in the detection of local recurrence and distant metastases of pediatric sarcoma. Pediatr Blood Cancer. 2007;49:901–5.

Babyn PS, Wihlborg CE, Tjong JK, Alman BA, Silberberg PJ. Local complications after limb-salvage surgery for pediatric bone tumours: a pictorial essay. Can Assoc Radiol J. 2001;52:35–42.

Bjordal K, Kaasa S. Psychometric validation of the EORTC Core Quality of Life Questionnaire, 30-item version and a diagnosis-specific module for head and neck cancer patients. Acta Oncol. 1992;31(3):311–21.

Costelloe CM, Kumar R, Yasko AW, et al. Imaging characteristics of locally recurrent tumors of bone. Am J Roentgenol. 2007;188:855–63.

Costelloe CM, Macapinlac HA, Madewell JE, et al. ^{18}F-FDG PET/CT as an indicator of progression-free and overall survival in osteosarcoma. J Nucl Med. 2009;50:340–7.

Daut RL, Cleeland DS, Flanery RC. Development of the Wisconsin Brief Pain Questionnaire to assess pain in cancer and other diseases. Pain. 1983;17:197–210.

Davis AM, Wright JG, Williams JI, et al. Development of a measure of physical function for patients with bone and soft tissue sarcoma. Qual Life Res. 1996;5:508–16.

Enneking WF, Dunham W, Gebhardt MC, Malawar M, Pritchard DJ. A system for the functional evaluation of reconstructive procedures after surgical treatment of tumors of the musculoskeletal system. Clinic Orthop. 1993;286:241–6.

Eustace S, Tello R, DeCarvalho V, et al. A comparison of whole-body turboSTIR MR imaging and planar ^{99m}Tc-methylene diphosphonate scintigraphy in the examination of patients with suspected skeletal metastases. Am J Roentgenol. 1997;169:1655–61.

Healey JH, Nikolic ZG, Athanasian E, Boland PJ. Quality of life as defined by orthopedic oncology patients. Ann Surg Oncol. 1997;4:591–6.

Karnofsky DA, Burchenal JH. The clinical evaluation of chemotherapeutic agents in cancer. In: MacLeod CM, editor. Evaluation of chemotherapeutic agents. New York: Columbia University Press; 1949. p. 191–205.

Keogh CF, Munk PL, Gee R, Chan LP, Marchinkow LO. Imaging of the painful hip arthroplasty. Am J Roentgenol. 2003;180:115–20.

Lansky SB, List MA, Lansky LL, Ritter-Sterr C, Miller DR. The measurement of performance in childhood cancer patients. Cancer. 1987;60:1651–6.

Ma J, Costelloe CM, Madewell JE, et al. Fast dixon-based multisequence and multiplanar MRI for whole-body detection of cancer metastases. J Magn Reson Imaging. 2009;29:1154–62.

Marchese VG, Ogle S, Womer RB, Dormans J, Ginsberg JP. An examination of outcome measures to assess functional mobility in childhood survivors of osteosarcoma. Pediatr Blood Cancer. 2004;42:41–5.

Miller TT. Imaging of hip arthroplasty. Semin Musculoskelet Radiol. 2006;10:30–46.

Ohashi K, El-Khoury GY, Bennett DL, Restrepo JM, Berbaum KS. Orthopedic hardware complications diagnosed with multi-detector row CT. Radiology. 2005;237:570–7.

Pfeilschifter J, Diel IJ. Osteoporosis due to cancer treatment: pathogenesis and management. J Clin Oncol. 2000;18:1570–93.

Reuther G, Mutschler W. Detection of local recurrent disease in musculoskeletal tumors: magnetic resonance imaging versus computed tomography. Skeletal Radiol. 1990;19:85–90.

Suh JS, Jeong EK, Shin KH, et al. Minimizing artifacts caused by metallic implants at MR imaging: experimental and clinical studies. Am J Roentgenol. 1998;171:1207–13.

Viano AM, Gronemeyer SA, Haliloglu M, Hoffer FA. Improved MR imaging for patients with metallic implants. Magn Reson Imaging. 2000;18:287–95.

Völker T, Denecke T, Steffen I, et al. Positron emission tomography for staging of pediatric sarcoma patients: results of a prospective multicenter trial. J Clin Oncol. 2007;25:5435–41.

Ware Jr JE, Sherbourne CD. The MOS 36-item short-form health survey (SF-36). I. Conceptual framework and item selection. Med Care. 1992;30:473–83.

Weissman B. Imaging of hip replacement. Radiology. 1997;202:611–23.

Zubrod CG, Schneiderman M, Frei E, et al. Appraisal of methods for the study of chemotherapy of cancer in man: comparative therapeutic trial of nitrogen mustard and triethylene thiophosphamide. J Chronic Dis. 1960;11:7–33.

Index